Computers in Health Care

Kathryn J. Hannah   Marion J. Ball
Series Editors

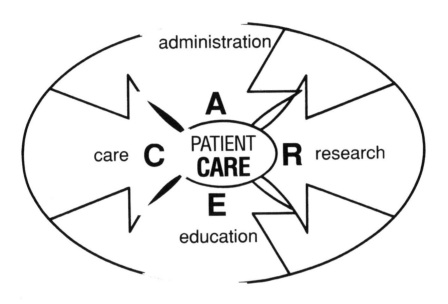

Computers in Health Care

Series Editors:
Kathryn J. Hannah   Marion J. Ball

Nursing Informatics
Where Caring and Technology Meet
M.J. Ball, K.J. Hannah, U. Gerdin, and H. Peterson

Healthcare Information Management Systems
A Practical Guide
M.J. Ball, J.V. Douglas, R.I. O'Desky, and J.W. Albright

Knowledge Coupling
New Premises and New Tools for Medical Care and Education
Lawrence L. Weed

Forthcoming Volume

Dental Informatics
Integrating Technology into the Dental Environment
Louis M. Abbey and John Zimmerman

Lawrence L. Weed

Knowledge Coupling
New Premises and New Tools for Medical Care and Education

Includes Works by
Louis M. Abbey   Kenneth A. Bartholomew   Charles S. Burger
Harold D. Cross   Richard Y. Hertzberg   Philip D. Nelson
Richard G. Rockefeller   Stephen C. Schimpff   Christopher C. Weed
Laura Weed   Willie Kai Yee

Springer-Verlag
New York Berlin Heidelberg London
Paris Tokyo Hong Kong Barcelona

Lawrence L. Weed
Problem-Knowledge Coupler Corp.
10 Mary St.
South Burlington, VT 05403

Library of Congress Cataloging-in-Publication Data
Weed, Lawrence L.
    Knowledge coupling : new premises and new tools for medical care
and education / Lawrence L. Weed.
        p.   cm. — (Computers in health care)
    Includes bibliographical references and index.
    ISBN-13: 978-1-4612-7815-3   e-ISBN-13: 978-1-4612-3150-9
    DOI: 10.1007/978-1-4612-3150-9
    1. Medical informatics. 2. Medical records. I. Title.
II. Series: Computers in health care (New York, N.Y.)
    [DNLM: 1. Diagnosis, Computer-Assisted. 2. Education, Medical.
3. Medical Informatics. 4. Medical Records, Problem-Oriented. W
26.5 W394k]
R858.W44   1991
616.07'50285—dc20
DNLM/DLC
for Library of Congress   91-4851

Printed on acid-free paper.

Camera-ready prepared by the author.
Printed and bound by Edwards Brothers, Inc., Ann Arbor, MI.
Softcover reprint of the hardcover 1st edition 1991

9 8 7 6 5 4 3 2 1

ISBN-13: 978-1-4612-7815-3 Springer-Verlag New York Berlin Heidelberg

To Laura, and Linc, Dinny, Jon, and Becky

Foreword

Richard G. Rockefeller, M.D.

Associate Professor of Family Medicine
Portland, Maine

"Larry Weed is absolutely right—he's just 20 years ahead of his time." Twenty years and more have passed since this refrain was first raised. As in fairy tales where the slighted witch returns to claim the child or the piper to demand his due, perhaps Dr. Larry Weed's time has arrived.

Some of his methods and ideas have already found their way into the mainstream of health care: the Problem Oriented Medical Record is widely employed, though often diluted or modified beyond recognition; the flowsheeting of multiple variables on patients is a well established component of his problem oriented system in both hospital and ambulatory care; and he provided much of the intellectual background for the movement toward patients' engagement in and responsibility for their medical care. Over three decades his tireless refinement and articulation of a new paradigm—a patient centered, problem oriented rational humanistic approach to medicine—has influenced the thoughts and actions of many.

Despite these achievements, however, the greater potential of Larry Weed's work is yet to be realized. Alhough this is hardly surprising (change is painful), it must be felt as a loss considering the quagmire into which our health care system continues to descend.

Today, hardly anyone touched by the health care system is unscathed by a woeful and burgeoning litany of ills. Taxpayers and employers stagger under intolerable and growing medical tithes. Many of the uninsured find even primary medical attention beyond their means. Patients are upset with doctors for the same reasons they always were, only more so: they indict physicians for a lack of interest in their personal concerns, a perceived attitude of arrogance or overcertitude, excessive charges, and overspecialization, to name just a few.

Today doctors are as distraught as anyone: we are angry with patients for suing us and for seeming to demand omniscience; we *have had it* with government and thirdparty payers for shackling us with bureaucracy and stripping our autonomy. We do not enjoy the dismantling of our professional stature in the public eye. And we are increasingly frustrated (though this is not so often nor so clearly articulated as our other grievances) by an ever expanding knowledge base that long ago outgrew our capacity to apply it comprehensively or consistently to the clinical problems of our trade.

This book sets forth an approach, a set of methods, and a description of computerized information tools[1] which offer a coalition of power, efficiency, and humanity never before achievable in the practice of medicine. Taken together, I believe these do provide a means to transcend our predicament.

Rather than recapitulate, let us highlight a single theme which informs the entire work. This constant, the *uniqueness of the individual patient,* serves as a still point around which the many facets revolve and competing goals are brought into harmony. Consider how two such goals, the betterment of science and the restoration of the humanity of medicine, are so served.

With regard to the science of medical practice, emphasis on the individual serves to redress an overemphasis on the role of *general* vs. *patient-specific* knowledge. The knowledge base so painstakingly accrued over this century is an achievement of extraordinary power and potential. But general knowledge alone is insufficient; many of the most important clues to an individual's health are to be found in what makes him unique. Weed understands the significance of this realm and his information tools make its exploration possible.

In practice, orientation toward the individual contributes to the science of medicine as follows: knowledge couplers are employed to gather and efficiently determine to what degree the patient's locus of findings *fits* a diagnostic or treatment category within the general knowledge base. Although occasionally the fit is perfect (and the work complete, almost independent of physician involvement), more usually several options are partially supported but none definitively. This is because, in the earlyy phases of any illness, insufficient findings may be manifest to implicate any one pattern. Problems of a more chronic nature become *personalized,* sometimes beyond recognition. The pattern of pathology may be unique to this patient or not yet recognized and named by medical science. But even where adequate fit is lacking, knowledge coupling has still performed an invaluable service, demonstrating at the *outset* what can and cannot be gleaned from the medical literature.

For the unaided human mind, the achievement of completeness in regard to the general database has been all but a hopeless dream, even as the endpoint of the clinical encounter. Like most objects beyond our reach, its

---

[1]   A computerized medical record as well as problem solving and decision-support software, the *Problem Knowledge Coupler system.*

value may have been exaggerated. Problem knowledge coupling allows us to achieve this end in predictable and consistent fashion; thereupon, seeing its limitations, we can move beyond, into the realm of the patient's uniqueness. This quest is for new knowledge, not just application of the old, and as such it is scientific work in the deepest sense. It is exacting work, finding and weaving the fine threads—details *of this* patient at *this* time under *these* circumstances—onto the sturdy warp of a complete general database, and it requires time and skills the physician alone cannot supply. However Weed's new premises assume (and his tools and methods allow) that each participant, human and electronic, will contribute whichever piece of the task for which he, she or it is best equipped. The result is a garment of better fit and fabric than general knowledge will allow or physicians alone can craft.

Outcomes of clinical medicine are improved as the science of practice is thus advanced. At the same time orientation toward the unique individual promises to make the experience of medicine more humane and satisfying for both patients and doctors. In the prevailing medical paradigm, orientated as it is toward general knowledge, patients feel appreciated and well cared for to the extent that their problems are generic, that is, match population based classifications of pathology. When the dimensions of their suffering and needs extravasate beyond these borders, as commonly happens, patients discover their idiosyncracies to be sources of frustration and anger. They often find themselves alienated not only from a system which fails to meet their needs but also from themselves, to the extent they identify with the system's implicit devaluation of their uniqueness. Weed's approach obviates such sources of disease because it takes the set of attributes, historical circumstances, and preferences which differentiate one individual from the next as central to, rather than as a troublesome distraction from, the important work of the therapeutic encounter. Patients' satisfaction is enhanced as their aptitudes and contributions—self-knowledge, willingness and ability to gather data pertaining to the problem, among others —are appropriately valued. Finally, as a reward for relinquishing the comfortable (but also dangerous, increasingly untenable, and ultimately unfulfilling) illusion of being wholly provided for by an omnipotent parent, patients are afforded the human rewards of collegiality, including equal stature in the patient/doctor relationship and control over decisions affecting their health.

Redirecting some attention from general knowledge to the unique patient can enhance the physician's gratification from medicine as well. For one thing our sense of worth and competence is better served by improved outcomes in the realm of the possible than by compensatory fantasies of omniscience. Further, the combination of realistic expectations by all parties, shared responsibility for decisions, and predictably better outcomes will make for more congenial relationships among participants in the health care system. As physicians relinquish the spurious stature which Weed has jocularly termed MDeity, we may also be freed of the acrimony and suspicion of charlatanism, shadows which have always dimmed medicine's lustre and now conjure the specter of litigation.

Finally, focus on the uniqueness of the individual highlights the importance to effective healing of a host of abilities beyond mere information storage and retrieval. These include among others: pattern recognition; judgment; the ability to lead patients when necessary from dependence to collegiality and self reliance, and into the making of difficult choices; self knowledge, especially the ability to recognize and withdraw the constant stream of projections we cast upon our patients; honesty and integrity; humility; compassion and comfort with suffering and death; humor; perseverance, and teamwork. These attributes are strictly human, and as such offer the rewards of irreplaceability as well as of breadth. Oliver Sacks includes many of these under the rubric *heart* as he writes, "...the peculiar joy I have known...for the past fifteen years, has been the fusion of scientific and 'romantic' penetration, finding my mind and my heart equally exercised and involved, and knowing that anything different would be a dereliction of both" (Sacks 1983).

Larry Weed offers, among many other things, the reagents for a fusion of this sort, not just to those so gifted and fortunate as Dr. Sacks, but to all physicians willing to venture into a new world of possibility.

Stephen C. Schimpff, M.D.

Executive Vice President
University of Maryland Medical System
Professor of Medicine, Pharmacology and Oncology
University of Maryland School of Medicine

There is a saying that managers do things right; leaders do the right thing. Dr. Larry Weed has the characteristics of a leader. One can disagree with him, and many do; one can question his logic, and some do. A leader pulls by example, by his enthusiasm and vision for the future. A leader is a change agent who must align constituencies to agree to the vision and develop the motivation to achieve the vision. Dr. Weed clearly outlines his vision of medicine; then he moves ahead to explain the use of computerized knowledge couplers as a tool to assist the clinician become a quality expert.

Dr. Weed points out that any great task requires four elements: philosophy, tools to get the job done, leadership, and users who perform the tasks. He believes that the philosophy must be determined before we decide on the tools. He strongly believes that we cannot achieve our noble task of quality patient care because our philosophy is incorrect. He suggests that we use one of our most important tools, our brain, inappropriately. We use it inappropriately because we have the wrong philosophy of medicine. Our philosophy began with the concept that physicians, to be effective, need to be well grounded in the sciences which make up the basis of current health care. Added to that must be a deep knowledge of individual diseases, their manifestations, causes, and treatment. The assumption is that if individuals have that basis of information, then, when faced with a clinical problem, they can make the appropriate decisions and create an action plan for resolution of the problem. But the database is enormous, and no one individual, no matter how intelligent, no matter how great a memory, can store it. Perhaps more importantly, it is just simply not possible for the human brain to process immense numbers of complex operations of the numbers and complexity involved in a rapid time frame allowing one to act immediately.

Weed suggests that medicine, not wanting to change its philosophy, has instead specialized, subspecialized, and then still further specialized so that the individual practitioner can be more expert by holding a fair sized knowledge base related to fewer clinical problems within his brain. Unfortunately, the physician does not choose the patient's medical problem. The patient presents with a problem, and if the problem is not within the knowledge scope of the specialist, the subspecialist, or the sub, subspecialist, then it is simply not reasonable to expect that individual to function effectively. Dr. Weed proposes we change our approach, which currently consists of cramming the brain with greater and greater amounts of data (which it cannot store) and then expecting the brain to process enormous amounts of complex information over a short timeframe (which it cannot do) so as to arrive at a decision for action. This is a requirement Dr. Weed states the brain cannot match. Rather, a more appropriate approach is to utilize the computer for both the enormous memory bank required and for the complex multiple processes of making combinations and permutations. The individual clinician, rather than spending time on vast memorization processes, should spend time honing his or her skills in taking a history, doing a physical examination, reviewing laboratory results, and developing an interpersonal relationship with the patient and the patient's family. Physicians should not be made to feel guilty and inadequate because they have, in fact, inadequate storage and processing capacities within their brains.

I first met Larry Weed in 1966 on a cold, snowy December day. I was applying for an internship at Cleveland Metropolitan Hospital, one of the two major teaching hospitals of Case Western Reserve Medical School. Dr. Weed met me on the ground floor with "Hi, let's walk up to my office." What followed was Dr. Weed conducting an interview as we dashed up six floors while I tried to catch my breath. His enthusiasm for medicine was infectious. He was not at all interested in what I had memorized over the last four years, but he was interested in my abilities to think logically, solve problems, and access information appropriately. He also cared about my personal value systems and the philosophy of medicine I was then developing. I chose to stay at Yale for housestaff training where, as in medical school, problem solving was valued over memorization; I didn't see Dr. Weed again until November 1990, when he was a guest speaker at a University of Maryland at Baltimore

Informatics Symposium organized by Dr. Marion Ball. He had the same energy I remembered from 24 years earlier, the same intensity of purpose, the same dynamic commitment to a vision or, as he called it, a philosophy of medicine.

I witnessed the use of his Problem Knowledge Couplers in action. It was a unique experience and quite humbling. It was a clear example of the validity of his concept. It was also obvious that once one is familiar with the equipment (he was using a laptop computer for this demonstration in a lecture hall) the process itself is essentially simple. Any individual with the most minimal of personal computer knowledge can work with his program. The key, of course, is in obtaining the data to be entered, and this relates back to Dr. Weed's philosophy that physicians need to spend more time honing their abilities at history, examination, and review of laboratory and imaging data rather than in pattern recognition based on a vast store of knowledge that will inevitably be incomplete. Fortunately, the knowledge couplers prompt the clinician to go back and obtain additional information where necessary or appropriate.

Weed's approach is akin to the knowledge based systems or expert systems coming into use in industry. Integral to these systems is the act of entering all data, once, at the point of origin. The computer then directs the users, allowing them to focus on what they do best. This approach, called "knowledge based systems," has been developed to improve the quality of decisions that require a substantial database in order to arrive at the best judgment. The idea is that decisions will be consistent, individuals will perform better, training time will be reduced, and response time will be not only fast but accurate. Industries in which such systems work, from automobile plants to bakeries, may seem light years away from clinical medicine, and they are. But the concept of knowlege based systems to assist the human brain to function more effectively is the real point.

Medical informatics (bringing knowledge and caring together) requires both machines and brains. When it works best, it integrates the two together; when it works poorly, Weed suggests, we end up with a Tower of Babble. The time students and physicians currently spend memorizing material for Board examinations would be better used studying problem solving, interviewing, and learning to negotiate ambiguities after the computer helps sort the data and hook up the knowledge coupler.

A visionary and, like Tom Peters and Robert Waldman, a change agent, Weed believes that the practice of delivering health care must undergo dramatic change. His philosophy is radically different from the norm of medicine today. His vision will probably not be rapidly accepted, because it will not be easy to align constituencies and motivate key individuals needed to achieve acceptance.

Larry Weed expands our vision and challenges us to rethink our basic philosophy. Ultimately, I have no doubt, much of what he suggests will be accepted. In this book, he shares with us that vision of the future.

From the Editors

It is with pride that we introduce this remarkable book by Larry Weed. His is truly a visionary mind, unafraid of pursuing ideas, regardless of the controversy that may surround them. Student and then staff at some of our most prestigious medical schools, he excelled in our medical establishment and found it lacking. For Larry Weed, the shattering conclusion was that the very premises of medical education and practice were flawed. But he refused to rest among the ruins and proceeded to construct a new approach. In 1969, he first set forth his philosophy in *Medical Records, Medical Education, and Patient Care*. He has worked ever since to test and refine his concepts.

This book is the culmination of that work and comes at a time when the medical establishment faces intense public and professional scrutiny. The Joint Commission on Accreditation of Healthcare Organizations (JCAHO) has set forth its Agenda for Change, and public and private sectors alike struggle with questions of cost and quality of care. There is no question that health care faces fundamental changes amounting to no less than a paradigm shift, a total transformation of the medical establishment which has served us so well until the last decades of the 20th century.

Publication of this book is strategically timed to coincide with the release of a major study completed by the Institute of Medicine. As a member of the committee that produced the report and co-chair of its subcommittee on technology, Marion Ball shared in its deliberations. Its recommendations for the next ten years call for a totally electronic patient record as the standard for health care in the United States. Although Larry Weed is still perceived as a controversial figure, the groundwork he laid with the concept of the Problem Oriented Medical Record underlies all the committee's work and every attempt to computerize the medical record. Absolutely, without any doubt whatsoever, Larry Weed's vision will be the catalyst which makes changes in health care possible well into the next century.

Understanding this vision, so different from that which we are trained to see, is a difficult task indeed. The extensive front matter helps to put the book into a number of perspectives. In the Foreword, Richard Rockefeller gives the insights he has gained in using Larry's Problem Knowledge Couplers in his medical practice, and Stephen Schimpff adds the vantage point of a physician/administrator who sees how Weed's approach can change the way medical care is delivered. In the Introduction, Larry explains the philosophy which underlies the text. To further aid the reader of this challenging book, an overview by Christopher Weed highlights key concepts; brief summaries appear before each chapter. The Appendix includes samples of introductions to individual couplers as well as the introduction and preface which appeared in *Medical Records, Medical Education, and Patient Care* (1969), where Larry Weed first advanced his new premises and new tools.

Practicing physicians may choose to focus on the chapters on the database and on flowsheets, while nonphysicians concerned with health care policy may concentrate on implications and interdependencies. Still other readers may be especially interested in the contributions of Bartholomew, Burger, Cross, Nelson, Abbey, and Yee, health care practitioners who have implemented Weed's philosophy.

As editors for this book and for the *Computers in Healthcare* series, we welcome the controversy which this book will bring, for it is through controversy that issues will be clarified and changes will be born—changes so profoundly needed in our health care system. We know that Larry Weed's vision will be questioned and attacked, but it cannot be ignored. We are honored indeed to have worked with Larry to help bring this vision into print and thus, eventually, into reality.

Marion J. Ball, Ed.D.
Judith V. Douglas

Overview

Christopher C. Weed

PKC Corporation
South Burlington, Vermont

In the years since *Medical Records, Medical Education, and Patient Care* was published in 1969, there has been an extraordinary growth and elaboration of the services and technical capability of the American health care system. There has unfortunately been a concomitant growth in the complexity and costliness of the system, which has become a major burden on American society. The purpose of this book is to outline a set of new premises and tools upon which the operation of the system must be based.

This is not to say that no other resolution whatsoever is possible. The current health care system is a relatively recent development, and one can easily imagine contenting ourselves with much more modest expectations of what biomedical research can make available at a sustainable cost to the general population. In conjunction with this, we would need to put far more emphasis on the responsibility of individuals and various social institutions to promote and sustain our people's health and well being, and accept a reduced availability of expensive remedies for the results of neglect and irresponsible behavior. There is no doubt that substantial movement in this direction is taking place in any case, and deserves to be encouraged.

Nevertheless, there are some fundamental systemic defects in the health care system, which may be seriously undercutting the potential benefits of whatever scientific and technological advances we choose to put into practice. This cannot help but affect our judgments as to what advances are worth pursuing, or what the prerequisites of their practical application really are.

The nature of these systemic defects, which are closely interrelated, may be presented as follows:

- The current practice of medicine relies far too heavily on the uncontrolled and unsupported exercise of human judgment extemporaneously applied at the time of decision making and action.

- Our confidence in our innate human capacity to make judgments as sound and reliable as our collective knowledge theoretically allows is simply unsupported by over 30 years of intensive research in clinical and cognitive psychology. Furthermore, there is extensive, often polemical as well as careful medical documentation that testifies to rampant nonapplication or misapplication of medical knowledge to everyday clinical situations. Perseveration on these past revelations has not really succeeded in changing the root causes nor is it likely that change will come with further investment in such studies (clinical efficacy or outcome studies) so long as inputs (the product of idiosyncratic decisions and actions of providers) remain uncontrolled.

- The difficulties follow from the limitations of unaided human minds in applying a very large body of knowledge, when any portion of that knowledge base is intermittently and unpredictably relevant in day to day work. Specialization represents an attempt to deal with this problem. Unfortunately it runs afoul of the persistent failure of real problems to fit within the socially and historically defined boundaries of medical specialties. Medical knowledge, viewed as a whole, is as highly interconnected as the minds and bodies of its subjects. Tracing these interconnections wherever they lead in response to a real problem, as if following a map, is what medical problem solving requires.

- The medical record, viewed as a scientific document and medium of communication between patients and health care professionals, suffers from neglect, disregard, and an almost complete lack of standards in structure and content. The principle, central to the Problem Oriented Medical Record, that the medical record should convey why things are done as well as what is done, speaks directly to this defect. Many providers, particularly specialists, regard medical record keeping as a clerical task, unworthy of their concentrated attention.

- Medical education has encouraged as well as evolved to accommodate these systemic problems in medical practice. Physicians in particular are indoctrinated with an unwarranted estimate of their capacities by social and financial pressures that are often extreme. This unfounded confidence, and the economic status quo based upon it, then serve to impede necessary changes in the premises and tools of medical practice.

- The patient's potential role as a unifying and coordinating participant in the management of his or her own health care has not been adequately explored and developed. In chronic problems, and in ambulatory care, the self defeating effects of patients being poorly informed have often been ignored. Until recently, the public has not been encouraged to understand the processes and enabling factors of medical decision making, and the role they can and must play in medical decisions.

This book is not specifically about the application of computers to the practice of medicine. Inexpensive, versatile information storage and retrieval mechanisms are probably vital and certainly helpful in implementing the changes called for in this book. Nevertheless it must be emphasized that the required tools do not demand massive storage capacity or computing power by the standards of the modern computer industry. Effective coupling of medical knowledge to action can be greatly facilitated by simple associative mechanisms, working with a large body of medical content appropriately represented and stored in an efficient database structure. An implementation of such a mechanism is described, called the Problem Knowledge Coupler System. Also described is a prototype of a microcomputer based medical record system, designed to help implement the problem oriented medical record in office practice.

The notion that simple associative mechanisms can actually address the problems outlined will seem heretical to many people. Medical decision-making is normally seen as a complex, irregularly structured, iterative process. This view provided an early inspiration for the development of expert systems. In this book, we argue that much of the apparent complexity arises from efforts to accommodate the limitations of the human mind, and to minimize time spent in data collection. If all options are to be given due consideration, in light of a patient's unique situation, and neither ignored nor prematurely dismissed, then the crucial relevant factors must be checked. Low prior probability of any one factor or option is not an adequate justification for neglecting this. The probability that something unusual will be going on is substantial, even if the probability of any one such factor is low. Furthermore the cost of neglecting the unusual or unexpected in a patient's case can be very high later on.

Admitting what has just been said, is it not true that additional reasoning with the data, which is often quite intricate, may be required? The first thing to understand is that the essential complexity of the intellectual processes involved in day to day medicine, as in many other areas requiring so called expert judgment, is greatly exaggerated. Like most of us, physicians have a lot of problems to worry about, and limited time in which to do the worrying. Like most of us, they look for simplifying assumptions and formulas, and various other ways to make their work more automatic and mindless, and less stressful. This is not inherently bad; in fact it is necessary to the maintenance of mental and emotional health, and personal productivity, under the circumstances. Given this natural tendency toward routinizing and simplifying medical practice, it is reasonable to consider the pitfalls of doing so in a system based upon human memory, and how such pitfalls might be avoided.

Psychological studies have demonstrated that the pitfalls of informal decision making behavior are legion. It has been unequivocally demonstrated that in many decision making contexts a simple scheme, known as a linear decision model, will give results as good or better than human judges making a decision on the basis of the factors used in the model.

A Problem Knowledge Coupler can be thought of simply as a set of coupled linear models. The crucial problem in building a coupler module for a specific presenting problem (complaint or prominent manifestation) is identifying the available options for the decision and identifying and choosing the crucial factors that bear upon those options. This often requires an extended struggle with the voluminous, redundant, and frequently inconsistent medical literature. The actual mechanical construction of a coupler database is comparatively trivial, given well designed software tools.

Problem Knowledge Couplers do not and should not recommend definite decisions in individual cases. Instead, they are meant to ensure that the patient and the provider are not only confronted with a full set of diagnostic or management options for the problem, but are also informed which options best match the patient's unique situation. In light of this, how valuable are conventional information sources? One need only ask what effort is being made in the current health care system to get the best medical knowledge to every patient by way of the minds of practitioners. Enormous expenditures of time and money are devoted to primary medical education, continuing medical education, seminars and teaching rounds, the writing and publication of journal articles and medical textbooks, and production of numerous ancillary sources of information (information bulletins, prescription drug information source such as the *Physician's Desk Reference*, or PDR) and more. All this effort in information distribution involves a great deal of redundant content and duplicated effort. Little effort is being made at present to help providers relate the information to unique patients. Nevertheless practitioners are expected to know whatever is needed to address the problems with which their patients present, or to make prompt contact with colleagues who possess the required knowledge. (In fact this latter avenue is often the preferred approach to information acquisition.)

It is argued in this book that centralization and unification of medical knowledge ought to be accomplished by incorporating it as guidance embedded in the very tools that providers use in everyday practical decision making. This is consonant with the belief that the published medical literature ought to be more directly relevant to practice than it currently is. This is what we mean by the metaphor of "voltage drop." Otherwise, as is too often the case, individual practitioners might just as well continue to rely on their own creative intuition, experience, and informal and random contacts with other concerned people. Without specific linkages of the knowledge base to practical decision-making, scientific medicine affects practice primarily through new procedures and associated technologies, while the application of such procedures and technologies is left to a sort of cottage industry or folk art based on something approaching oral tradition.

What would be some of the secondary benefits of the widespread, standardized use of such tools? A major issue in medical information handling these days is the control and standardization of medical vocabulary. Outcomes evaluation is handicapped by lack of control of inputs—including the medical knowledge relied upon when people make decisions, and what they mean by the terms they use. It is now possible to embed the definitions and the knowledge needed to fully address problems in tools used for everyday practice. Indeed, it is important that the standardization of terminology be carefully assessed and tested by use in decision support tools like PKCs, as generally should medical knowledge. (It should be noted here that the integration into such tools of graphic representations of the objects and processes named by medical terms would greatly facilitate their correct and consistent use.)

Another major potential benefit of standardized knowledge coupling and medical record storage and retrieval tools is increased patient understanding and involvement. As a matter of principle, the Problem Knowledge Coupler System is oriented around problems as they initially present themselves. This also makes couplers particularly suitable for conveying the scope and requirements of a diagnostic or management problem. They can also provide a means of conveying this information in writing for the patient's ongoing use. The key point is that the system combines a standard knowledge base with a capacity for *adaptively* extracting and presenting information for each patient, so that relevance is assured.

One might pose the question, "How many coupler modules are needed as a basis for practice, and what resources are required for their construction and maintenance?" Whether we are talking about the 15 to 20 modules that would be used in a highly specialized practice or the number necessary to accommodate any conceivable diagnostic or management problem in clinical medicine, how many is not the crucial question. The important point is that we know the number is reasonably finite, that 27 couplers have already been completed and are available, and once the initial set is completed, the updating and maintenance of the couplers can be the focal point for making the efforts of all workers in the field of medicine collaborative and cumulative. Without the new premises and new tools, and a deep commitment to changing the way we practice medicine, the massively expensive and often irrelevant "clatter of the knowledge industry" will go on.

Acknowledgments

Since the philosophy and detailed implementation of the ideas expressed in this book have their roots in my experiences over 45 years in seven different medical schools (both the basic science and clinical departments), a community hospital in Maine, a large city hospital in Cleveland, national medical record associations, nursing organizations, veterinary schools, and many other valued contacts in the field of medicine, it is almost impossible to truly acknowledge all the benefits I have received from so many people. The efforts of the recognized leaders along the way have been invaluable, but also, looking back, I recognize more and more how important the insights were that I gained each day from the nurses, the social workers, the students, the house officers, and the patients. And of course none of the technical advances would have been possible without the generous support of the granting agencies in Washington in the 1970s.

For much of the recent work described in this volume, there are several names that stand out, and that I would like to mention them at the risk of omitting some other very important contributors. First of all, there is the creator of the computer software that has made this extensive discussion of new premises and new tools possible, Richard Hertzberg. He has been a unique resource. As a software designer and programmer, he is a problem solver of uncommon ability and speed who turns out solutions of unusual elegance. But of equal importance has been his understanding of the philosophy and his commitment to its implementation. My wife, Dr. Laura Brooks Weed, through her work as a practicing physician and as a main contributor to Problem Knowledge Coupler development, and as an editor of all the writings over the years, has made an ongoing contribution that cannot be measured. In the past eight years, Christopher C. Weed has not only been the operational backbone of the PKC organization, but has also done much to guide the philosophy and basic understanding of our efforts. I have tried to recognize his exact writings in the text where I can, but there are many paragraphs that I am sure came from his mind and pen that have been woven into the whole final fabric. Both he and Laura Weed refused co-authorship because they did not actually write the full text, but the reader should know how basic their contribution has been. Without the combined and cooperative efforts of Laura, Chris, and Richard at many critical junctures, this book and the work it describes would not have been possible.

The final chapters of this book by Drs. Bartholomew, Burger, Cross (general practice), Yee (psychiatry), Abbey (dentistry), and Nelson (veterinary medicine) speak for themselves. Anyone who appreciates how difficult it is to paint, let alone remodel, the boat while you are sailing in it will be particularly appreciative of their efforts, since all of them are engaged in either full time practice or combined practice, education, and research. Zelda Gebhard (Faulkton, South Dakota) and Chris Weed have been invaluable in providing continuous support and insights at both the technical and medical levels. I have been most appreciative of Dr. Richard Rockefeller's steady support and constructive insights as he has used couplers in the practice of medicine.

A wide variety of students, residents, and practitioners around the country have to varying degrees contributed to the coupler building effort that has been based in Vermont.

In conclusion, Marion Ball, who has played a pivotal role in the field of medical informatics, by her encouragement, support, and very concrete work, has been invaluable in getting this publication underway. I want to express my gratitude to Marion Ball, Judy Douglas, Marilyn Burnett, and all the capable people who have worked with them on this manuscript. The combination of their extraordinary understanding of the field of medicine and the experience, competence, and enthusiasm they have brought to the editing and publication of this book made everything not only possible but pleasant and easy.

Contents

Contributors

LOUIS M. ABBEY, D.M.D.
Professor of Oral Pathology, School of Dentistry, Medical College of Virginia, Virginia Commonwealth University, Richmond, Virginia 23298

KENNETH A. BARTHOLOMEW, M.D.
General Practice, Chief of Staff, Faulk County Memorial Hospital, Faulkton, South Dakota 57438

CHARLES S. BURGER, M.D.
Family Practice, 650 Evergreen Woods, Bangor, Maine 04401

HAROLD D. CROSS, M.D.
Family Practice, 71 Dudley Street, Hampden, Maine 04444

PHILLIP D. NELSON, D.V.M.
Professor, School of Veterinary Medicine, Tuskegee University, Tuskegee Institute, Tuskegee, Alabama 36088

RICHARD G. ROCKEFELLER, M.D.
71 Foreside Road, Falmouth, Maine 04105

STEPHEN C. SCHIMPFF, M.D.
Executive Vice President, University of Maryland Medical System, Baltimore, Maryland 21201

CHRISTOPHER C. WEED
PKC Corporation, South Burlington, Vermont 04444

WILLIE KAI YEE, M.D.
Staff Psychiatrist, Ulster County Mental Health Center, New Paltz, New York 12561

The purpose of the examples used in the flowsheets and medical cases cited is to denote concepts and facilitate the auditing of the quality of care. The actual data present were developed in real time and have not been modified. They may not represent current medical practices or even the best quality that was achievable at the time.

Introduction

Lawrence L. Weed

This book is about a journey from an old tool to a new tool, to new premises, and finally to *knowledge couplers*, another new tool that emerged from what the early days of the journey had revealed.

The *premises* that underlie our daily activities lie quietly for years underneath the surface of our lives, unarticulated and unchallenged. The *tools* we employ to perform everyday tasks are used for long periods with very little thought given to changing and improving the tools themselves. Many, in the practice of medicine, have not only neglected one of the most potentially powerful tools in the provision of high quality care, *the medical record*, but have considered it a nuisance to be completed after the fact. But the record is far more than that. It was in the reshaping of that tool, the medical record, and the sharper focus on the logic of our actions that led to a challenge of the basic premises upon which the whole medical enterprise has been based (Weed 1964, Weed 1969).

We would all like to live in a society where the logic and actions of everyone are based on the best available knowledge and analyses of the day. A physician diagnosing and treating a patient, a farmer planning his crops, or a diplomat negotiating a complex political agreement would not only mobilize all the relevant current information, but, without error or crucial omissions, would integrate the information with the set of variables unique to the problem situation.

We know that this does not happen most of the time. Furthermore, we tend to blame it on the fact that people are not sufficiently *well educated*. Our basic premise has been that it is *education* that enables us to couple the best available knowledge and thought to everyday action. We *learn* by being *taught* in school, and we then expect the unaided human mind to recall and process vast amounts of information, all in the *same breath*, at the time of action. Proctored examinations in schools, and credentials based upon them, reinforce our educational notions and the illusions they perpetuate. We have focused so much on the difference between the *educated expert* and the *uneducated* that we have failed to focus on the difference between what the *educated expert* knows and does and what the problem ideally requires. But as we examine this difference critically, it dawns on us how misplaced is our confidence in the present premises of education, a confidence which leads us to trust the unaided human mind in the face of many variables at the time of problem solving.

In the middle 1950s, when I was engaged in basic research, *basic science* teaching, and clinical teaching, I was struck by the differences in the way we approached the teaching of a graduate student in basic research and a medical student engaged in solving the problems of patients. The medical record, it seemed to me, should be not only the physician's laboratory notebook for the recording of observations and investigations, but also his final manuscript. The physician, thereby, would make available to other scientists, other providers of care, and the patients themselves the logic of the conclusions as they emerged from highly organized data about each of the patient's problems. My thesis was that in order to accomplish this, we needed to restructure the medical record. By converting it from a *source oriented* record (all the data filed according to its source—all the laboratory data together, all the nurse's notes together, etc.—to a *problem oriented* record, we would automatically have a record not only of *what* was done, but *why* it was done. Within such a framework, a fair audit can be accomplished, outcomes can be rigorously interpreted, and a disciplined approach to problem solving can develop in the system of medical care and medical education. Over the last 20 years, beginning with the two volumes edited by Hurst and Walker (1972, 1973) and the book by Bjorn and Cross (1970), much has been written about the problem oriented system. But, right from the very beginning, the system emphasized what laymen have always known as they have shopped for doctors, that when they go to different physicians or institutions with the same complaint, very different things happen. Indeed, one of the patients of Bjorn and Cross worked with them to document in a small way what they called this *legendary variation* among physicians. The patient simply picked names of professionals from the yellow pages in the phone book, went to each of them with the same problems and request for a workup, and recorded what happened (Bjorn and Cross 1970). For many years, innumerable scholarly studies have confirmed and reconfirmed this great variation at many levels of *outcome* in the medical care system [see the extensive bibliographies of Gaummer 1984 and Inlander et al 1988]. The problem oriented system has provided a framework for understanding why such variations might occur. The time is long overdue for major corrective surgery on the medical care system itself. Over the years, the problem oriented system has *required* and has *revealed*:

Database

Required: A defined database from which a complete problem list can be derived.

Revealed: The unaided minds of multiple providers of care, working with dictaphones or blank sheets of paper, rarely achieve this first step in a consistent, thorough, and reliable manner.

Problem List

Required: A complete list of problems that accounts for all the abnormalities in the database.

Revealed: A complete problem list is not achieved in most environments. This may be due to an incomplete database. But also the data that are in the database may not be used to achieve the maximum synthesis that is possible; the unaided mind does not see many of the significant relationships among the various bits of data. And what synthesis there is may be unjustifiably biased by the specialty training and parochial experiences of the providers. Furthermore, since a complete list of problems is not made available to all providers, and to the patients themselves, on all clinical encounters, medical care activities are not coordinated and cumulative.

Problem Oriented Plans

Required: Organized planning for each problem acknowledges
- the other problems of the patient
- the best known options from the literature for solving the problem
- the needs and goals of the patient and the family.

Revealed: The unaided human mind using current methods is often unable to recall all the relevant data on the patient and all the relevant diagnostic and management options from the literature, and is often unable to take those two bodies of information and integrate them systematically to come up with the best course of action for a unique individual. Furthermore, the patient's role in his or her own behalf has been grossly neglected.

Problem Oriented Progress Notes and Flowsheets

Required: Titled and numbered progress notes on each problem that coordinate multiple providers and provide feedback on the actions taken.

Revealed: Frequently there has not been disciplined implementation of a plan once it has been formulated; frequently, there has been no appropriate modification of a plan based on new data as they are accumulated. Providers do not consistently communicate effectively and parameters are not followed meticulously and recorded accurately on every occasion. Clinicians try to deal with many variables extemporaneously, without flowsheets, at the time of action, and they frequently fail to see all the trends and make all the correlations that are possible and all the changes that are indicated.

From the above it became apparent that there is a great *voltage drop* from the knowledge in libraries to the actions on patients. Providers are continually making judgments without a thorough knowledge of the options that the literature offers and the factors bearing on these options that should be checked in each patient. They are trying to make decisions in the face of avoidable ignorance. Distorted clinical experience biases and corrupts their judgment over time and impairs their ability to estimate the soundness and usefulness of medical knowledge.

For many patients the flow of coordinated, error free, undistorted knowledge becomes a poorly channeled trickle, and for some patients it is nothing at all. This is well documented in the standard medical literature (Gaumer 1984; Inlander et al 1988). How can so much information be dissipated and distorted on its way to its final destination? And if the best knowledge is not applied to every patient every time, how can outcome analyses be used to set priorities, ration resources wisely, and correct the errors in the original medical knowledge? Until we learn to have control over and understanding of the *inputs* of the medical care system, we will not be able to rigorously interpret the *outputs*. But once we do gain such control over the inputs, *outcome* analyses will be automatic byproducts of the system for care, and costly, separate studies after the fact will not be necessary.

The Voltage Drop

If the information transfer from DNA to the working machinery of the cell were as disorganized and chaotic as it is across human minds and actions in the medical care system, many organisms would not survive, and those that did would be beset with malfunctions. Up until now, basic science for students has mainly been involved with understanding how nature runs its information system; scientists are beginning to try to affect that system when errors, such as genetic defects, arise. In medical practice, we must not only understand, but also conceive and implement, our own information system, one that rigorously couples the fruits of scholarly effort and research to the everyday actions of us all. We ourselves are the engine of our own extrasomatic evolution. Physical man has changed little over thousands of years. It has been his tools and beliefs that have enabled our civilization to develop. The present premises and tools of medical education and medical care cannot support or even allow the proper evolutionary steps to take place.

Much of the frustration felt by so many hard working people in the medical profession has its roots in flawed premises and inadequate tools. We can no longer survive on pride in brilliant focussed efforts in research or specialty practice; we cannot take refuge in phrases such as *pure science*, dismissing the system of everyday medical care as *applied science* for lesser minds working in an environment of less intellectual rigor and discipline. The most difficult of intellectual challenges now lies ahead—developing a framework in which the brilliant pieces of understanding are routinely assembled into a working unit of social machinery that is coherent and as error free as possible— a challenge in which we ourselves are among the working parts to be organized and brought under control. As Bertrand Russell said,

> Not only will men of science have to grapple with the sciences that deal with man, but—and this is a far more difficult matter—they will have to persuade the world to listen to what they have discovered.

The first step in persuading others is to be clear in our own minds about what the problems and the solutions are. What, in concrete terms, are some new premises and some new tools, and what are some of the old beliefs and premises that should be replaced?

Old and New Premises

OLD: A core of knowledge must be taught and memorized.

NEW: A core of behavior, not a core of knowledge, must be inculcated. A person must be thorough, reliable, capable of defending the logic of his actions, and efficient in completing the tasks for which he or she is responsible in a well defined system of medical care. As John Ruskin said a century ago, "Education is not teaching people to know what they do not know. It is teaching them to behave as they do not behave."

OLD: It is possible, after exposure to a core of knowledge, to recall and process all the necessary variables at the bedside or in the clinic at the time of clinical action.

NEW: It is necessary to use electronic extensions of the human memory and analytical capacity at the time of action, just as we need x-rays to extend the human eye. Physicians should rely on such tools just as a traveler relies on maps instead of memorizing trips in geography courses. A central facility should have the responsibility for keeping the tools up to date.

OLD: National Board and Specialty Board examinations are an adequate basis for credentials which in turn should be indicators of one's capacity over a lifetime to fulfil one's responsibility to patients.

NEW: Good medical practice can only be assured through random audit of performance in the real world; such an audit requires a defined system of care and the availability of up to date information tools.

OLD: Knowledge can be divided into academic packages or courses; defects in performance such as unethical behavior or failure to consider all the determinants of health, such as nutrition, environmental contaminants and influences, genetics, abuse of drugs and medical procedures, can be remedied by adding a new course to the curriculum.

NEW: Whether practical or theoretical, real problems in the real world do not fit neatly into academic boundaries, and it is dangerous for professions serving real people to try to make them do so. Academic boundaries and specialties make us focus on the few things that patients with a given disease have in common, whereas the thousands of things they do not have in common may have far more to do with what action should be taken and what the outcome will be. Defects in the care process should be corrected by updating the information tools provided for use at the time of care and by demanding a more disciplined use of the proper tools at the time of action. The knowledge in the information tools will be determined by what the problem requires, regardless of the old classification system for knowledge, such as science, humanities, nutrition, sanitation, surgery, medicine, psychiatry, social work, ethics, etc.

OLD: Medical personnel, on an ad hoc basis, should be the principal force in defining, allocating, and prioritizing society's limited resources in matters related to health. Physicians should then be the principal force in choosing among diagnostic and therapeutic options for individual patients.

NEW: Society as a whole should determine how limited resources are to be applied in matters of health; what therapeutic options are to be made available to individuals vs. what resources are to be applied to cover health determinants for populations of individuals (schools, sanitation, prenatal clinics, etc.). Patients and their families should be the principal force in choosing among options made available to them by society. Up to date information tools (guidance systems) should be the concrete means whereby options are articulated and offered by society and whereby specific options are then chosen by patients in partnership with all medical personnel. Patients should always have a copy of their own problem oriented medical records to facilitate their role in the partnership.

Roots of the Old Premises and Limitations of the Unaided Human Mind

Once the entire premise of a core of knowledge is questioned, we can think back to the medical school experience and remember how little if any discussion went on in the presence of the students about the very nature of the vast reservoir of medical knowledge. Who defined the boundaries? Who decided on the content of courses and what should be omitted or discarded? And where was the evidence that what had been selected for courses related rigorously to the care of patients? And, even if it did, what evidence was there that the tired and bewildered minds of students could recall and process the infinite variety of facts and variables that highly specialized faculty members were forever pouring into student brains? Why was there a basic science course in biochemistry filled with intricate details about metabolic cycles, but no such course in basic psychology in most medical schools? The majority of patients, to say nothing of students and faculties themselves, are beset with psychological problems and with normal limitations to what the human mind can actually achieve. It is in the psychology literature (Tversky and Kahneman 1974; Kern and Doherty 1982; Wason and Johnson-Laird 1972; Dawes et al 1989) that we find the basis for the following assertions:

- The human mind will start generating hypotheses in the earliest moments of encounters with patients and thereby prematurely bias the remaining steps in the search for data.

- The human mind will limit the number of hypotheses to a number far smaller than the problem requires. We therefore do not fulfil our responsibility to the patients with the rare disorders. As Wason and Johnson-Laird state, "When the individual mind's logical ability is restricted, it will operate within heuristic or hit-or-miss procedures which do not guarantee a solution."

- The mind will underestimate the complexity of problems and overinterpret the data it does collect. It will indulge in the categorical reasoning of the expert.

- The mind will take the probability information based on the studies of a very small number of variables on large populations and let it supersede highly improbable but correct information on a very large number of variables in a unique patient, thereby shortchanging, if not actually endangering, the patient. The mind also applies inappropriate prevalence data in many of its calculations, placing a patina of quantitative and numerical respectability on to a not so respectable foundation of misguided and inaccurate estimations.

As Wason and Johnson-Laird (1972) have said,

We like to think the educated human mind is capable of thinking in terms of propositions which take into account the possible and the hypothetical, and that the mind will be able to isolate variables in the problem and subject them to combinatorial analysis which nicely exhausts the possibilities.

But this, of course, as they point out, is exactly what most of their subjects failed to do. And not only psychologists, but poets were warning us. Edna St. Vincent Millay wrote in one of her sonnets:

Upon this age that never speaks its mind,
This furtive age, this age endowed with power
To wake the moon with footsteps, fit an oar
Into the rowlocks of the wind, and find
What swims before its prow, what swirls behind—
Upon this gifted age, in its dark hour,
Rains from the sky a meteoric shower
Of facts...they lie unquestioned, uncombined.
Wisdom enough to leech us from our ill

Is daily spun, but there exists no loom
To weave it into a fabric.

Although we do not explicitly recognize these natural limitations of the human minds as we drive students through the process of memorizing, regurgitating, and forgetting, we do so implicitly as we choose faculty to preside over this tyranny of memorized knowledge. Specialists with command of small parts of the knowledge base are hired. For the basic sciences, the specialists are often PhDs, who not only may have very little idea of exactly how the knowledge they are imparting is to be used in the lives of physicians and their patients, but even more importantly, who cannot, on the basis of their own experiences, help the student comprehend and prepare for the problem solving conditions that confront a physician. In the life of a PhD, time and tasks are the variables, and achievement the constant. One or two tasks at a time and the necessary time and grant money are made available until peers review the work and it is published. Experiments can be carefully designed and variables can be controlled. In contrast, a physician or a medical student does not choose the problem: the patient may have any problem. There is not one problem at a time to work on: one patient might have five or ten problems and there can be 30 patients on the ward and hundreds in the ambulatory care setting. Nor can the timetable be set by the doctor. The appendix will rupture on its timetable, not the physician's.

In spite of the above realities, many faculty members have come to believe that if each of them could somehow get his or her collection of specialized facts into the student's head, the student would always be able to recall them and integrate them properly into the multiple complex problem situations confronted day in and day out. Medical students are being stuffed with the facts of basic science, but could it be that the behavior of a scientist is escaping them? Indeed, would it not be impossible for anyone to exhibit good scientific behavior under the conditions of modern medical education—multiple PhDs and MDs converging on the single mind of a medical student, all under the premise that a mind so exposed can store, recall, and process all the appropriate variables at the time of problem solving in the real world?

Educational Malpractice and Quality Control in Medicine

The above realities help explain why not only physicians, but also professionals in business and other fields and the interested public are having difficulty with the problems of defining and assessing the quality of medical care. For most nonphysicians, quality has always been defined as the excellence with which a well defined function is fulfilled. In medicine, however, quality has been defined as that which people with credentials do, and only others with credentials have a right to judge it—even though everyone knows that those credentials represent nothing more then a passing grade on an examination taken years ago. Furthermore, examination results have not been shown to consistently reveal what the examinee would do when confronted with a real problem in the real world under all sorts of conditions. Suppose some regulatory agency had scrutinized the credentialing process of the human mind with the same rigor that the Food and Drug Administration (FDA) looks at a new drug or a new instrument. Had they done so, they would have found that the production standards and the requirements for ongoing quality control of the output of the credentialed human mind are far below any standards we use for any drug or instrument. How ironic, for it is the educated, credentialed human mind that orders the drugs and makes all the decisions that set all the various technologies into motion.

The implications of this state of affairs for those who are expected to practice high quality medicine are enormous. A bad system, false premises, and inadequate tools may not yield what the public expects no matter how hard the people within the system work. And in the absence of well defined, achievable goals and in the presence of malpractice threats and lawsuits, hard work may embitter and demoralize everyone involved. Patients will continue to receive less than optimum care, and physicians will continue to be badgered and frustrated if the basic system of care and licensing does not change. Unfortunately, it is also true that a bad system, skillfully manipulated, can yield great economic benefits to suppliers, administrators, lawyers, and all types of medical practitioners. And those who control and profit from the present system will resist new premises and new tools no matter how logical and powerful they might be. Ian Lawson, in a commentary on the problem oriented medical record he wrote some years ago, captured the essence of much that is becoming apparent in the presence of new tools (Lawson 1974):

> The POMR [problem oriented medical record] sets out to affect the basic attitudes of professionals toward people-problems, as well as their formal logic in patient care. It compels relationships and interdependences as conditions of physician conduct. And now, through computer technology, it draws us into a thorough-going consistency, which is unfamiliar to most natures and threatening to our tolerated caprices.

Political Structure Confronted by Change

Before discussing the new premises and the new tools, let us review the political structures that are being confronted with change and, also, review the state of problem solving in the current establishment.

Memory based, credentialed specialists have been persons of departments and deans. Over the years, they have established their own ways of keeping records, doing research, setting fees, and teaching students and residents. Undeniable benefits, indeed remarkable achievements, have come from this concentrated, highly specialized approach. But to this day, specialists have not worked together to establish a single problem oriented medical record system throughout an institution and a community, with the patient at all times having a copy of that record in his or her own hands. It resembles the situation that existed over 150 years ago, when the great railroad barons and tycoons had trouble agreeing on a single gauge track that would have effected enormous efficiencies in the transportation of all sorts of materials over a broad geographic area. Like the railroads, medicine faces a political problem, not a technical one. In *Medical Records, Medical Education, and Patient Care* (Weed 1969), I set forth my hopes that development of the computerized *p*roblem *o*riented *m*edical *i*nformation *s*ystem (PROMIS) would help both to coordinate the many providers working with a single patient, and to overcome the memory limitations of the providers of care. The PROMIS system soon revealed that solving the memory problem of the human mind uncovers a *processing limitation* that is even worse than the *memory limitation*. That is to say, with 55,000 displays of medical details accessible with the stroke of a finger, the physician could be overwhelmed by the task of integrating the relevant details from the unique patient with the relevant details now instantly available on the computer screen. We came face to face with the realities and complexities in decision making that had been hidden under such terms as *clinical judgment, intuition,* and *experience.* The hallucinatory fulfillment for students and faculty alike was rudely interrupted. How could we make sense out of the situation we found ourselves in? (See PROMIS references.)

Basic Issues in Problem Solving

We all knew in a common sense way that decisions in medicine can go wrong if we make them without enough information or if the *facts* in the situation are not accurate. A decision can also go wrong if we do not know how to interpret the facts. Medical training, as most of us have known it, has not equipped us to come to terms with these decision making situations in a well defined manner. Some have turned to mathematicians, psychologists, and computer scientists for help. Many of these people, in turn, focus on the intelligent manipulation of the facts that their medical colleagues give to them, paying little attention to the inaccuracies, incompleteness, and highly provincial nature of the data flowing from a deeply flawed medical care system. The data come from a memory based, credential oriented group of medical providers, who are often specialists not linked to one another in a highly disciplined fashion and who in many cases keep inadequate medical records. Such records, along with a medical literature system severely criticized for its lack of quality control standards, have been the underlying basis for specialists' "expert" opinions and uninhibited intuitive leaps to conclusions about diagnoses and management options. All of this has led to much magnificent navigation to the wrong port. In some decision support systems, there have been calculations of probabilities before many relevant and easily available variables have been isolated and taken into account. Many seem to be disregarding the idea that probabilities are used in direct proportion to the ignorance of the uniqueness of a given situation. *Combinatorial thinking,* on the other hand, seeks out the uniqueness of a situation and exhausts all the possibilities in a complex diagnostic or management situation; such thinking is as much beyond the unaided mind as modern astronomy is beyond the unaided human eye (Wason and Laird 1972). And yet here we are in 1991 still examining students on what they know instead of on how gracefully and effectively they interface with the areas of their ignorance when others are trusting them to solve a problem.

The Role of Patients in Problem Solving and in Managing Their Own Health

Patients are not interested in what is probable among large numbers of patients based on a few variables, nor are they primarily interested in what the expert knows. They are interested in what is wrong with them, no matter how improbable and unique their situation might be. And knowing the power of taking into account uniqueness in making wise choices among diagnostic and management options, we realize how serious have been the consequences of the neglect of all the details in the lives of patients. We realize how easy it was to rely and operate on the meager set of facts that we could hold in the memory or elicit from an incomplete and disorganized medical record—and how easy it was to neglect the role of patients in their own behalf. If the patients and the families do not understand and do not have the right tools to work with, then the most sophisticated efforts in the information sciences may come to naught (Weed 1975).

To illustrate, I remember the day in a medical center on a ward with a modern information system when they wanted to present a patient to me on rounds. I said, "Do not present a new patient; tell me who is going home today." The nurse volunteered the name of a middle aged woman who had had lupus for ten years. I suggested that they give me 15 minutes with the patient and then return for discussion. I asked the patient to tell me all about each of her problems. She knew very little about the medical problems.

"Do you have a copy of your own medical record?"

"No."

"Are all your medications in the bedside stand, and does the nurse come around at regular intervals to see if you are taking the right ones at the right time?"

"No. The nurse just comes with little paper cups with pills in them, and I swallow whatever is there."

"Do you know what a flowsheet is? What parameters we are trying to follow? What endpoints we are trying to reach?"

"No."

At this point I called the staff back together and told them what I had found. Their reactions were as follows:

"We never give patients their records."

"We do not have the time to give the medicines that way. It would not be safe to leave her with them unattended. She is on many powerful drugs."

"The patient is not very well educated, and I do not think she could do all the things your questions imply."

"But," I said, "you said she is going home this afternoon. She lives alone. At 2 pm you will put her in a wheelchair, give her a paper bag full of drugs, and send her out the door. Are you going home with her?"

"No. Is her management at home our problem?"

"You just said she could not handle it. Who will do it? The patient may not seem well educated or very bright to you, but what could be more unintelligent than what you are doing?"

We must consider the whole information system and not just infinitely elaborate on the parts that interest us or fit into a given specialty. Patients do not specialize, and they or their families are in charge of all the relevant variables 24 hours a day, every day. They must be given the right tools to work with. They are the most neglected source of better quality and savings in the health care system. After all,

- They are highly motivated, and if they are not, nothing works in the long run anyway.

- They do not charge. They even pay to help.

- There is at least one "caregiver" for every member of the population.

The Evolution of Our Present Difficulties

As we reflect upon how the present situation evolved, we can see that the very conditions that produced it tend to sustain it. The process of memorizing, regurgitating, and forgetting in order to acquire legal credentials to function, coupled with the physical exhaustion of meeting the unending demands sick people can make, leaves physicians little time to reflect upon the flaws of the system, let alone design and implement a new one. Most of us were not schooled in the nature of medical knowledge, the epistemology that is the basis of a whole career. In the whole matter of making a diagnosis, there was little time to reflect upon the word itself—that it involved a specialized classification system, that great minds had struggled for decades, even centuries, over the underlying principles of taxonomy. Premedical students may have been required to memorize a few names in organic chemistry and biology, but the whole field of evolutionary biology was the intense preoccupation of a very few. Little time was given to truly understanding the writings of such as Darwin, and still less to read recent authors like Sneath and Sokal (1973), numerical taxonomists, who wrote,

> It is the self-reinforcing circular arguments used to establish categories, which on repeated application invest the latter with the appearance of possessing objective and definable reality. This type of reasoning is, of course, not restricted to taxonomy...but it is no less fallacious on that account. ...A group assumes a degree of permanence and reality quite out of keeping with the tentative basis on which it was established.

Tolstoy seemed to understand the essence of what they were saying when he wrote (1942) in *War and Peace*,

> She could not eat or sleep, grew visibly thinner, coughed, and as the doctors made them feel, was in danger. They could not think of anything but how to help her. Doctors came to see her singly and in consultation, talked much in French, German, and Latin, blamed one another, and prescribed a great variety of medicine for all the diseases known to them, but the simple fact never occurred to any of them, that they could not know the disease that Natasha was suffering from, as no disease suffered by a live man can be known, for every living person has his own peculiar, personal, novel, complicated disease unknown to medicine— not a disease of the of the lungs, liver, skin, heart, nerves and so on, mentioned in medical books, but a disease consisting of one of the innumerable combinations of the maladies of those organs. This simple thought

cannot occur to the doctors, as it cannot to the wizard who is unable to work his charms.

Medical students are made to feel stupid; in the midst of complex medical situations, patients are often made to feel guilty when they overhear themselves being identified as "neurotic" or "turkeys." Both patients and students struggle with the inconsistencies among experts and are baffled when a given unique situation does not match textbook pictures and averages, or does not yield neatly to mathematical manipulations based on flawed premises and inadequate or unreliable data. In training, professionals are always so busy meeting the demands of superiors and assigned workloads that those individuals being trained often do not demand logical and rigorous connections between what they are memorizing and what they will someday do in the context of their own patients' lives. Many just assume that somehow a complete and evenly working system will evolve out of a group of scientists and specialists of all sorts making their living out of their chosen specialized part of the human body. We all need to be reminded of the cynical belief of Malthus (Heilbroner 1972) that we would always be victims of the insensible bias of situation and interest. Medicine has had, and will always have, its counterparts to the Jay Goulds, the Andrew Carnegies, and the Whitneys of the business world (Heilbroner 1972). They had, and physicians have, their apologists who translate unconscionable and even cutthroat behaviors and unbalanced distribution of resources and rewards into words and phrases such as *thrift*, *dedication*, and *pure science*. All people in medicine are subject to that passion which Kar' Marx said was the most violent to inhabit the human breast—the passion of self interest. As we now grapple with the relevance of the efforts of each individual to the whole health care enterprise with all of its humanitarian and scientific aspects, it is in the articulation of new premises for medical care and education and in the creation of new tools and information systems that all the pieces can be brought together into a meaningful whole, into a framework for creative and productive activity in a science of medical practice. We no longer need to be in le Corbusier's phrase, "A spectacle of fragments of intention." We are now in a position to move much of medicine from the "World 2" of the philosopher Karl Popper to his "World 3," from the world of our notions, our intuitions, our judgments, and our mystique, to a world of objective reality that is open to criticism and logical correction of defects as they appear. Memory based, credential oriented systems, with their "habits of certainty" and obscure dark corners of mystique, must now be abandoned. Without competence and accountability, compassionate concern is always in danger of becoming fraud and malpractice.

Once we stop examining health care workers on what they know and start examining them on how effectively they operate with modern information tools that have built into them the parameters of guidance and the currency of information for doing each job correctly and in the context of the individual's life, then will we be able to return to that era of a century ago. As the historian Sloan (1979) described it, "that was the era when moral philosophy was the most important course in the college curriculum; it aimed to pull together, to integrate, to give meaning and purpose to the student's entire college experience. Even more important, it sought to equip graduating seniors with the ethical sensitivity and insight needed to put their newly acquired knowledge to use in ways that would benefit both themselves and also the larger society. Intellectual unity was required as the essential safeguard against moral and cultural chaos." Sloan quotes Horace Mann as saying that schools are the "balance wheel of the social machinery."

But what happened as the last century came to a close and our own century began? Knowledge expanded, subject matter placed increasing demands on the curriculum, and fragmentation was underway. We think of Adam Smith as the first great economist, but he was, first and foremost in his day, a professor of moral philosophy. In our time, his career and the courses he taught have splintered into political science, economics, philosophy, philosophical ethics, psychology, anthropology, and sociology. Fewer and fewer educators could teach from the example of the breadth and moral concerns of their own lives. Sloan says, "Faculties became trained experts. And emphasis on ethics gave way to an emphasis on research and specialized training." "Scholarly" productivity consumed us all. And now what are some of the products of that objective, scientific, scholarly activity? We have a massive mixture of the good and the bad—thalidomide and penicillin, Three Mile Island and relativity, modern plastics and undrinkable water supplies.

If we are ever to recapture the intellectual unity that is "the essential safeguard against moral and cultural chaos" and still not be nihilistic about the advancing technology and ever expanding knowledge, we must change the premises of our educational system. The new tools for extending our minds at the time of action allow us to do that. But many of us just keep extolling the virtues of the modern information tools while we do nothing to change the premises, so the new tools are thereby prevented from fulfilling their real promise. Suppose they had given the new printing press only to the monks so they alone could copy their manuscripts faster as opposed to letting it, in Thomas Carlyle's words, "cashier in kings and senates and introduce a whole new democratic world." In many places, we have literally done little more than automate the chaos, or use the tools in ingenious ways to "pick up after" erratic, unaided human minds as they set all sorts of misguided clinical activities into motion, instead of giving proper guidance to those minds in the first place. And then for years, even decades, many have persisted in doing outcome studies without first doing what we needed to understand and control the inputs—all leading to masses of data that defy rigorous and meaningful interpretation. Our very use of phrases like *expert systems* and *artificial intelligence* suggested to many that we had yet to admit that many an expert and many an unaided intelligence cannot do what patients and third party payers had always assumed they could do. And knowing the studies in the literature that have already demonstrated the limitations of the unaided mind, we still hear demands for controlled studies to prove that new tools are better than what we are now doing. When we introduced the x-ray machine to extend the unaided human eye and ear, we did not talk about "artificial eyes" and evaluate the adequacy of the x-ray by comparing its results to the vision of experts in clinical medicine. Nor did we try to use x-rays alone without the added modalities of the stethoscope and histories and physical examinations. In contrast, recently one professor said he thought computerized knowledge coupling tools (C. Weed 1982; L. Weed 1983, 1985, 1986, 1987) might have some advantages, but he, with his broad experience, would only use them on the difficult case. How would we react if we heard a person say that he thinks the telescope is an interesting, even a powerful tool, but because of his years of experience of looking at the sky, he will use the telescope only on the nights he sees something unusual up there? When will we admit that the human capacity to recall and process many variables must be extended with new tools if the patients are ever consistently to receive the best that medical science has to offer? The veto power of the credentialed experts is awesome because we have vested in them the power to counter logic, not with evidence and more logic, but with authority.

Were I teaching biochemistry with these new information tools in place, I would not be overwhelming students with tricky exams involving multiple choice questions about a thousand metabolic pathways, but I would ask them to stand back and notice all the things that a single *E coli* can make (vitamins and amino acids, etc.) with just a little salt water and minimal nutrients thrown in, something that no human can do. I would also point out that the civilization of *E coli* is not very sophisticated, just a division every 50 minutes. No single cell of a multicellular human being can stand alone quite as well an *E coli*, yet human cells working together in a highly organized environment form a higher organism which in turn has developed a higher civilization. As the cells came together to do bigger things, each gave up some of its autonomy in order to do its specialized functions better, but do them in the context of the other cells of the organism. Now the time has come to think in more precise terms about how the single cells of society, human individuals, communicate to accomplish larger goals. Complexity demands that we have the right combination of people, tools, and philosophy to deal with that complexity in an effective and productive manner. Whole systems must be thought out in advance. One individual cannot, all at the same time, be the cartographer who makes maps and the busy traveler who uses them. In medicine, the options on the medical landscape must be laid out in great detail and then made available to patients and providers alike at the time of action. Modern knowledge coupling (C. Weed 1982; L. Weed 1983, 1985, 1986, 1987) tools are now available to do that, and the subsequent chapters will deal with their construction and their use. The expert cartographer cannot tell travelers what their trips should be, but neither can travelers make the best possible trip without the cartographer's map. There are almost an infinite number of trips on the map, but each of them must be made within the restrictions of the rules of the road and the traveler's destination.

For society to grapple with its problems and with problem solving in all areas where complexity is overwhelming us, we need to evolve a nervous system that can precisely connect the parts. That is exactly what our computer information systems are beginning to do. If the professors of moral philosophy of 150 years ago had had our tools, they would have been able to master and control details and construct corrective feedback loops without being swallowed up by the ugly, noncumulative, stultifying process of memorizing, regurgitating, and forgetting, all in the name of higher education and credentials. We should at least call it lower education, reminding ourselves daily of just how backward we are. Students should be colleagues using these modern tools to build with us, recognizing by their daily efforts, as John Dewey did, that "There is an inseparable relationship between knowledge and action, research and its consequences, science and ethics, the natural world and human values." He proclaimed against the fallacy of selective emphasis.

We are now in a position to heed Whitehead when he says that it is a misconception, particularly among educated people, that we can think about what we are doing at the time we are doing it in a complex task, or that civilization rises in direct proportion to its capacity to put complex tasks at the unconscious level.

It is true, as Boorstin (1983) has said, that often the enemy of new knowledge is old knowledge. Scholars who knew Ptolemy's maps had greater difficulty recognizing a new continent than those who never learned that America cannot be there. And since modern information tools can do things that the unaided human mind cannot do, when we use such tools we may see a picture of medicine that we have not seen before. The most experienced, the most highly credentialed experts may be the ones who find it most difficult to accept the new ambiguities and the contradictions to our present knowledge. John Milton found it difficult to accept the telescope; it presented a picture of the universe different from his own (Boorstin 1983). Pride in our knowledge can be our worst enemy, particularly too much pride in the knowing itself. For when we become proud of what we know, we are in danger of becoming imprisoned by the boundaries of what our limited minds can know, and we do not get on to the business of building, and using consistently, the tools we need to mobilize crucial knowledge at the time of problem solving in the real world. Never again should we judge people or empower people purely on the basis of what they know or once did know. We all should be judged on what we do. Nor should time and tasks be the constants and achievement the variable in education. Each human being is unique, and if we are to reach the highest level of achievement in what each individual does, then:

- No two people can ever be expected to do the same number of tasks in the same amount of time and to the same level of quality.

- Every individual shall have at his or her disposal the best possible tools for doing his or her work correctly.

Implications of New Premises and New Tools

Given these new premises and new tools, how then do we define a physician or nurse? First of all, we should recognize that no one, no matter what the education, can acquire all possible technical skills in medicine, even with the best information tools available. Nor can the provider be born with the patient, move out of town with the patient, or be available 24 hours a day, seven days a week, all year round. The care of a human being over time requires the efforts of many people. The patient or the patient's family should have a central role in coordinating all care. For many of the tasks in medicine to be done at a high level of quality, there is no alternative to specialization, although we all recognize its evils. The problem has been that the efforts of specialists have not been coordinated within the context of the whole life of the individual. As Wendell Berry (1977) has said in the context of farming,

> Specialization is thus seen to be a way of institutionalizing, justifying, and paying for a calamitous disintegration and scattering-out of the various functions of character—workmanship, care, conscience, responsibility.

Berry thinks of the modern single crop farmer as an exploiter, not a nurturer like the old fashioned complete, ideal farmer. For Berry, the standard of the exploiter is efficiency, whereas the standard of the nurturer is health—of the land, the family, even the community and the country. Our goal must be to develop a system of medical care whereby all individuals are the nurturers of their own health care and have available to them the guidance of an information system and the skills of providers who have demonstrated competence in performing specific tasks that patients cannot perform for themselves. Until such a framework is in place and the patient is in charge, our situation can only grow worse. The exploitative nature of the specialist will get out of control. In Berry's view,

> The specialists are profiting too well from the symptoms to be concerned about cures (prevention of the situation in the first place). The problems become the stock in trade of the specialists.

Competent performers of specific tasks in a well-defined system should legally be able to compete in the marketplace and not be a excluded by guilds of credentialed professionals whose actual performance of specific tasks can remain unevaluated and unchallenged for years. The economic implications of such a change could be enormous. Certainly until such a change is instituted, the costs of medical care will continue to skyrocket.

The exploitative nature of the generalist, though perhaps more subtle, may become an equally serious problem. It is one thing for those advocating more holistic approaches (programs in family practice, psychosomatic medicine, Oriental medicine, psychoimmunology, etc.) to inveigh against the mistakes of the specialist and relate remarkable examples of healing attributed to all sorts of spiritual forces and mind/body interactions, but it is quite another thing for them to help concerned patients to know precisely when it is wise and effective to choose and rely upon such approaches. We all know instances when precious time was lost in the case of a ruptured appendix, a confusing brain abscess, or an unusual metabolic disorder because the patient relied too heavily on anecdotes at conferences or bestsellers on healing. Only an organized system of care, executed with great discipline, can provide the best of both worlds to each patient on every encounter.

Conclusion

Once a defined system of medical care and education, based on new premises and new tools, is in place, the following advantages may become apparent, and we can hope for and, in fact, expect the following results:

- Patients and students will become productive members of the system as they move from a dependency state to being informed partners in the process. The energy that went into memorizing and regurgitating can now go into thoughtful analysis, useful work, and suggested improvements in the system.

- As Problem Knowledge Couplers immediately map the patient's unique problem and situation against known diagnostic and management options, students and all providers will learn to ask the question, "How well do present arbitrarily defined classification systems and therapeutic interventions accommodate the unique combination of findings presented by the patient?" The focus will be as much on the fallibility and inadequacies of current knowledge as it will be on failures and inadequacies of patients and students.

- Students and providers will shed their habits of certainty and associated intolerance, and instead cultivate a capacity to tolerate and to negotiate the ambiguities that inevitably appear when natural situations are honestly confronted. Each patient problem becomes a research challenge and not just another case to be run through a diagnostic mill.

- Creative people from all walks of life, as they interact with the medical care system, may offer very concrete suggestions for improving a given step in the well defined processes of care. No longer will improvement of the system be the province of only medical researchers and members of the medical industries.

- Since everyone will eventually be an informed, knowledgeable member of the medical care system, priorities can be fairly set and the economics of care openly discussed. No country's economy would ever be able to support the expectation of the best of medical care for all people, in all age groups, at all times.

With this Introduction, we are now prepared to discuss how the new premises and tools facilitate the development of a system of care and education that enhances the patient's role in his or her own care, that allows an assessment of quality, and that provides corrective feedback loops.

Throughout, the structures of the Problem Oriented Medical Record (POMR) shall be the basis for organizing our thoughts, implementing our premises, and applying the new information tools.

The four parts of the POMR upon which the discussion may proceed include

- *The Database.* Those facts on how an individual lives and functions from an emotional and social, and physical point of view. In the present system, this sort of information resides in the present illness, chief complaint, systems review and physical examination of physicians, notes of nurses, social workers, and physical therapists, psychologists, etc.

- *The Problem List.* The abnormalities in the database expressed at the highest level of synthesis and abstraction that is consistent with the evidence at hand.

- *The Titled Plans.* For each problem, there is stated the following:

    - Goal
    - Basis for the problem statement
    - Status of the problem
    - Disability from the problem
    - Parameters to follow (both symptomatic and objective) and the treatments
    - Investigate further—to rule out what diagnoses and by what means
    - Complications to watch for

● *The Titled Progress Notes for Each Problem.*

      S: Symptomatic and subjective data
      O: Objective data
      A: Assessment
      P: Plans for the next steps

Chapter 1 Summary

This chapter defines the goal, rationale, and components of the database, the first phase of the Problem Oriented Medical Record. In so doing, it describes the new information tools—Problem Knowledge Couplers and the computerized Problem Oriented Record—that accompany the new premises set forth in the Introduction.

The database, with all its detail, is the implementation of the philosophy that is the heart of this book. In sum, the very tools that health care providers use to do their work should have built into them the parameters of guidance and currency of information for doing that work in the best possible up to date manner. As maps guide the traveler securely through new and unfamiliar territory, so do these new tools guide providers through the medical landscape. Furthermore, the landscape made available by these tools to all medical travelers does not have the false boundaries that have grown up among a bewildering array of providers in the present system. Up until now, patients have been left on their own to negotiate and relate to the arbitrarily marked off territories of holistic health, family practice, specialties of all types, Oriental medicine, Western scientific medicine, public health medicine, and osteopathic, chiropractic, allopathic medicine—to say nothing of the turfs and territorial imperatives of physicians, nurses, social workers, psychologists, paramedical personnel, medical technicians, and administrators in ever increasing numbers.

A byproduct of this defined, broad, and organized database, the input into the medical care system, is an ongoing availability of interpretable output data at no great additional expense. Defined baseline data not only make more rational choices possible on unique individuals, but they also make the efforts of all patients and providers more collaborative and cumulative.

The combinatorial approach that the Problem Knowledge Couplers represent exploits the power of the details about unique individuals in solving problems. How it operates and its relationship to other structured approaches and what we call the *art of medicine* are elucidated. Detailed examples demonstrate how the tools are used to keep people well, discover problems at the earliest possible stages, diagnose new problems, and manage problems for which the diagnosis is known.

1
The Database: Its Definition and Present Status

Lawrence L. Weed and Christopher C. Weed

In the problem oriented system, the database is an organized collection of information on how an individual lives and functions from a physical, emotional, and social point of view. Its purpose is to discover any problems in their earliest stages and to organize them for analysis and solution. A total list of problems assures that each problem is dealt with in the context of all the other problems. In present paper based medical care systems and in many computerized systems, this information resides in notes on review of systems, chief complaints, physical examination, and present illnesses (largely written by physicians) and in the notes of nurses, physical therapists, social workers, and many other medical care workers. Today, portions of the information reside in hospitals, offices of all types of health workers, schools, etc. Individual patients may have little or none of it in their own possession. Furthermore, in the present system, some of the most important information related to wellness is nowhere, because it was never elicited in an organized manner in the first place.

Goal and Rationale of the Database

Our goal should be to have all the database information highly organized and accessible at any site where the patient is being seen and always available to the patient as well. The very tools for eliciting this information should have built into them the parameters of guidance and currency of information that assure standardization of *inputs* into the medical care system. Defined inputs allow meaningful study of *outcomes* and regular updating of the system of care itself.

Many of the mistakes in medicine have their roots in inadequate and uncoordinated information in the hands of all providers and the patients themselves. We cannot set a goal and complete the planning steps for one problem if we are not aware of all the problems and the conditions under which the person is expected to live and function. The Achilles heel of the specialist is intellectual isolation and the failure to take into account the whole person when dealing with part of the person. The specialist may be doing the thing right, but not be doing the right thing. The hip can be pinned perfectly, but the patient can die in heart failure. On the other hand, the development of great skill and the consistent production of high quality medical interventions require that individuals specialize. We need specialists, but we need them functioning together within a well defined system, all using a common database and all working from the same up to date problem list. Total care will always represent the efforts of many people over a long period of time. Those efforts must be highly coordinated or mistakes will be made.

We can no longer function effectively within a system where each physician does a separate workup without regard to what has already been done, and operates from a separate problem list. Nor should we collect data for the database mindlessly without having a system of care in which all of the data are used in an appropriate, integrated manner.

Components of the Database

Patient Profile

The patient profile is an explicit account of how the patient spends a routine day. Only this type of information permits the physician and patient to plan realistically for the practical welfare of the patient. The two examples cited in Figure 1 (A and B) illustrate the kind of patient profile, written routinely on actual cases, that will present some significant guidance to the physician.

Review of Systems and Physical Examination

The second part of the database is the traditional review of systems and physical examination. For a given facility, the baseline questions to be asked of, and the observations to be made on, each patient must be defined. The goal here is to get enough information to discover as many problems as possible at their earliest stages, but not necessarily enough to solve and manage each one. For example, the finding of an abnormally high blood pressure can be the first step in uncovering any one of 40 or more diagnoses.

Profile A
5/22

Intern's Readmission Note:

69-year old married white male with known lymphocytic lymphoma

was discharged 4/11, rehospitalized with comment: "I don't want

to croak at home."

Information:

Patient, and wife (reliable), old chart, Dr. ---- to be contacted.

patient Profile:

Mr. ---- is a 69-year old married white male, the father of three children

(with two daughters living, the son having been killed in World War II),

who worked in "structural steel" and as a truck driver. He is described

by his wife as a moody, somewhat self-centered individual whose main

interest in life involved keeping his car (Chevy) clean and polished

and going for drives in it-which he has been unable to during the last

few weeks of his illness. Recently he has been lying in bed at home,

doing essentially nothing-does not read, watch TV, etc.becoming

more and more depressed, complaining of feeling weak. He is a

meticulously clean person who·was disturbed by the lack of

cleanliness at the hospital during his previous admission, and

is the type of person who is overconcerned at the slightest

sign of physical illness (scratch on skin). Although he has

been said to have been told his diagnosis (according to wife),

he gave no evidence of knowing it during our interview (denial?).

Figure 1. Patient Profile A.

Profile B
7/11

SMS Admission Note

This is the first ---- Hospital admission for this 35-year-old white female admitted through the Gastrointestinal Clinic for therapy for a gastric ulcer. The patient's chief complaint is "my ulcer."

Source of Information: Patient (reliable), and Outpatient Clinic chart.

Patient Profile:

Mrs. ---- was born in Wilmington, Delaware- eldest of 2 children. She attended school through 2 years of high school. She has been married for 12 years and has no children. She and her husband lived in Wilmington until 3 years ago when they moved to Detroit so that her husband could find a better job. They left Detroit 1 month ago because they "hated it" and moved to Cleveland. Mr. ---- is currently employed at C------ and S------ Company as a supervisor. He works a night shift and is rarely at home. His income is sufficient to support them and they have hospitalization insurance. The couple lives in a 4-room rented apartment on West 25th St. Mrs. ---- describes herself as "a nervous person" who worries about "little things." She has been employed for 2 weeks at L--- K---- Mills and says she enjoys the work because "she can talk to the girls." Previous to this she spent most of her time at home reading, watching TV. She notes that it is very lonely with her husband at work most of the time and states that she doesn't know any of her neighbors because she "doesn't mix well with people." Up until 5 weeks ago she had a dog who was her constant companion and whom she loved "like a little child." Her dog "passed away" and she dissolves into tears each time she speaks about her pet. She is quite anxious about her hospital stay-she is worried that her ulcer will not heal, that she will need an operation, and that she won't be able to relax properly. She knows every detail about her illness and is extremely talkative. She does not drink alcohol but smokes 1 + packs of Camels per day for many years. Notes that unless she has her cigarettes at her bedside she gets extremely nervous.

Figure 1. Patient Profile B.

That one finding, therefore, should be in the database. The details that help us sort the 40 causes will be in the knowledge coupler, a new computerized information tool that will be discussed in the pages that follow.

Failure to define the initial database is like playing football with a different number of men on the team each time, on a field of no defined length. Individual plays may be perfected, but their value depends upon the context in which they are used. A poorly defined medical exploration of the patient, which may be incomplete in infinitely variable ways from patient to patient, damages the physician's ability both to determine what it is he or she ought to do and then to assess the quality of what he or she actually has done.

It should no longer be acceptable to say that the physician does not have the time to get or to study the data. Nor is it acceptable to say the physician could take the time, but the expense is too great considering the hourly rate of the average physician. It is better to explore nonphysician ways to get good data than it is to give up getting the data altogether. The analogy of rescue squads is appropriate here. When the need was defined, an economically and intellectually feasible way was found to get that service without expensive physician time for much of the effort. Good physicians may have done much in the way of design and training to ensure the success of that effort (a success that is now generally recognized), but nonphysician personnel keep the system going and keep the community involved. We should feel as responsible for preventing problems and discovering them early as we do for rescuing people in emergencies. Emergencies consume inordinate amounts of money and resources.

Constancy and Maintenance of the Database

Once the desirable database has been defined for a given practice or locality, unauthorized modifications in it should not be allowed. The pressure to ignore the broad view of a patient will be ever present. The economic gains to specialists and generalists doing episodic care on many patients in rapid succession can be enormous. For them, there is no way that prevention and care in the broadest possible context can be as financially rewarding as the present system and payment mechanisms. A specialist can easily become an exploiter of contextual chaos. Under the present system, physicians get paid for doing a procedure they can prove to be justified at the moment. The fact that an expensive procedure might have been avoided altogether if total overall care and maintenance had been provided from the beginning in no way prevents the physician from doing it and getting paid. Hospitals can be thought of in many instances as an intellectual and monetary harvest on delayed maintenance. The physician who requires three visits to unravel a problem that might have been solved in one visit with the right information tools still gets paid for all three visits.

Uniformity in the database is among the important factors tending to permit accurate comparability and generalization. This uniformity is essential to the welfare of the whole patient. Both for the sake of our science and the sake of our patients, the standard database must be conscientiously sought on each patient, even if paramedical personnel must ultimately be relied upon to procure it. Failure to utilize nonphysician personnel in the past is not, I believe, related to any intrinsic lack of ability on their part; rather it stems from our failure to define specific goals for them and to perfect the techniques that should be applied to reach those goals. In this latter regard, much has been accomplished, using the computer, to facilitate the efficient acquisition of a defined database.

Summarizing our discussion thus far on the database:

- We must acquire and act upon information first to keep people well.

- We then must discover problems in their earliest stages and organize them for solution. It is at this stage that we are prepared to create the first problem list on the patient, one that includes or accounts for every abnormality detected thus far in the database.

- We must then get more detailed information on the patient's chief complaint and on each of the problems that has been discovered in preparation for the diagnosis and management of each.

The Computer in Coupling Medical Knowledge to Action

The implementation of the above three steps and subsequent steps in the problem oriented system in a complete and rigorous manner implies a great deal of medical knowledge and a capacity to organize and apply that knowledge to unique problem situations under pressures of time and circumstance. We have called this the knowledge coupling problem. We are just now beginning to admit how deficient the unaided mind has been in this regard and how much the computer can help.

Before proceeding further, we should pause and place the computer in the proper perspective because its effects can be profound and far reaching. New approaches are practical right now and no further delay should be tolerated in getting out of the present paradigm and into a new one.

To point out more precisely at what points in the medical care process the unaided mind has been deficient, we shall use the framework of the problem oriented record that I first set forth in *Medical Records, Medical Education, and Patient Care* (1969). Certain assumptions were made about what the mind could and was doing as it progressed through the four phases of medical action: from database to problem list, to the titled plans for each problem, and to the titled progress notes on each problem.

It was assumed that the problems would be properly prioritized as the problem list was generated from examining the database. In the third major portion of the database, the present illness/es, where the physician gets more detailed information on each complaint or abnormal finding, it was assumed that the details about the complaint or a finding (onset, duration, findings associated with the abnormality, etc.) were acquired. It was further assumed that the reasons why these details were pursued and what they pointed to in the doctor's mind in terms of diagnosis and management were precisely known and became the basis for a highly organized pursuit of the problem. But it has not been possible in most records to discern unambiguously how each detail (each positive finding) of the present illness and physical examination was interpreted and used. For example, the term *crescendo* may appear as a descriptor after a systolic heart murmur in a routine physical examination, yet the person who wrote it may not have in mind a list of all the causes of a systolic murmur and a clear idea of which of the causes the finding crescendo may suggest (i.e., "vote for") and how it should be used in other interpretations. Even among physicians who can explain how they used a bit of information from a present illness or physical examination to make a diagnosis or choose a management option, there may be striking variability in the way they interpret the same bit of information.

In other words, there is no way of knowing from the medical record itself how or whether much of the information in a record has been processed by the human mind. Nor is it evident from the record what the original universe of details consisted of, from which the positive findings on a given patient were derived. If a given association is not recorded, it is impossible to know whether it is because it was never asked or done on physical examination or whether it was asked or done and was not present in the patient, or whether it was done, was present, but never recorded. Of course, the way the complaint is represented on the problem list may suggest the kind of thinking that went on. For example, if a complaint is simply stated as abdominal pain, then the person writing the present illness did not use the details to carry the problem to a higher level of abstraction. On the other hand, the use of the descriptor *cholecystitis* on the problem list supports inferences regarding the interpretation of the details about and associated with the abdominal pain. Even then, there is no strict accounting of the universe of diagnoses considered or of the details that "voted for" and "voted against" each diagnostic option. It is this precise level of accounting that is required in order to identify and correct faulty or incomplete reasoning in the diagnostic or management process.

Knowledge couplers enable every user of the record (providers, patients, or epidemiologists) to know why every bit of information was elicited and precisely how each bit was used or could be used for interpretation and action. The reviewer will no longer be in the position of not knowing whether a critical item is absent because the patient did not have it or because it was not observed or asked about even though the patient had it. Nor will there be doubt as to how the information was used to formulate the problems or define specific diagnostic or management actions. In other words, we will no longer be in the position of saying that the process of progressing from the database to the problem list or from the problem list to the plans for each problem was one of "informed clinical judgment." Moreover, with printout capability, patients can immediately have a copy of the whole transaction and leave the physician's office without wondering what their responsibilities are or what is going on in the mind of the physician.

And so, when we are in the database, phase 1 of the POMR, much is being done with the data as they are acquired to organize them into a list of problems stated at the highest level of abstraction possible and to lay the basis for the plans in very concrete terms. The precisely stated plans for each problem become the basis for problem oriented progress notes that reveal to all what progress has been.

The Knowledge Coupling Problem

The knowledge coupling problem can be simply put this way: Given a decision making problem in diagnosis or management, what do we need to do to assure that

- All relevant diagnoses or management options known to medical science are readily available for consideration?

- The unique features of the problem situation bearing on the discrimination among these options are appropriately checked and assessed?

- The appropriate associations are made between the unique features of the situation and the many diagnostic or management options?

In a diagnostic problem such as memory loss and/or confusion, where the number of distinguishable potential causes may approach 100, and where the number of relevant details about the specific patient may be many more than that, it is clear that the unaided human mind is not up to the task. Individual experience is of limited value, since it is always somewhat parochial. This is notably true of the specialist, since the knowledge required to deal rigorously and completely with real patients' problems usually crosses specialty boundaries. In managing essential hypertension, for example, the array of drugs and nonpharmacologic approaches and the enormous variety of patients with the problem present equally overwhelming numbers of details to be considered and related to one another.

Effective and thorough knowledge coupling is a necessary part of sound medical decision making, and can be considered as a substantial problem in its own right. Certainly medical decision making involves additional elements some might hope to emulate in computer software and hardware. However, our position is that the difficulties and failures of medical decision making in everyday practice are largely failures in knowledge coupling, due to the over-reliance on the unaided human mind to recall and organize all the relevant details. They are not, specifically and essentially, failures to reason logically with the medical knowledge once it is presented completely and in a highly organized form within the framework of the patient's total and unique situation.

Reliance on human memory and processing capability is not the only obstacle to an effective solution to the knowledge coupling problem as we have defined it. Individual practitioners are also confronted with the task of "loading their memory" from the medical literature, which is not a concentrated source of the easily accessible, current, and clinically relevant answers needed in the effective application of knowledge. We have concluded that practitioners should not have to digest large and growing bodies of literature in training or in the midst of practice to couple effectively medical knowledge to their actions. This process of digestion can be done in advance by a central library or repository, which captures its results in knowledge coupling tools. These tools should then be used routinely in the practice of medicine. The tools themselves can contain all the important options to be considered, the observations to be made on the unique patient, and the significant associations or linkages among them. The tools can be responsive and flexible in their presentation to the user because the logical structure of the data to be presented and the useful modes of presentation can be quite simple. Such a structure lends itself to implementation with efficient and well understood database design techniques for small computers.

Structuring Medical Knowledge for Effective Coupling to Action

The logical structure of the envisioned knowledge coupling tool can be outlined as follows:

- *A present illness*, such as memory loss (a problem to be diagnosed) or essential hypertension (a known diagnosis to be managed). The problem can be expected to turn up either as a chief complaint or in a routine screening history and physical examination.

- *Primary options*, a complete set of diagnostic possibilities or management options for the problem. Each option and its precise linkage to the problem under consideration should be referenced to the medical literature in the form of specifically relevant excerpts.

- *Potential findings*, a set of them to be looked for in the patient together with linkages of those findings to the diagnostic or management options. These findings and their linkages should also be referenced to the medical literature. All the findings must be checked for in each case. With their linkages they provide a basis for discriminating among the primary options. The linkages can be thought of as defining an associative matrix.

- *A structured questionnaire*, including all the potential findings should be used to interrogate the patient and those examining the patient.

- *Secondary options*, those invasive or expensive treatments or further diagnostic measures that should be considered if the initial positive findings and their linkages indicate particularly likely diagnoses or appropriate management options.

- *Commentary*, associated with the potential findings or the primary or secondary options, which provides additional information of potential clinical value about all the above mentioned components.

The comment section, although just one of the four basic building blocks of a coupler, has proved to make a unique contribution to the system. It allows the builder of the coupler to convey, and the user of the coupler to understand, useful details about the entities and linkages in the coupler. When confronted with ambiguities and disagreements in what appears to be reliable literature sources, the builder can make the user aware of them through a comment rather than arbitrarily choosing one point of view over another without informing the user. Interesting information in case reports, and other material in studies that statisticians would frown upon, can be placed in the proper perspective as opposed to ignoring or denying it altogether. Quantitative details about timing, frequency, and severity of findings and their relationships to causes or management options can be concisely stated and presented to the user when most needed—when weighing one cause or one management option against another as presented by the coupler. These capabilities of the system enable the provider and the patient to be both more productive and better informed in the decision making process. And their relevance to the patient is assured by the match of findings on the patient that elicited the comments in the first place.

In short, we have examined above the nature and significance of the knowledge coupling problem, and defined what the logical structure of the tool requires in order to *couple* the details of *knowledge about a patient with a problem* to the *relevant knowledge from the medical literature*, hence the name for the tool—the *Problem Knowledge Coupler*. The number of details from each of the knowledge sources can be so numerous, and the process of matching the details from the patient to the details from the vast medical literature so demanding, that a new tool to extend the capacity of the unaided mind was necessary.

It will be apparent from the foregoing that the structure of a Problem Knowledge Coupler is quite simple. The coupler system generates its results by a highly regular, repeatable process, which is driven in a straightforward manner by the associations or linkages encoded in a coupler database.

The rules for display of a primary option can be stated as follows:

Rule D1: If one or more of the primary (diagnostic or management) option's associated findings occur in a patient, display the option.

> That is all that is involved in deciding to display a primary option. The remaining display rules have to do with the ordering of the primary options in a selection index displayed by the coupler system. These rules are also very straightforward.

Rule D2: Sort the primary options into groups according to their assigned display weights—from highest to lowest.

> The display weights are assigned by the person who builds a coupler. Refer to the introductions to the various couplers for discussions of precisely how these display weights are used.

Rule D3: Within a group, sort the primary options in descending order by the absolute number of findings observed in the patient.

There are a few simple rules concerning the display of information associated with each primary diagnostic or management option.

Rule P1: In a diagnostic coupler, display all the potential *findings* associated with a primary diagnostic option in the coupler database. Sort the findings into a group of findings present (in the patient) and findings not present. In a management coupler, display only the findings present.

Rule P2: Display all elements of coupler commentary (*comments*) associated with the primary option in the coupler database, which are flagged to appear with the findings.

Rule P3: Display a menu choice for accessing secondary options (tests, procedures, treatments) that are associated with the primary option in the coupler database, if such data exist.

Rule P4 (triggered by Rule P3): When secondary options are accessed for a primary option, display them in a list. Display below them all coupler *comments* associated with the primary option in the coupler database, which are flagged to appear with the secondary options.

Rule P5 (triggered by Rules P1-P4): When displaying information associated with a primary option, display its associated reference numbers when the coupler system is in "with references" display mode.

Rule P6 (triggered by Rule P1): When displaying findings associated with a primary option, display the number of additional primary options associated with each finding when the coupler system is in "with # of other Causes/MgtOpts" display mode.

Finally, there are a few simple rules concerning the display of all the observed findings in a coupler session (the first part of the session results). The rules are:

Rule F1: Sort the *findings* by their assigned *display weights*, and display them in groups, with the highest weighted groups appearing first.

Generally, these groupings roughly correspond to the traditional way of organizing medical database information in the present illness and the systems review of the patient.

Rule F2: Under each of the *findings*, display the *comments* associated with each finding in the coupler database, along with their associated reference numbers.

With this formulation of the central functions of the coupler system, we are now prepared to ask how these functions relate to what is ordinarily thought of as reasoning with a medical knowledge base.

Step 1: Medical reasoning, at times intricate, is required during the compilation and editing process when the coupler is built. This is done by human beings. These human beings are supported by computer based development tools and a central database of medical knowledge, called a knowledge network.

Step 2: Associative and organizing power is then required of the computer to take the positive findings, elicited from the patient at the time of coupler use, and relate them in a highly organized manner to the most appropriate diagnostic or management options for the unique patient of the moment.

Step 3: The patient and the provider then reason with what is presented to them and make the choices most appropriate to their values and goals.

The above three steps, then, summarize what is going on when knowledge couplers are used in everyday problem solving. When clinicians function on their own without knowledge couplers or any other external aid, there is considerable psychological evidence that they rely heavily on associative responses to situations, based on their factual knowledge, to solve problems quickly, especially under pressure. Except in the most probable and easily anticipated instances, people may fail because their factual knowledge and their associative powers are limited and often unreliable. This is true even of so called experts. They may outperform the nonexpert because their factual knowledge in a given area is greater, but probably not because their associative powers are greater. An individual's associative powers are dependent on the amount of factual knowledge that an individual has to work on. Although couplers are not necessarily perfect or complete, they do provide a defined and reproducible way of coupling knowledge to action. This reproducibility constitutes the basis for corrective feedback loops.

Experts can fail miserably when a patient enters their care whose history or physical examination contains relevant details that are unknown to them or whose problem has a cause outside of their specialty or knowledge base. This happens all too often since real problems always cross the manmade specialty boundaries of the expert. Patients, on the other hand, automatically have available to them a great deal of factual knowledge about their own problem situation, which is never exploited to the fullest when operating under the old premises.

In other words, to get everyday work done, most people try to develop a store of usefully associative information on what works and what is important. Careful logical reasoning from basic principles is often either inapplicable or impractical. The difficulty is that people can only do this well with respect to the particular diagnostic or management options for problems that they have thought about or experienced repeatedly. There is, therefore, a strong tendency to respond to problems in terms that are familiar to the problem solver, rather than appropriate to the problem. This can be avoided only with an external aid like the coupler, combined with appropriate attitudes towards its use, and through a more active role of patients in their own behalf.

Thinking then in terms of the three steps mentioned above, we may have, in the past, seriously overestimated the human mind's knowledge base and associative capacity at the time of problem solving, and seriously underestimated each individual's capacity to do Step 3, that is, to reason effectively with the diagnostic and management options and associated comments that the system presents to both the provider and the patient.

All this raises the question, How does the Problem Knowledge Coupler System differ from other approaches to making medical knowledge more accessible and effective in application? The alternative approaches, most of them better known, can be classified as follows:

Online medical literature retrieval. This provides a vast reservoir of factual knowledge, but it leaves it to the user to decide what information should be elicited from and about his or her patient. It also limits providers to their individual associative powers and their individual powers to present the appropriate options to their patients so the latter can place all the details in the context of their own values and goals. It does not do Step 2 above as the knowledge coupler does.

An online literature search is like giving a hungry woman a bushel of wheat. She would like you to at least give her a loaf of bread. A knowledge coupler is like giving her a sandwich. To use another analogy, providing a large unprocessed literature base is like giving a tired man a very large, well equipped shop and a load of lumber, when what he needs and wants is a chair.

Approaches based on Bayesian decision theory. Medical decision analysis can be considered the immediate theoretical background for these approaches. These approaches operate far more on the basis of probability information on large populations (much of it averaged over the whole course of an illness and without regard to precisely where the patient is in the course of the illness), with a few fragments of information on "pretest likelihood" (details about the unique patient). The knowledge coupler, on the other hand, elicits hundreds of details about the patient and then matches them in a combinatorial sense to all the diagnostic or management options that can be legitimately extracted from the medical literature. Every time another relevant detail is extracted from a patient, the probabilities for each option are changed. In a very short time, almost any prior estimate of probabilities becomes totally irrelevant. Again, providers use probabilities in direct proportion to their ignorance of the uniqueness of the problem situation.

Approaches which are not strictly Bayesian but that roughly attempt to emulate the analytic thought processes of an expert physician, using computations based on significance weightings and weighting functions, also, various rule based or so called expert systems. The knowledge coupler does not even attempt to model what experts do when confronted with a specific problem. It tries, rather, to avoid the pitfalls of human judgement that are so well documented in the psychology literature.

Pattern recognition approaches, some based on neural network technology, which are more or less explicitly probabilistic.

More conventional approaches based on various theories and techniques of modern engineering, typically used for fairly specialized applications, such as automated EKG interpretation. These approaches are also typically used in situations that conform at least in part to an industrial process control model.

Wherever possible, the results of some of these highly successful and well engineered approaches to getting crucial data should be used as input to the knowledge coupler.

In summary, the Problem Knowledge Coupler can be thought of as standing midway between the first class (online literature retrieval) and the remaining classes. It was designed, as we have shown, to be very simple and regular in its structure, and quite limited in its demands on computing resources. However, the coupler system also possesses some singular methodological and epistemological virtues closely related to this simplicity of structure. It provides a supplementation and support of human capabilities, not a replacement or a simulation of them, even in principle. Coupler results, while providing a necessary basis for decisions, contains no determinate decision rules. We conceived the problem as one of structuring, sorting, and filtering the literature so that what remains is always of potential clinical relevance and can be most easily coupled to the actual presentation of clinical problems. We wanted our solution to be potentially applicable to most of the literature, and to be compatible with and perform well on the most inexpensive and widely available computers.

We concluded that effective access to the clinically relevant medical knowledge must be problem oriented and must provide systematic guidance in data collection from both the patient and the literature relative to a problem. It must then organize and present the relevant bits of knowledge that were extracted and relate them to one another in patterns that are easily negotiated by the user.

Having described the approach outlined, we can now review some additional virtues in it.

First, the coupler system does not condition the collection of data (findings) on tentative or preliminary choices of primary options (diagnoses or management options). In other words, it does not attempt to imitate uncritically a hypothetical-deductive or iterative mode of arriving at decisions. This has two notable advantages:

- The system facilitates discovery of the limitations of existing criteria and classification schemes as a byproduct of everyday clinical work. Much of medical knowledge is conventional and arbitrary, conditioned by accidents of history and the parochial outlooks of particular investigators. Disease processes have certain expected features, expected outcomes, and expected responses to various interventions. We need to continuously check the strength of the correlations these expectations imply. The coupler system supports this when all the potential findings are checked before considering any of the suggested options (in the coupler results).

If current knowledge and thought, the currency of educators, are not rigorously coupled to everyday action, and if rigorous records and feedback loops are not employed to follow the results of those actions, then misconceptions can go uncorrected and the whole knowledge base and educational process are corrupted; medical education and patient care become a fragmented collection of uncoordinated parts that never add up to wisdom—they are never "woven into a fabric." As the great justice Learned Hand expressed it at the time the Hooper Doctrine emerged as part of our body of law: At times a whole profession or industry can be held liable.

- The system reduces the likelihood of overlooking temporal aspects of an illness, by not eliminating options from consideration based on a few criteria, and by explicitly informing the user (in comments on the primary options) of the potentially misleading temporal aspects of specific situations.

Second, the coupler system does not require, or even allow, failure to present a primary option based on supposed relationships of mutual exclusion with other primary options. If evidence for multiple diagnoses, or indications for multiple management options, exists, this will be clearly presented. Information on relationships of mutual exclusion can be provided in comments for the user to consider. A well known weakness of the simplest Bayesian diagnostic approaches is their requirement of mutual exclusion of diagnoses, and conditional independence of potential findings. These requirements are commonly violated in practice. Various strategies have been developed for mitigating these weaknesses, which substantially complicate the approach. (It should be noted that Bayes' formula can be generalized to eliminate the requirement of mutual exclusivity, at the price of a great increase in its complexity. The strategies mentioned can be regarded as techniques for approximately implementing the principle in its general form.)

Third, the coupler system, because it does not fully model decision making with the use of definite decision criteria, does not have do the computation involved in implementing such criteria. As a corollary to this it does not require the numerical input data that Bayesian and other probabilistic techniques require. This is important, because such data are often either not readily available or of dubious quality. Also, as previously alluded to, statistical decision analytic techniques are generically inadequate in dealing with the temporal aspects of illness, if only because these aspects promise to add substantial additional complexity to an already complex field.

The intended primary mode of presentation of the content of a knowledge coupling tool is as follows:

- The user goes through the questionnaire, performing the indicated data collection, observations, or examination procedures in order to thoroughly characterize the patient's case.

- The user requests a presentation of results, which should include

  - A review of the findings made in the case

  - An index of the primary diagnostic or management options associated with findings made on the patient (NOTE: The primary options are not mutually exclusive and can be grouped in various ways to distinguish classes of options or convey different views of the situation. In a diagnostic context, the index is roughly comparable to a differential diagnosis for the given findings.)

    - Detailed information associated with each primary option on the index to aid in its evaluation: Associated findings, possibly including potential findings that did not show up in the patient, potentially useful commentary on the primary option, and a list of relevant secondary options.

- The user studies the results and makes decisions about the options presented—whether to pursue them, and if so, how.

- The user records his or her decisions, along with the supporting information from the literature provided by the knowledge coupling tool.

The user and the patient are free to incorporate additional considerations of the unique situation into the decisions, just as they would in using any source of medical information. Knowledge coupling tools should be thought of as providing a map of the medical territory into which a patient has been led by the unique course of his or her life. The information in maps cannot be a complete basis for all travel decisions, because maps cannot deal with all the nongeographic information and transient circumstances that may bear on those decisions. They nevertheless provide an essential framework for those decisions. The availability of maps liberates individuals, making it possible for them to navigate in and explore with confidence and flexibility regions they have never encountered before.

The creation and maintenance of geographic maps is a specialized and quite centralized function, based on widely accepted standards for representation and communication of geographic information. We do not expect all travelers to carry a copy of the world's store of geographic information in their heads, and we do not expect them to create and maintain their own maps of a region, country, or the world. We expect them to acquire the modest and uniform knowledge and skills needed to use maps, and to judge when maps are needed to supplement their own store of geographic information.

It is unlikely that anyone could create an initial set of diagnostic and management couplers that would be complete, up to date, and satisfactory from everyone's point of view, but if we all agree upon the goal of achieving a set useful to all, it can rapidly be achieved. A central repository open to communication from all users can make the necessary changes and additions at regular intervals, referencing each as it is made. Such a mechanism makes the efforts of all providers in the medical care system collaborative and cumulative. To those who suggest that such an approach robs the system of a valuable diversity, we can point out that diversity in action that is based on mutual ignorance of the experience of other workers in the field is not necessarily valuable. Rather, it is misleading, unfair, and confusing to the patient who deserves the best that our collective intelligence can provide. The valuable diversity will manifest itself in the information that flows from the records of all the unique individuals who use the system. Ultimately that knowledge from usage should be the most powerful influence on the content of the couplers themselves. It is, after all, clinical research on large numbers of people in the broadest possible context with guaranteed relevance to the actual practice of medicine.

In his recent thoughtful editorial, Edward J. Huth (1989) observed, "What an irony! As medicine knows more and more about how to recognize disease and its nature and how to relieve patients of its burdens, each of us has become less and less able to offer competent care for all the problems that patients might bring to us." Covell and Manning's article in the *Annals of Internal Medicine* in 1985 said essentially what the 1989 article and editorial stated. Knowledge coupling tools were conceived and designed in the early 1980s to meet the problems these authors are discussing.

The Role of the Computer in Implementing the Three Steps of the Database

Step 1: Wellness

We must acquire and act upon information first to keep people well.

Not only does the computer provide guidance as to what data should be acquired, but it takes the positive responses keyed in by the user and automatically organizes them. In the case of wellness the coupler on the microcomputer, the computer provides immediate guidance as to what the management of a given finding might be.

As users of the wellness coupler, patients answer many questions on a computer screen or from a booklet designed to have its results entered into the computer. The details of these questions are under such categories as nutrition, habits and lifestyle, living arrangements, major life events, environmental exposures, drugs and alcohol, attitudes and feelings, interpersonal relationships, personal care (sleep, exercise, etc.), immunizations, and risk factors.

Figure 2 is the first display on the computer screen that we see after choosing the wellness coupler. If we make a choice from this display by typing one of the numbers in front of the choices, a display similar to Figure 3 appears. We then make choices from this latter display, and an arrow appears in front of the choice that is made. After having gone through the whole coupler, we return to the original display (Figure 2) and make the choice "C:Couple." A total list appears of all the choices that were made (the positive findings). Figure 4 shows some of the management options that those choices suggest. Figure 5 is what we will see if we select one of the management options seen in Figure 4. The two displays on Figure 5 are expansions of two of the management options for the patient, representative examples of what this patient takes home and uses as a basis for keeping well. Everything the patient takes home is tailored to his or her needs, because it was the patient's original choices that elicited the unique set of management options.

Step 2: Discovering Problems

We then must discover problems in their earliest stages and organize them for solution. It is at this stage that we are prepared to create the first problem list on the patient, one that includes or accounts for every abnormality detected thus far in the database.

Systems Review and Physical Examination. In the case of the systems review and physical examination, the user again answers many questions on a computer screen or from a booklet designed to have its results entered into the computer. The microcomputer takes the positive responses and organizes them into prioritized work lists in addition to providing some specific guidance for certain positive items. To assure that a very sick patient requiring immediate attention for a serious physiological derangement, such as shock, severe bleeding, or rapidly progressing neurological findings, is not compromised by a long data gathering process, the first displays on the computer go directly to the basic parameters that should be checked before embarking on the complete data gathering process. If any or several of these are positive, as users, we are advised to stop the routine workup, initiate all necessary emergency measures, and stabilize the patient. After these things are accomplished, the complete database is acquired if possible.

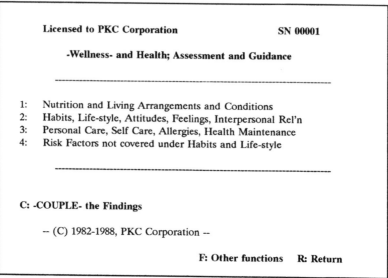

Figure 2

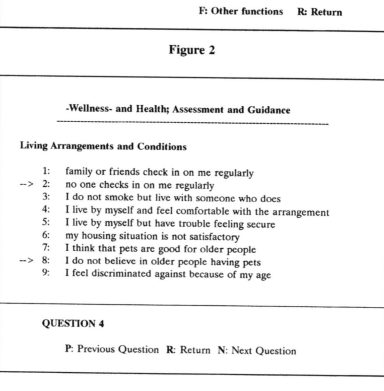

Figure 3

```
+-------------------------------------------------------------------------+
|                   -- Suggested Management Options --                     |
|                                                                         |
| 1:COMMENDABLE HEALTH HABITS AND BELIEFS YOU HAVE AND                     |
|    SHOULD MAINTAIN                                                       |
| 2:INCREASE FIBER IN YOUR DIET - There is increasing evidence it is im... |
| 3:AT BREAKFAST ON A REGULAR BASIS. Even if you do not feel like eat...   |
| 4:FISH SHOULD BE IN YOUR DIET 2-3 TIMES WEEKLY. There is evidence        |
|    tha...                                                                |
| 5:HAVE SOMEONE CHECK IN ON YOU ON A REGULAR BASIS AT A                   |
|    REGULAR TIME -...                                                     |
| 6:A TRY at HAVING A PET should be CONSIDERED - Evidence is               |
|    accumulati...                                                         |
| 7:AVOID DRINKING ALCOHOL EXCEPT IN MINIMAL OR MODERATE                   |
|    AMOUNTS - that...                                                     |
| 8:NEVER BORROW A MOTORCYCLE OR EVEN A BICYCLE IF                         |
|    POSSIBLE. If you use...                                               |
| 9:TRY TO READ ONE BOOK A MONTH - It is important to keep up this         |
|    habi...                                                               |
|    (17 more ...)                                                         |
|                                                                         |
| 1..9: Display MgOpt information                                         |
|     D: Change display mode -- [ normal ]                                 |
|                   M:More   P: Print Results   F: Findings   R: Return   |
+-------------------------------------------------------------------------+
```

Figure 4

```
+-------------------------------------------------------------------------+
|                                                                  Page 1 |
| A TRY at HAVING A PET should be CONSIDERED - Evidence is accumulating that|
| both person and pet benefit. Blood pressure is lowered, stress reduced, self worth|
| increased. Have someone who cares for pets help you find the best kind for you.|
|                                                                         |
|     I do not believe in older people having pets . . . . . . . .        |
|                                                                         |
| One study showed that heart attack pts. with pets have 1/3 the death rate. Blood|
| pressures fall when one greets and pets an animal. The pet shifts attention from anxious|
| thoughts and helps depression and self esteem problems.                 |
|     [Refs: 2883]                                                        |
|     F: First          P: Print          R: Return                       |
+-------------------------------------------------------------------------+
```

```
+-------------------------------------------------------------------------+
| NEVER BORROW A MOTORCYCLE OR EVEN A BICYCLE IF POSSIBLE. If you         |
| use a motorcycle, become very experienced in its use under the safest possible conditions.|
|   I use bicycles or motorcycles - even borrow them from others          |
|                                 [Refs: 2004 2799 2805]                   |
|                                                                         |
| 37% of cycling injuries occur on borrowed bikes. 3/4 of the injuries involving passengers|
| occurred on borrowed bikes. 1/2 of the riders in fatal and non-fatal injuries were under|
| 15. 90% of fatalities occurred in collisions with motor cars            |
|                                 [Refs: 2799 2804 2805]                   |
|                                                                         |
| Bicycle/motor vehicle collision injuries might be reduced by 11% by helmets. 70% of|
| head injuries fall within the area covered by most helmets designed for bicyclists. Bikes|
| put together at home are particularly dangerous.                        |
|                         [Refs: 2799 2804 2805]                           |
| The majority of motorcycle crashes involve inexperience, failure of another driver to|
| perceive the 2-wheeled vehicle, or use of alcohol.                      |
|                         [Refs:2799 2804 2805]                            |
|     F: First          P: Print          R: Return                       |
+-------------------------------------------------------------------------+
```

Figure 5

The prioritized work lists are organized according to the findings, as follows:

Findings requiring

- *Immediate or emergency attention*, for example, vomiting blood

- *Attention* on the *day of discovery* at least to the point of explaining it to the patient and outlining the first steps to deal with it

- *Long term problems*, for example, psoriasis that needs attention for optimum care, but there is no danger from a few days delay if that is necessary

- *Risk factors*, for example, a family history of polyps of the colon, a factor that should lead to certain procedures in following this patient that would not be appropriate in a patient without this history.

Together with the patient, we as providers go through the displays as in the Wellness Coupler. Figure 6 is the beginning display of the systems review. After making a choice on this display, we see specific questions (Figure 7). After making choices from the questions and after coupling, we first see all the positive findings as shown in Figure 8.

The screening history elicits and prioritizes the positive findings under four headings (Figure 9, Items 1 to 4). The findings under all four headings taken together add up to the first problem list on the patient. We may examine this total list and immediately combine some findings under a single heading, thereby condensing the problem list. Other findings will go on the list as a separate problem, often requiring a diagnostic or management coupler to clarify the situation further.

For example, if three findings, such as shortness of breath, leg edema, and hepatomegaly, all appeared at approximately the same time, and we as providers recognize them as manifestations of heart failure, then we place that problem on the problem list. On the other hand, if they seemed to occur independently or if we do not have enough evidence or experience to combine them, then each finding can be a separate problem, Once a complete set of couplers is available, and each finding is persued through its respective coupler, then a synthesis should emerge. If several findings have an obvious temporal relationship and appear to be manifestations of a single problem, then before bothering to do couplers on each, we as users should begin with the finding that is the most objective and reproducible and localizes to a single body system.

Licensed to PKC Corporation SN 00001

      -HISTORY-   **Screening to Discover Patient's Problems**

1:    EMERGENCY FINDINGS-MANAGE STAT (abort routine work-up)

2:    Body Systems Review

3:    Habits, Life-style, Allergies, Health Maintenance

4:    Previous Surgery and X-Rays

5:    Risk Factors not covered under Habits and Life-style

    C: -COUPLE- the Findings

In the Hx and Px "Couplers", each response is "coupled" to one of the standard Systems Review headings (e.g. rash under Skin) as well as to the appropriate Management Options which set priorities for the management of abnormal findings.

          -- (C) 1982-1988, PKC Corporation --

            F: Other functions   R: Return

Figure 6

         -HISTORY-   **Screening to Discover Patient's Problems**

Skin and hair:

--> 1:   mole or pigmented lesion that is changing size/color/border
    2:    rash on skin - new and unexplained
    3:    skin changing texture: eg shiny, stiff, coarse, dry, scaly
    4:    new mass or growth on skin other than a mole
--> 5:   psoriasis has been diagnosed
    6:    acne that is troublesome

QUESTION 2

        P: Previous Question   R: Return   N: Next Question

Figure 7

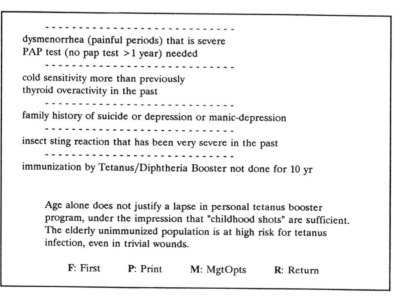

Page 1

***> OBSERVED FINDINGS

BREATHING DIFFICULTY - progressive and/or severe

- -
mole or pigmented lesion that is changing size/color/border
psoriasis has been diagnosed
- -
eye pain (frequent or recurring) within the past year
- -
tonsillectomy in the past
- -
moldy hay exposure
- -
hypertension (known) or elevated blood pressure
- -
swallowing is painful
hernia surgery in the past
rectal pain
- -
kidney stone history

        N: Next   **P:** Print **M:** MgtOpts **R:** Return

- -
dysmenorrhea (painful periods) that is severe
PAP test (no pap test >1 year) needed
- -
cold sensitivity more than previously
thyroid overactivity in the past
- -
family history of suicide or depression or manic-depression
- -
insect sting reaction that has been very severe in the past
- -
immunization by Tetanus/Diphtheria Booster not done for 10 yr

Age alone does not justify a lapse in personal tetanus booster
program, under the impression that "childhood shots" are sufficient.
The elderly unimmunized population is at high risk for tetanus
infection, even in trivial wounds.

      F: First   **P:** Print   **M:** MgtOpts   **R:** Return

Figure 8

--**Suggested Management Options**--

1:   IMMEDIATE MANAGEMENT required for:
2:   EVALUATE NOW AND INITIATE WORK-UP IF APPROPRIATE:
3:   LONG TERM OBSERVATION AND MANAGEMENT may be required
     for:
4:   RISK FACTOR - requires recognition and management:

5:   DEPRESSIVE DISORDER should be considered as a possible
     explanation ...
6:   Allergies and Drug Reactions:
7:   OBTAIN SCREENING LUNG FUNCTION TESTS NOW: (FVC, FEV-1,
     PEAK FLOW/M...
                         (21 more ...)

1:   SCHEDULE PELVIC/PAP TEST APPT., if not completed at time of
     complet...

2:   PAST MEDICAL HISTORY - Write opposite each the Date, MD, Place,
     Rea...

3:   LIST PREVIOUS X-RAYS - record date, type of study and where done...
4:   LIST or BRING ALL MEDICATIONS to doctor's office. Write opposite
     e...

5:   BOOSTER TETANUS/DIPHTHERIA IMMUNIZATION (with Td)
     because:
6:   PATIENT TO READ and SIGN INFORMED CONSENT FORM re
     Immunization befo...
7:   MAINTAIN PERSONAL IMMUNIZATION RECORD from now on,
     on file with val...
8:   Immunization status:
9:   OBTAIN BENEFIT/RISK INFORMATION PRIOR to administration of
     Vaccine.
                         12 more ...)

1:   GET INSECT-STING KIT AND PREVENT STINGS BY: destroy nests,
     periodic...

2:   CONFIRM ON PHYSICAL EXAMINATION OR GET MORE
     INFORMATION prior to fu...

1..A: Display MgOpt information
   D: Change display mode -- [normal]

          T: Top   M: More   P: Print Results   F: Findings   R: Return

Figure 9

SCHEDULE PELVIC/PAP TEST APPT., if not completed at time of complete P.E. Doctor's office will report results: both normal/abnormal to patient, within ____ days.

PAP test (no pap test >1 year) needed. . . . .

Screening for cancer in the pelvis should include PAP smear and a bimanual pelvic examination. In a DES daughter, such screening should begin at age 14 or at menarche and be done on an annual basis thereafter.

PAP test annual screening should begin annually after the onset of sexual activity. Exceptions to the ACOG recommendation for an annual PAP are: virgin, hysterectomy for benign disease, monogamous sexual relationship.

The ACS and the ACOG differ in their recommendations concerning frequency of PAP test screening: ACS - screen all pts. q. 2-3 yrs. following a series of 2-3 normal years; ACOG - screen all women with an annual PAP test.

BOOSTER TETANUS/DIPHTHERIA IMMUNIZATION (with Td) because:
immunization by Tetanus/Diphtheria Booster not done for 10 yr

CDC Immunization Advisory Committee recommends Td (Tetanus Toxoid/reduced diphtheria toxoid) q 10 yrs. throughout life. The elderly unimmunized population is at high risk for tetanus infection in even trivial wounds.

A previously immunized person, with an injury, whose last Tetanus Booster was > 10 years prior injury, should get a Booster. If last Booster was < 10 years, NO Booster, UNLESS wound is tetanus-prone, and has had no Booster within 5 years.

Official personal immunization record cards are available from every state. Important Information Statements are available thru the CDC in Atlanta, but no benefit-risk information has been universally and legally adopted.

If a wound is dirty and fairly severe, and a history of primary tetanus immunization is uncertain, give 250 U Tetanus Human Immune Globulin IM and also - into a separate site - ADSORBED tetanus toxoid.

Page 2

If a primary series of tetanus/diphtheria has been completed, but there is no history of tetanus booster within the PRECEDING 5 yrs., the Td adult toxoid should be administered in the presence of a severe contaminated wound.

If a primary tetanus/diphtheria series has been completed in the past, toxoid booster every 10 years is sufficient protection for MINOR UNCONTAMINATED WOUNDS.

Page 1

GET INSECT-STING KIT AND PREVENT STINGS BY: destroy nests, periodically inspect, avoid bright clothing and perfume, cover skin (hat, gloves, avoid bare feet and sandals) when among flowers, etc. HAVE KIT AVAILABLE AT ALL LIKELY SITES.

insect sting reaction that has been very severe in the past.

1% of the general population is allergic to stinging insects. Each year 25,000 have severe reactions and as many as 30 die. Some references say that accurate figures are not available. Most people are aware of their problem; some are not.

Desensitization with venom of one species may not protect against another. Wholebody extracts are not as effective as venom. Stinging insects include ant, honey bee, yellow jacket, hornet, and wasp. Allergies occur with other insects also.

Hypersensitive people may have any of the following after an insect sting/bite: anaphylaxis (an emergency), nausea, dizziness, wheezing, abdominal discomfort, hives, itching, labored breathing, confusion, cyanosis, anxiety, collapse.

Epinephrine is the only effective Rx for anaphylaxis. GET THE KIT AND learn the dose and how to administer it and about the use of tourniquets, antihistamines, oxygen, IV fluids, corticosteroids and close monitoring.

Optimum regime for venom immunotherapy is not established. Venom preparations

Figure 10

For example, if a patient presents with a cough, a rapid respiratory rate, abnormal physical findings in the chest, a high fever and a headache, we should pursue one of the specific respiratory findings first, and the coupler will often accommodate and explain the more general system findings of fever and headache. On the other hand, if headache is a prominent, persistent finding without other objective clues, we would then use the Headache Coupler at the outset. In such a system, the experienced person, capable of early synthesis, can immediately develop a problem list at a high level of abstraction, whereas the beginner may reach it by a series of well defined steps. But even experienced providers, if they have any doubt at all, should take the time to use the necessary couplers, and thereby avoid misguided intuitive leaps. A small amount of time at the outset to mobilize and relate all the simple facts in the case may avoid expensive, time consuming, and even dangerous use of unwarranted procedures and unnecessary anxiety for the patient. Whenever a mistake occurs in the use of such a well defined system, it can be immediately determined whether a coupler was defective (in which case it is fixed) or whether the system was used improperly (in which case the provider can be educated). In this way, all the efforts in the medical care system are cumulative and collaborative. In a memory based system, the same mistakes can be made over and over again: the system itself does not improve as it is used.

After the first four items on Figure 9, there are specific management options that grow directly out of some of the findings. Figure 10 shows an expansion of three such management options. By coupling original data to very specific actions and giving the patient a copy, we are less likely to have important findings left dangling or lost in some medical record, ignored by the specialist and neglected by the patient who may never have known of their existence or their significance. At all times, our goal should be to empower the patient and the family.

Step 3: Solving and Managing Problems—The Present Illnesses

On each of the problems that has been discovered, we must get more detailed information for diagnosis and management.

For each present illness, there should be a separate knowledge coupler session unless temporal relationships or other data suggest several findings are all part of the same problem. For example, if a person had been feeling well and suddenly developed a headache, followed by some diarrhea, then several hours later became confused, then we should write a single present illness or use a knowledge coupler titled the same as one of the principal manifestations of the overall illness. On the other hand, if two complaints seem totally unrelated, temporally or otherwise, such as an acute low back pain and earache, then we might logically use two couplers or write two present illnesses.

We should write present illnesses on relapses in well established chronic illnesses such as diabetes, heart failure, Parkinson's disease, etc.

The Art of Medicine and Its Relationship to Structured Approaches and Technology

Before going through an example of a diagnostic knowledge coupler, we should confront the concern of many that modern western medicine is too technical and too structured and that the science of medicine is overwhelming the art of medicine. The healing touch, they fear, is being lost in our preoccupation with logic and scientific details.

To many the art of medicine is exemplified by the open ended, free wheeling discussion between patient and physician without those structured inputs that may interfere with the empathy and humaneness of the personal encounter. The assumption is that an unstructured approach will be maximally holistic, that between the patient and the physician no important stone will be left unturned, and that all relevant relationships among the findings will be perceived and acted upon.

In discussing Oliver Sacks, Wasserstein (1988) defines romantic science in Luria's terms as one "that preserves the wealth of living reality" and contrasts it with classical analytical science which reduces "living reality with all of its richness of detail to abstract schemas."

Others say that any language appropriates and inevitably alters reality by representing it and making it a reflection of the speaker's or writer's perspective. They quote Derrida as saying that language may be an activity of violence. They talk about the artificiality of language and the ways it can manipulate reality. Poirer and Brauner (1988) are particularly concerned about summaries and case reports and about presentations on rounds in the absence of the patients. The reports may be based on material elicited by physicians whose cultural background, imagination and judgment determined the questions they asked, the tests they chose to run, and the details they finally organized and put into the patient's medical record. They wonder whether the story being told is the story of the patient's life or the story of the physician's relationship with the patient's illness. Putsch and Joyce (1990), in their discussions of cross cultural care, have emphasized that "cultural boundaries are a major source of discrepant view of reality."

Telling a patient's story (to say nothing about interpreting it in diagnostic and management terms) is a tricky business. Not only in medicine, but in other fields, as Eudora Welty suggests, we must be careful. She writes, "Sometimes in the middle of story I have the illusion that I've closed it. But never more than a minute. Your common sense tells you that you haven't done it. When you see yourself in proportion—as you are bound to do when you get some sense—then you see how much greater what is real is than anything you can put down"(Welty 1983).

Recognizing that we, in medicine, run the risk of distorting and altering the patient's reality in the medical record in all kinds of ways, there are certain considerations that should guide us as we establish and use a database on a patient:

- There should not be sole dependence upon the human mind to recall and organize all the relevant variables for discovering and analyzing problems.

- The required portions of the database should be considered as minimal, not restrictive. Contributions from the patient over and above what is required should always be carefully considered.

- Open ended interviews and structured approaches are not mutually exclusive.

- Patients should have copies of their own records and should be present at as many events as possible where their cases are being discussed. They should be encouraged to correct any misconceptions they hear or see in the record, and they should demand explanations for expectations of them that they do not understand. The presence of the patient and their consciousness of the reality they have to deal with is the best antidote we have to the alleged dehumanized schemes of scientists and to possible distortions and omissions in narrative approaches that attempt to "preserve the wealth of living reality."

Example of a Diagnostic Knowledge Coupler

We shall take the Vertigo/Dizziness Coupler to illustrate the ease with this tool allows us to approach a complaint or problem.

Figure 11 shows the large number of causes that are present in this coupler. There are many relevant potential findings, which we as clinicians might check for in the patient that favor some causes over others in this unique individual. A simple principle in coupler building guides us in our selection of findings. First we choose those relevant findings on history, physical examination, and routine laboratory that are available at minimal expense, danger, and discomfort to the patient. *In the combinatorial, nonalgorithmic approach to problem solving, we are taking advantage of the power of simple, reasonably discriminatory findings in the aggregate to yield recognizable patterns of disease.*

The software matches *findings in the patient* to *causes in the literature* and makes those matches immediately visible to us. At this point, as clinicians, we can make judgments and choices and then proceed selectively and analytically into the territory of the more expensive and more invasive acquisition of information from and about the patient. Until now, the power of simple observations in the aggregate in solving problems has never been fully exploited. The human memory is not capable of remembering all the findings that should be checked for. Nor is it capable of organizing instantly and accurately all the positive findings into all the possible patterns. Because of the uncertainty that these human limitations lead to, it was natural for some to mobilize the probablistic approaches that had been designed to deal with uncertainty. In other words, *we use probabilities in direct proportion to our ignorance of the uniqueness of the situation*. But we can first reduce uncertainty to a minimum by using computers to help us overcome not only our ignorance of what findings we should seek, but also the significance of those positive findings that grow out of an organized search. In the case of the coupler on vertigo/dizziness, approximately 170 such findings should be systematically checked for and the positives matched to potential causes. Figure 12 shows the sequences on history, physical examination, and routine laboratory work under which these findings are organized.

As large as the number of 170 findings may seem, it is quite easily negotiated when they are logically organized into digestible groups such as nature of the dizziness or vertigo, factors associated with the development and/or precipitation of the problem, factors that make the problem worse, systemic derangements (e.g., fever), drugs and environmental hazards that may be relevant, and findings in each body system to which the patient made no conscious association but which may be useful clues in unraveling the problem.

The actual time required to implement this systematic approach may turn out to be less in the long run than our present sketchy initial approaches followed by endless iterations in the form of rounds and consultations and often unnecessary expensive and time consuming procedures of a catch-up and trial and error nature.

Returning to the example of an application to a patient's clinical problem, let us assume all the proper choices have been made from sequences 1, 2, and 3. The computer brings us back to the first display (Figure 12) which provides the opportunity to couple the choices (the positive findings) to the causes they may signify. Once this is done, the first display that appears is a summary of the positive findings (Figure 13).

We next proceed to an index of causes (Figure 14). Opposite each cause are two numbers. The first is the number of findings in the patient that actually match that cause, and the second number is the total number of findings for that cause stored in the computer's knowledge base for the coupler being used. There is, of course, by definition, one finding, vertigo or dizziness, that matches every cause in this coupler. In many cases, dizziness can be the presenting finding, albeit unusual or unheard of or unlikely in the experience of a particular user, as in a hyperviscosity syndrome, for example.

In the specific example shown in Figure 14, we shall review each group of causes in terms of how the user of the system would negotiate the index of causes in an efficient and easy manner. Group I, in this coupler, contains those causes requiring immediate consideration, since each cause that appears there is a disorder in which time is of the essence and unnecessary delays in management are unacceptable if the cause is at all likely. In this case, the actual findings on the patient resulted in only three causes appearing; none of them has more than one matching characteristic. To determine exactly what that characteristic is, we merely choose the number in front of the cause, and the details appear (Figure 15). In the case of hypoglycemia, the one finding of a low blood sugar is all that we need *if* it consistently coincided with the dizziness complaint. Other findings are added for this particular cause because we may have missed getting the blood sugar at the critical moment. The history of other findings, if many are present, can alert us to the possibility. At any rate, it takes but a moment of time to check the causes in this group and get on to the next group. In group II, the findings are organized in terms of location of the lesion in the nervous system or in terms of a physiological grouping. In this particular case, there are bits of evidence for several locations. Again, by choosing the number in front of each, we can determine what that evidence is. Group III contains those causes which require only one finding to make it a serious suspect, i.e., the presence of a single drug, an environmental hazard, etc. In this case, two drugs which could be the culprit have appeared. This does not mean that they actually are the cause, but only that they are a strong possibility as a cause or contributing factor. It is this sort of ambiguity that we must learn to deal with in working with complex problems. Like group I, group IV contains specific diseases. However, these diseases allow us a greater margin of time to pursue the problem with care and deliberation. As we examine this last group, we can see that most of the causes on the list do not match well at all and so the first few can be reviewed quickly with a touch of the keyboard, and a choice made which immediately becomes the basis for a discussion with the patient.

(Other groupings occur in other couplers. In a busy medical practice, a physician may be required, when dealing with certain problems, to set into motion particular management options (e.g., "Hospitalize") or diagnostic procedures (e.g., "Blood culture") on the basis of a few early observations and before there has been time to collect and analyze the initial history and physical findings. In such cases, the first group or groups to appear on the index of causes are actions to take as opposed to diagnoses to consider. By reviewing the section of the book that contains the introductions to each of the couplers now available, we can see how groupings on the index of causes are used to achieve thoroughness without compromising efficiency and common sense in the busy practice of medicine. The introductions to the couplers presented elsewhere illustrate these issues in a very concrete manner.)

Causes and Physiological Groups in the "Vertigo & Dizziness" Coupler

A BRAIN STEM lesion	[3]	Hypoglycemia	[79]
A CENTRAL vestibular lesion	[1]	Hypotension, including postural	
A MIDBRAIN lesion	[4]	hypotension	[43]
A non-organic problem - perhaps		Hypothyroidism	[44]
hysteria	[77]	Hypoxia	[45]
A PERIPHERAL vestibular lesion	[2]	Industrial solvents	[46]
A PROPRIOCEPTIVE		Influenza	[47]
DISORDER	[140]	Labyrinthian concussion	[50]
Acoustic neuroma	[10]	LABYRINTHIAN DISEASE	[6]
Alcohol related	[12]	Labyrinthitis - suppurative	[49]
Allergy	[147]	Lermoyez syndrome	[51]
An EYE DISORDER	[142]	Leukemia	[52]
Anemia	[13]	Meniere's syndrome	[53]
Aortic stenosis	[15]	Mercury exposure	[54]
Apophyseal joint disease	[17]	MIDDLE EAR disease	[5]
Arrhythmia	[16]	Migraine	[56]
BASAL GANGLION LESION	[7]	Migraine - basilar artery type	[55]
Carbon monoxide exposure	[24]	Multiple sclerosis	[57]
Carotid artery stenosis	[67]	Neck trauma (including	
Carotid sinus syndrome	[148]	Whiplash Injury)	[63]
Cataracts	[19]	Osteitis deformans	[58]
Cerebellar artery (posterior inf.)		Otolith disease	[60]
syndrome	[22]	Otosclerosis	[59]
Cerebellar cortical nuclear		Pellagra	[145]
degen. or tumor	[20]	Perilymph fistula - internal ear	[61]
CEREBELLAR		Pernicious anemia	[144]
HEMORRHAGE	[21]	Platybasia	[62]
CEREBELLAR LESION	[9]	Positional nystagmus - benign,	
CEREBRAL ANOXIA	[141]	paroxysmal	[64]
Cervical root compression	[25]	Positional nystagmus - central	[65]
Cervical spondylosis	[26]	Skull fracture	[66]
Cholesteatoma	[23]	Subclavian steal syndrome	[69]
Cogan's syndrome	[27]	Surgery (particularly on the ear)	[70]
Decompression sickness	[28]	Syphilis	[72]
Depression	[29]	Takayasu arteritis	
Developmental dysplasia		(a giant cell arteritis)	[73]
of the ear	[30]	Temporomandibular joint	
Drugs	[31]	dysfunction	[78]
Epilepsy	[34]	Vertebral-basilar artery	
Glaucoma	[143]	syndrome	[74]
Head trauma	[38]	Vestibular epilepsy	[35]
Heat stroke	[37]	VESTIBULAR LESION	[8]
Herpes zoster	[39]	Vestibular neuronitis	[75]
Hyperlipidemia	[40]		
Hyperventilation syndrome-			
Anxiety Stress	[14]		
Hyperviscosity syndrome	[42]		

Figure 11

```
┌─────────────────────────────────────────────────────────────────────┐
│                                                                       │
│     Licensed to PKC Corporation              SN 00001                 │
│                                                                       │
│                         Vertigo & Dizziness                           │
│                                                                       │
│   ─────────────────────────────────────────────────────────────      │
│                                                                       │
│         1: History                                                    │
│                                                                       │
│         2: Physical Examination                                       │
│                                                                       │
│         3: Laboratory                                                  │
│                                                                       │
│   ─────────────────────────────────────────────────────────────      │
│                                                                       │
│          C: -COUPLE- the Findings                                     │
│                                                                       │
│   Many older people with gradually increasing dizziness/vertigo and   │
│   deafness may not match well to any of the specific diagnoses of     │
│   this coupler. They are often said to have a "disequilibrium         │
│   syndrome" or aging balance system. It is common.                    │
│                                                                       │
│             -- (C) 1982-1988, PKC Corporation --                      │
│                                                                       │
│                              F: Other functions    R: Return          │
│                                                                       │
└─────────────────────────────────────────────────────────────────────┘
```

Figure 12

```
┌─────────────────────────────────────────────────────────────────────┐
│                                                                       │
│   ***> OBSERVED FINDINGS                                              │
│                                                                       │
│   decreased vision or changes in vision (blurred eg)                  │
│   nystagmus                                                           │
│   limited/abnormal eye movements - bilateral or unilateral            │
│        - - - - - - - - - - - - - - - - - - - - - - - - - - - -        │
│                                                                       │
│   paresthesiae in arms and/or legs                                    │
│   ataxia                                                              │
│   Babinski positive                                                   │
│                                                                       │
│           - - - - - - - - - - - - - - - - - - - - - - - - - - -       │
│                                                                       │
│   valium                                                              │
│   cymetidine                                                          │
│                                                                       │
│                          P: Print  C: Cause  R:Return                 │
│                                                                       │
└─────────────────────────────────────────────────────────────────────┘
```

Figure 13

```
                -- Possible Causes --                 Obs/Tot

    1:   Hypoglycemia                                 1:9
    2:   Glaucoma                                     1.5
    3:   Hypotension - inc. postural hypotension      1:8

    4:   CEREBELLAR LESION                            2:8
    5:   An EYE DISORDER                              1:5
    6:   A BRAIN STEM lesion                          1:5
    7:   A MIDBRAIN lesion                            1:5
    8:   A PROPRIOCEPTIVE DISORDER                    1:3

    9:   Drugs                                        2.14

   10:   Multiple sclerosis                           6:7
    A:   Migraine - basilar artery type              3:6
         (20 more ...)

    1..  A:   Display Cause information
         D:   Change display mode -- [ normal ]

               M: More   P: Print Results   F: Findings   R: Return
```

```
                -- Possible Causes --                 Obs/Tot

    1:   Acoustic neuroma                             2:7
    2:   Migrain                                      2:15
    3:   Cerebellar artery syndrome                   2:7
    4:   Apophyseal joint disease                     2:4
    5:   Vertebral-basilar artery syndrome            2:16
    6:   Cere. cortical nuclear degen. or tumor       2:4
    7:   Pernicious anemia                            2:4
    8:   Meniere's syndrome                           2:9
    9:   Syphilis                                     2:7

         (10 more ...)
```

Figure 14

In the particular example we are discussing here, the best match is *multiple sclerosis*. To examine this more carefully, we type the number before it, and the display shown in Figure 16 appears. The comments under this cause are appropriate to the user's needs when confronted with this type of patient. If, in a given coupler, further steps are needed either to pursue a given diagnosis further or to treat, a choice at the bottom of the screen, designated "Option," can be made. It is at this point we see the secondary options described above. If we are curious as to why *acoustic neuroma* is on the index of causes, we merely type the number in front of it and a display similar to Figure 17 appears. It shows which findings fit with a diagnosis of acoustic neuroma and which ones are and are not present in this particular patient. This figure exhibits a number associated with each finding and comment; it is the number of the reference in the knowledge network that supports the relationship or the evidence in the comment (a discussion of the network follows below). On the index of causes (Figure 14), we see the opportunity to type the letter "D." If we type "D," the reference numbers appear as they do in Figure 17. If we type the letter "D" again, we get opposite each finding a number that tells how many of the other causes in this coupler that have the same finding. If we then type "D" again, we return to the usual state in which no numbers are associated with the findings or comments.

Applying this same coupler to another patient, we may get an entirely different picture (Figure 18). In this case, the index of causes is short, and the match is very good for the hyperventilation syndrome/anxiety/stress (Figure 19).

We may choose a series of eye findings that may lead us quickly and precisely to the midbrain. Busy general practitioners or internists may never have elicited such findings without the guidance of the coupler. If they had elicited them, they may not have realized their full significance.

The above examples demonstrate the amount of detail we should cover if a problem is properly pursued. The examples also illustrate how the total list of causes encompasses many body systems and specialties. The full understanding of all the diagnostic or management options of a real problem usually involves a body of knowledge that crosses specialty boundaries. We cannot expect a single physician to have command of all these areas. Consequently, what happens to a patient depends not only on whether he or she goes through the neurology door, the ENT door, the family practice door, the internal medicine door, or the emergency room door, but also on the memory, attitudes, and background of the individual practitioner in any one of those places. In spite of the odds against them, many providers do try to recall, from extensive and costly years of training, all of the following:

- all the different types of dizziness and vertigo

- the basic science aspects of all that is known about the stato-kinetic system with the role of the eyes, the proprioceptive system in muscles and joints, the role of the labyrinths, the brain stem, etc.
- the endless details about each syndrome
- the drugs
- the ten to 12 different types of nystagmus
- the factors that distinguish central from peripheral vestibular function, etc.

Frustrated by such an overwhelming information load, providers, to varying degrees, abandon a complete and systematic approach. Instead, the patient is referred or labeled with one of the four or five most common causes of dizziness with the hope that it will all go away or will evolve into something obvious on the next visit. Not only is the patient at risk and the process inefficient and expensive, but the provider is not without hazard. A staggering load of fear and guilt may overcome those who are conscientious. "Did I ask and do all the right things?" The articles and editorials mentioned earlier document the seriousness of the information problems of the practicing physician (Covell 1985; Huth 1989; Williamson 1989). These cold, hard realities are what we should be constructively dealing with instead of oscillating between horror stories of the increasing malpractice crisis and romantic hero stories of the all knowing family doctor or the occasional brilliant, intuitive diagnostic leap of the experienced clinician.

Patients have to come to terms with the fact that, on any single medical encounter, they may fall into the hands of personnel who are the lowest common denominator of the system. We all, therefore, should focus more on how the system runs. There will be more than enough room for the mystical aspects of human interactions in medicine to flourish once a sound base for those interactions is consistently and uniformly established. In fact, the art of medicine will be moved to a much higher plane.

As Beryl Markham said in her reminiscences about flying, "After this era of great pilots is gone, as the era of great sea captains has gone—each nudged aside by the march of inventive genius, by steel cogs and copper discs and hair-thin wires on white faces that are dumb, but speak—it will be found, I think, that all the science of flying has been captured in the breadth of an instrument board, but not the religion of it" (Markham 1983).

Let us now summarize what a knowledge coupler can do for practitioners:

- It reminds them of the appropriate items to elicit on the history and physical examination, given a specific problem.

- It makes a list of the positive findings immediately available on a screen or on paper for both provider and patient.

Suggested Cause: Hypoglycemia

-- **Findings Present** --
decreased vision or changes in vision (blurred e.g.) . . . . .

-- **Findings Not Present** --
palpitations . . . .
generalized headache . . . .
drowsiness and/or stupor . . . .
change in mental function. . . . .
excessive sweating . . . .
hypoglycemia . . . .
personality change occurring at time of dizziness/vertigo.
insulin. . . . .

An anginal like chest pain may develop with hypoglycemia and palpitations
are not uncommon. The neurological manifestations of hypoglycemia are
extremely varied.

F: First   P: Print   R: Return

Figure 15

Suggested Cause: Multiple sclerosis

-- **Findings Present** --

decreased vision or changes in vision (blurred e.g.) . . . .
nystagmus. . . . .
limited/abnormal eye movements - bilateral or unilateral . . . .
paresthesiae in arms and/or legs . . . .
ataxia . . . .
Babinski positive. . . . .

-- **Findings Not Present** --
incontinence . . . .

Multiple sclerosis may present with vertigo and nystagmus. Vestibular tests
are almost always abnormal. Abnormal eye movements (weak adduction III
N) bilaterally, whereas vascular brainstem lesions are usually unilateral.

F: First   P: Print   R: Return

Figure 16

Suggested Cause: Acoustic neuroma
[Refs: 1862 1870]

-- Findings Present --
nystagmus. . . . .
    [Refs: 1870]
ataxia . . . .
    [Refs: 1870]

-- Findings Not Present --
hearing loss - unilateral. . . . .
    [Refs: 1870]
ringing in the ears - tinnitus . . . .
    [Refs: 1870]
facial pain - unilateral . . . .
    [Refs: 1870]
facial weakness - unilateral . . . .
    [Refs: 1870]
unsteadiness feelings preceded development of vertigo prob . . . .
    [Refs: 1870]

Tinnitus is one of the most common Sx's in acoustic neuroma.
Any tumor of the cerebellar-pontine angle gives a similar picture
- e.g. meningioma, aneurysms, arachnoid cysts etc. Unexplained nerve
deafness in 1 ear suggests this diagnosis
    [Refs: 1870]

In acoustic neuroma, the vertigo develops slowly without paroxysms
except for 5%of pts. It is not as severe as neuronitis. A chronic
ataxia comes in the later stages but along period of unsteadiness
may have been an early symptom.
    [Refs: 1870]

             N: Next   **P:** Print   **R:** Return

Figure 17

-- Possible Causes --	Obs/Tot
1: Hypoglycemia	1:9
2: Drugs	1:14
3: Hyperventilation syndrome - Anxiety - Stress	8:9
4: Arrhythmia	1:2
5: Vertebral-basilar artery syndrome	1:16
6: Neck trauma (including Whiplash Injury)	1:9
7: Pellagra	1:6

Figure 18

Suggested Cause: Hyperventilation syndrome - Anxiety - Stress

   -- Findings Present --

mouth unusually dry and troublesome. . . . .
choking sensations . . . .
palpitations . . . .
shortness of breath. . . . .
heavy breathing without obvious reason (hyperventilating). . . .
diarrhea . . . .
frequent urination . . . .
sleep walking and night terrors have been a problem. . . . .

   -- Findings Not Present --
paresthesiae in arms and/or legs . . . .

23% of one series of dizziness patients had hyperventilation as the cause.
Patients may be able to hyperventilate without it being clinically apparent.
Also the patient may not even be aware that he is hyperventilating.

About 2/3 of chronic hyperventilators have a pCO_2 below normal.
Bicarbonate excretion may increase 3-4 fold. Cerebral blood flow
falls 2% for each 1 mm fall in pCO_2. Hypophosphatemia may develop
with many adverse physiologic effects.

The chest pain in pts. with a hyperventilation/anxiety/stress complex can
be a sharp, momentary, cutting pain or a precordial aching that lasts for
minutes to hours or a substernal oppression or constricting pain aggravated
by each breath.

   F: First   **P: Print**   **R: Return**

Figure 19

- It organizes the findings in terms of possible causes and, in some couplers, also in terms of physiological function.

- For each cause presented, it displays the findings present in the patient that support that cause, and the findings not present that might be expected for the cause (significant negatives).

- Linked to each cause are comments that help the user interpret the findings from temporal and severity points of view.

The knowledge coupler software does not do any mathematical manipulations or present the user with ordered probabilities. This is true because the exact weight to give to each finding for each cause is not known. In medical practice we have not consistently kept records of sufficient quality to do this meaningfully. Furthermore, we do not know the prevalence of each of the possibilities in the population from which our patient comes, and finally we do not know where in the course of the disease the patient is. For example, in early appendicitis, there may be epigastric pain but no right lower quadrant pain. Later in the disease the reverse may be true. No human expert could know such details beforehand to insert into any computer program. In fact, differential weighting may be inappropriate in many cases if the findings and set of possible causes have been well chosen. Powerful support for this conclusion can be found in Dawes' work on "Linear Models in Decision Making" (1974).

A Problem Knowledge Coupler can be thought of as a set of linked linear models (one linear model per primary option). The models are linked in the sense that in general any two of them will employ some of the same finding variables, and in the sense that all the primary options stand in a specific common relationship to the topic of the coupler.

Many physicians and other health care professionals approach the Problem Knowledge Coupler with a preexisting point of view, which can be roughly conveyed by a series of questions and assertions:

- What problems of the sort that motivated the development of the Problem Knowledge Coupler System are really too large to be handled by a human being equipped with the usual support (books, journals, online databases, etc.)?

- Isn't it a distinguishing characteristic of genuine experts that they can confront a problem of apparently overwhelming complexity (the so called combinatorial explosion) and approach it in a way designed to reduce the number of options to a manageable number at any stage of the analysis?

- What about statistical considerations? Most options are really not that likely to be relevant in a given situation. Experts should have at their command methods of successive elimination that tell them the few questions to ask first in order to eliminate many possibilities with minimal effort.

- If people have trouble keeping these methods at their command, then shouldn't the primary focus for developers of decision support systems be to provide automated interactive versions of the successive elimination methods that real experts use?

- Reduction of the number of options that need to be pursued is really the fundamental problem. Suppose, for the sake of argument, that we decide to assume that a patient has one or more of several possible conditions, to play it safe. Each of these possibilities entails certain treatment strategies and requirements for monitoring. Can we really afford to carry forward with all these possibilities? The expenses, complications, and risks of management would become overwhelming. We need to narrow the list of possibilities fast. The iterative process of medical care will offset the danger of neglecting something. We investigate and deal with problems that our current assumptions cannot account for, regardless of whether those problems were originally overlooked or are new to appear.

As a preliminary response, we would assert that the above questions and assertions do not address how genuine expertise is identified, or alleged expertise is evaluated, in terms of objective criteria for the adequacy of the solution to a problem.

Nor do they deal with the incidental motivations for using the successive elimination approach, that are distinct from, and may actually conflict with, the requirements for a disciplined approach to a problem. Specifically, human decision makers suffer from severe and well documented limitations in reasoning with many variables, especially under the pressures often encountered in medicine. The successive elimination approach is in many cases quite clearly motivated by a desire to keep a problem psychologically manageable, in the face of what otherwise would be manifestly unreasonable human performance requirements. This can make the approach very attractive, in spite of its pitfalls.

Moreover, the above questions and assertions do not deal with the possible theoretical limitations of the successive elimination of alternatives approach, and of other approaches that might do as well or better. In other words, it is implicitly assumed that a successive elimination approach can always be more effective and efficient than other approaches.

Principles of Coupler Building

A fundamental and practical principle of coupler building is that at the outset we should restrict ourselves to findings that are individually easy to check, at minimal cost and risk to the patient. Many simple findings can be informative in the aggregate if they are elicited consistently and if their relationships to one another (unique patterns) are properly presented to the human mind. This is precisely what knowledge couplers are designed to do.

There are many examples, even in the best medical centers, where costly and unnecessary delays occurred in making "improbable" diagnoses such as hypopituitarism or intermittent porphyria because the simplest of clinical observations were not made and organized into obvious patterns right at the outset. On the other hand, simple observations may not have such power in certain cases, even when we expect them to on the basis of established diagnostic methods and approaches. When this is so, Problem Knowledge Couplers can immediately reveal it and provide a sound empirical basis for relying on more sophisticated diagnostic procedures. Without the routine use of such a tool, even experienced clinicians who try to keep up on the continuous flow of literature on a common problem, such as diarrhea, struggle vainly to apply all the details of that literature in a manner that minimizes the risk, cost, and discomfort to the patient. The struggle, when engaged in by an honest, conscientious medical student, can be devastating.

Another fundamental principle of coupler building is that we should try to learn as much as possible from the unique situation of the patient as we can (given what the medical literature has to say) before invoking prior information about the prevalence of particular causes. Indeed, this principle was a major motivation in the development of the Problem Knowledge Coupler System.

This principle is based on the following consideration. To the extent that we have any reliable information on the prevalence of various diseases at all, it is because we have checked for the relevant indicators and have identified the necessary confirmatory findings in many cases, in a way that was not prejudiced by anticipation of particular results. This does not mean that we disavowed any reason to expect certain results. Rather it means that we proceeded in a way designed to test or check our expectations, rather than merely confirm them.

If couplers are widely used, and certain diseases are much more common than others in a population, then this fact will be reflected in the statistical trends that appear in the accumulation of coupler results across that population. Suppose, however, that trends are identified for a given population. It might then be argued that, if certain causes for a particular presenting problem are much more common than others, the effort expended to check for the rare causes is unnecessary. A major and proper role for prevalence data, the argument goes, is to avoid such wasted effort.

The flaw in this argument, and the danger in the application of its conclusion, is the implicit assumption of the stability of the prevalence information. What we really want to know is why certain causes are much more prevalent than others, and to be alerted when prevalence patterns begin to shift. Of course, prevalence should be a central consideration in making many public health decisions. But it should not be central in assessing individual cases, and need not be if this assessment is done with adequate knowledge coupling tools and efficient and reliable methods of data collection.

The requirement that we learn as much as possible from the uniqueness of each case can be reformulated in light of these considerations. Even in the everyday application of medical knowledge, we should endeavor to check the soundness of the generalizations we are applying, rather than using them uncritically to draw as many conclusions as we can from meager information. One of the principal deficiencies of the current medical care system is the frequency with which it tries to evade this requirement. This is unavoidable if we continue to tolerate inadequate medical records and lack of support to care providers in coupling medical knowledge to everyday action.

Using Management Couplers

Thus far we have been discussing diagnostic couplers and the principles that underlie their use. The same principles apply to management couplers. Many problems suggest multiple management and specific therapeutic alternatives, and we should map the patient's unique needs and characteristics against these options.

We can now briefly review how knowledge coupling tools can be applied to a management problem. Let us assume that the diagnosis of essential hypertension has been made for the first time in a patient who now needs to choose among multiple options for the medical management of the problem.

The patient and provider again proceed through a series of displays on a personal computer, making choices as they go. The relevant issues in the patient's life are grouped under headings such as severity and nature of the blood pressure problem, relevant habits and lifestyle, demographic considerations, review of the relevant symptoms and signs for each body system, and basic laboratory findings. Let us assume some choices have been made and coupling of those choices to the relevant medical knowledge has been accomplished. Figure 20 shows the display of the findings present (i.e., the choices made). Figure 21 shows the management options appropriate for this unique patient. It will be noted that the options are in groups. The first group is lifestyle changes that do not involve drugs. By choosing #1 ("Abstain from Alcohol"), for example, we can see the details of that management option, as shown in Figure 22. The management options also include the *pros* and *cons* of various drugs for this particular patient. Figure 22 includes the example of "*cons* for a converting enzyme inhibitor," again for this particular patient.

When using such a management tool with patients, several things become apparent:

- All patients elicit a set of options that are unique to them as individuals, and the details for them to consider are immediately available as a basis for a complete dialogue between patient and provider on trade offs and actions to be taken.

- The direct connection between reliability of inputs and the reliability of outputs is apparent to the patients. Their care is only as good as the quality of information that is provided at the outset.

- The amount of time spent at the outset is more than compensated for by the following:

  - providing immediate command of crucial details

- providing immediate printouts that avoid costly and time consuming writing or dictating of records

- solving the patient education problem by giving patients their copy—having marked on the printout the choices decided upon.

- The ambiguity inherent in many, if not most, of diagnostic and management decisions can be honestly confronted in a manner that does not paralyze everyone with confusion as would a verbal, off the cuff discussion if this much detail were covered.

Quality of care can now be assessed in terms of the logic of choices made from a defined knowledge base and *not by the credentials of a provider whose exact knowledge base is unknown to others at the time of action*. In other words, quality is now the excellence with which a well defined function is fulfilled and not that which people with credentials do, which only other people with credentials have a right to judge.

The extent to which we use a patient's uniqueness to choose among options leads to the questions of where and when we should employ statistical information on populations of patients in the management of single individuals. This latter type of information can be used to create the diagnostic and management options and the comments in the couplers. To return to the travel analogy, statistical information is used to improve, close and open new roads, but the traveler's unique needs and goals determine which path is chosen from among those roads once they have been created.

Professionals have to be on their guard against unwisely using such statistical information to manage individuals: "The flu is going around. Take an aspirin and I'll see you tomorrow." A meningococcemia may overwhelm the patient before tomorrow ever comes. A few simple details properly elicited and interpreted can make all the difference.

Once the basic framework is established for thinking about and using knowledge couplers, we can elaborate on some features of the coupler system that not only facilitate their usage, but also increase our understanding of them and their potential. We shall use specific different couplers to explain these features and what they reveal, beginning with the Low Back Pain Coupler.

The question is often raised; "What is the universe of causes covered by a particular diagnostic coupler?" To answer this question, we access the causes list by making a choice on the first display of the coupler different from the usual one we make when working directly with the patient. We select "F: Other functions" from the bottom of the screen (Figure 23); this leads us to the next display (Figure 24), which offers us the choice "C: -Review- Coupler cause info." This choice gives us a complete list of the causes in a coupler listed alphabetically. If we want to go directly to a cause, we type the first couple letters of that cause, and the appropriate alphabetized list appears with our choice at or near the top of the list. We can then choose the cause and see a display similar to Figure 25, which presents the findings associated with that cause, the comments, and the choice "O: Options" for further diagnostic action or management."

At this point we should pause and further elaborate on the issue of options for further diagnostic effort or management. In a diagnostic coupler, the user goes through a series of queries concerning easily elicited details on history, physical examination, and routine laboratory work that are relevant to the problem. The user is asked to cover every point regardless of what the response has been on previous points. In other words, there is no "if-then," algorithmic branching type of logic. It is wise to avoid branching systems whenever possible for two reasons:

- For the sake of progressing through an algorithm, the user will often make arbitrary choices at branching points in the face of ambiguity or ignorance of certain details. These easily forgotten passing bits of ambiguity may accumulate and mislead more than one realizes in a system where long term followup in a broad context is not done.

- A branch may be clear and accurately taken, but it prevented consideration of other points raised on the untaken branch, points which may have great significance in a multifactorial situation.

With branching, in short, a user may end up with a far more definite answer than a truly complete accounting would allow. In contrast, in combinatorial thinking, as is used in the couplers, every point is covered, all possible combinations revealed, and any ambiguity held to the end of the process, forcing the user to face it and discuss it honestly with the patient.

```
                                                                    Page 1
  ***> OBSERVED FINDINGS


  stomach ulcers - gastric acid secretion rate increased
  nephrotic syndrome
  - - - - - - - - - - - - - - - - - - - - - - - - - - - -
  smoking
  overweight
  alcohol usage
  oral contraceptives are being used
  - - - - - - - - - - - - - - - - - - - - - - - - - - - -
  Initial therapy is required - no drug has been used yet
  - - - - - - - - - - - - - - - - - - - - - - - - - - - -
  cimetidine
  - - - - - - - - - - - - - - - - - - - - - - - - - - - -
  cholesterol and/or other blood lipids elevated
  leukopenia and/or neutropenia
```

Figure 20

```
                    -- Suggested Management Options --

  ABSTAIN FROM ALCOHOL for several weeks before initiating any drug t...
  CONTRACEPTIVES should be DISCONTINUED
  SMOKING SHOULD BE DISCONTINUED
  WEIGHT REDUCTION PROGRAM should be instituted: CALORIC
       RESTRICTION...
  LOW CHOLESTEROL, LOW FAT DIET should be instituted because:
  GO THROUGH THE HYPERLIPIDEMIA COUPLER

  CONVERTING ENZYME INHIBITOR-CON's or CAUTIONS
       in THIS patient...
  CONVERTING ENZYME INHIBITOR-PRO's (1st tier) in THIS pt. (see...

  CALCIUM CHANNEL BLOCKER-PRO.S (1st tier) in THIS pt. (see 1st...

  ALPHA ADRENERGIC BLOCKER-PRO's (1st tier) in THIS pt. (see 1s...

  DIURETIC THERAPY-PRO's (2nd tier) in THIS pt. (see 1st commen...
  DIURETIC THERAPY-CON's or CAUTIONS in THIS patient...

  BLOCK TRANSPORT OF NOREPINEPHRINE
       INTO STORAGE GRANULES-CON's...
  BLOCK TRANSPORT OF NOREPINEPHRINE
       INTO STORAGE GRANULES-PRO's in ...

  POTASSIUM SPARER and/or ALDOSTERONE ANTAGONIST-CON's...

  BETA ADRENERGIC BLOCKER-CON's or CAUTIONS in THIS patient
  BETA ADRENERGIC BLOCKER-PRO's (2nd tier) in THIS pt. (see 1st...

  CENTRALLY ACTING ALPHA AGONIST - PRO's in THIS patient ...
```

Figure 21

ABSTAIN FROM ALCOHOL for several weeks before initiating any drug therapy for hypertension. Drugs may prove unnecessary. Even if drugs are needed, they may be more effective at lower doses if alcohol is avoided.

alcohol usage. . . . .

2 ounces of alcohol a day may elevate the blood pressure. As many as half of those who drink 80 ml (2.6 oz) of alcohol a day may be hypertensive (i.e., in the range of 4 beers or 1-2 glasses of wine). This type of elevation is reversible.

There is some evidence that blood pressures are lower among those who have 2-4 drinks a week than those who abstain completely. Among heavier drinkers, however, alcohol may be the commonest cause of reversible hypertension.

CONVERTING ENZYME INHIBITOR - CON's or CAUTIONS in THIS patient

Captopril, enalapril

cimetidine . . . .
leukopenia and/or neutropenia. . . . .

CEI drugs may cause hyperkalemia, especially if Na intake is limited, K-sparing diuretics or non-steroidal anti-inflammatory drugs being used, or heart failure or diabetes present. Mood elevation may occur. A dry cough occurs in some pts.

Side effects from CEI drugs may have seemed excessive at first when larger doses were used unnecessarily. Side effects may be less with enalapril than captopril because no SH group. CEI's DO BLUNT a compensatory response to volume depletion.

CEI drugs may cause: a maculopapular rash - usually self-limiting and occurs in 1st 2-3 mos. (10% in 1 study); angioedema can be dangerous but is rare & usually occurs in 1st month (more with long acting drugs); exfoliative dermatitis rare.

Neutropenia is rare (exact frequency not known) - may be more with collagen or renal dis. or immunosuppressive agents. Taste may be sour or metallic or lost.

Some estimate that side effects overall cause the drug to be discontinued in 6%.

Neurological disturbances under captopril treatment should be watched for if the patient is also taking cimetidine. Enalapril may cause dizziness and headaches in 4-5% of pts. Proteinuria in 2% (? prev. dis); BUN rise is minor & reversible.

Figure 22

Acute Low Back Pain and/or Leg Pain of not > 2 months durat.

   1: History
   2: Physical Examination
   3: Laboratory

C: -COUPLE- the Findings

Back pain may be the tip of an iceberg. Whatever specific disorder this
coupler may point to, it is worthwhile to review the results of the
screening history and physical (and wellness coupler) to be aware of poor
overall care and habits.

-- (C) 1982-1988, PKC Corporation --

F: Other functions   R: Return

Figure 23

- - - - - - - - - - **Other Coupler System Functions** - - - - - - - - - -

COUPLER: Acute Low Back Pain and/or Leg Pain of not > 2 months durat.

Number 9, Rev 8/13/89

Title for printouts of Coupler session results:
11/10/89 10:28 -- Coupler Session Results

T: -Edit- session title

                                C: -Review- Coupler cause info.

D: Change cause info. display mode

S: -Save- this Coupler session to disk

L: -Load- old Coupler session from disk

                                  E: -ERASE- all findings

1: -Add- to the set of positive findings

2: -Review/Delete- findings in set

Figure 24

Suggested Cause: Spinal stenosis or spinal claudication
-- Findings Present --

bowel and/or bladder function changed as problem developed .
leg pain on walking that is relieved by rest . . . .
leg pain on walking but not when pedaling a bicycle. . . . .
paresthesiae in both feet after exertion . . . .
plantar reflexes - exertion -> positive; rest -> normal . . . . . .
pain is relieved by spinal flexion and worse on extension. . . . .

-- Findings Not Present --
- < none > -
In spinal stenosis, bilateral paresthesiae and numbness occur in the majority
of patients. There may be feelings of weakness but not much objective
evidence. Straight legraising and range of motion of the spine are normal.

Possible bladder abnormalities are: 1. vesicular irritability 2. loss of desire
to void and unaware of need to 3. partial or total urinary retention. In spinal
stenosis, the problem may be intermittent; unlikely in monoradicular
involvement.

In spinal stenosis,, there may be mild sensory loss, whereas it is rare in
vascular claudication. Exercise may lead to absent ankle jerks and even
urinary retention - both returning to normal with rest in a pt. with spinal
stenosis.

In spinal stenosis, there may be vague pain in the back and legs that's relieved by sitting or lying down. Exertion combined with the lordotic position
make it worse (walking down hill eg), whereas riding a bicycle may be
symptom free.

There are differing opinions as to the lowest normal sagittal diameter of the
vertebral canal and on the exact role the various anatomical features play in
the intermittent claudication (lateral recesses, central stenosis etc).

Back pain that follows prolonged standing and relieved by sitting and lying
also occurs in spondylolisthesis. Spondylolisthesis also causes discomfort on
the out aspect of both thighs and paresthesiae in both feet relieved by
sitting/lying.
            F: First   P: Print   O: Options   R: Return

Figure 25

Nonetheless, there is a point when it is wise to switch to branching logic;
that is when the acquisition of a particular piece of data evidence involves
undue danger, discomfort, or expense to the patient. Data of this sort,
although often necessary to acquire, should only be gotten if there is already
evidence from combinations of simple, easy to get bits of data that a certain
cause is a reasonable possibility and there is danger associated with not

establishing and treating that cause. In this regard, the causes in a coupler vary greatly in what is required to diagnose and manage them. Some diagnoses can be made on the simple things alone, whereas others require more steps. The latter are handled by having an option choice at the bottom of the display (Figure 25) that leads the user directly to either the procedures that could be done to nail down the cause more securely, or to the specific step or steps in management that are now possible without any further diagnostic effort being necessary. In this sense, a single coupler can be both a diagnostic and management coupler.

When, then, is a management coupler a separate entity on its own? This occurs when there are so many management options that it is neither safe nor easy to choose among them without further detailed knowledge about the patient. If, for example, we decide the diagnosis is essential hypertension, we are confronted with a wide variety of drugs and lifestyle changes to choose from. Likewise, details concerning the severity and nature of various manifestations of a diagnosis, such as an acute asthmatic attack, may play decisive roles in choosing among options. It is impossible for the unaided human mind to elicit and organize such details so that the trade-offs can be rationally discussed. A knowledge coupler not only makes such an analysis immediately available, but it also becomes the vehicle whereby complicated matters and difficult trade-offs can be systematically reviewed with the patient and/or the family.

The choice "C: -Review- Coupler cause info" (Figure 24) can be used in several ways. First, it can be the route clinicians choose if they are confident of a diagnosis and just want to use the coupler as a means of getting a printout of the cause with its findings, comments, and options for the record and the patient. However, this approach is not recommended. Bypassing the questions of the coupler does not save that much time in the hands of an experienced user, and it subjects the patient to the unnecessary risk that crucial details may be overlooked.

Another use for the choice, "C: -Review- Cause info," is to pick a specific cause such as "Disc disruption - internal," notice the findings under it, and then enter those findings into the coupler to see what other causes give a similar or overlapping clinical picture. To enter the specific findings, users do not need to search through the questions of the coupler itself, but can choose "1: -Add- to the set of positive findings" (Figure 24) and type in the first couple of letters of each finding. An alphabetized list appears from which to choose the appropriate finding. After entering all the findings, the user returns to the main display (Figure 23) and types "C" for couple. The index of causes then appears (Figure 26). The disease for which findings were entered stands out as a very good match on a very short list of alternatives, whereas the other diseases (except for fracture) on the list match very poorly.

The diseases displayed (Figure 26) are in two different groups. The first group has two disorders suggested; both are disorders that, if present, are urgent and not to be missed. The user can in minimal time examine the match by selecting the disease and deciding whether there is enough evidence to take the possibility seriously, and if so whether there are any options suggested to follow-up on it. The *trauma* or *axial loading* finding that caused the fracture possibility to appear is also a finding that is very consistent with the diagnosis of *Disc disruption—internal* (Figure 27). After reviewing the match for this latter diagnosis, the user can immediately proceed to the options for pursuing this possibility further.The "Cauda equina syndrome" (Figure 28) may appear highly unlikely because of only one finding. However, the user has the means to keep it in mind as time progresses. The user also knows exactly which additional findings to be alert for to be on top of this diagnosis in the event that it is first being seen in the very early stages. Only one finding is required to have the possibility of fracture appear on the list and to be taken seriously and necessitating that further studies done.

Adding one more finding, such as "recent stress—divorce, job loss, etc.," to the example given above, and then choosing C:Couple adds two more items to the index of causes, one of which is in a group by itself. This latter group, the *risk factor group*, deserves comment.

It is important for the provider to distinguish between findings that place a patient *at risk* for a disorder and findings that are *evidence* for a disorder. When a patient has many risk factors, it is easy for a busy provider to jump to conclusions and make a diagnosis for which there is really very little evidence or to ignore a diagnosis (often an uncommon disorder) for which there is a great deal of evidence in the particular patient. The presence of many risk factors in a patient can lead to faulty, premature hypothesis formation, creating misguided courses of action from which it may be difficult to recover. Since patients often have many factors in their lives which may or not be related to the problem at hand, these added findings can result in a kind of background noise on the index of causes. In real clinical situations, the provider has to be alert to the presence of more than a single diagnosis, as well as the existence of "red herrings" in complex situations. Knowledge couplers provide the basis for dealing with complex issues in an organized manner without becoming hopelessly entangled in all of the data.

Another example (Figure 29) illustrates the issue of *risk vs. evidence*. In this case, a patient matches to the picture of spinal stenosis, but also fits into the risk factor group showing both lumbago and disc disorder. An examination of the findings under each of these three choices will show that the latter two appeared because the patient's history revealed significant exposure to vibrations such as a jackhammer or a great deal of time spent in a certain type of vehicle. That finding does not "vote" for spinal stenosis. The evidence for spinal stenosis appears in a patient who is at risk for the more common disorders of lumbago and disk displacement. In a busy clinic, it is easy to see why diagnoses are missed and wrong ones are made in what seems at the time like a rational manner.

Figures 30 and 31 are used to illustrate another type of information that may appear on an index of causes. The last group in each case here is characterized not by urgency, risk, or disease entity, but by localization of the lesion whatever the lesion is. Making the choice "5th lumbar root lesion" results in a display which provides the evidence (the findings present in the patient) for such a *localization of the lesion.*

It is apparent from the above that the style of a coupler and the format and groupings for presentation of the results are related to the nature of the problem being considered. There are further groupings, not discussed here, which will become apparent to both the patients and providers as they utilize specific couplers. The Memory Loss/Confusion Coupler is a good example of how a coupler can facilitate looking at a problem from several points of view, extracting a maximum amount of understanding and interpretation from a single set of observations. This is quite different from experts writing dense prose in specialized language for others to digest and extemporaneously integrate into difficult situations on ill defined cues.

To quote Beryl Markham again: "Everything those authors said was sound and sane and reasonable, but they went on the theory that truth is rarer than radium and that if it became easily available, the market for it would be glutted, holders of stock in it would become destitute, and gems of eternal verity would be given away as premiums" (Markham 1983).

After using his coupler on the management of depression regularly with patients, Dr. Willie Yee, a psychiatrist, wrote:

The most profound alteration becomes apparent the first time the psychiatrist sits down with the patient to review the results of a Coupler. This side-by-side posture can be seen as a metaphor for the alteration in the relationship that is taking place. The psychiatrist and patient are now involved in a collaborative relationship, with both parties having access to the information from which a decision could be made. Since Couplers are structured to present multiple options, e.g., less frequent diagnoses or less commonly used treatments, there is no longer a *treatment of choice* for a given condition. The ambiguity which physicians, including psychiatrists, face all the time is now confronted by both patient and provider. The hierarchical structure of medicine, in which a single diagnosis or treatment is authoritatively prescribed is replaced by a relationship which acknowledges uncertainty and the trade-offs which must be confronted when any decision is made.

Since the mind cannot accomplish what the coupler can, we must be wary of automating what the unaided expert minds have done in the past. We must look critically at what experts put into computer programs which are then employed to generate conclusions in realtime situations. Since the patient's values and goals and detailed quantitative knowledge can be so important at each step in the problem solving process (information which can never be put into a computer program for general use), and since informed follow-up by an ever present observer can only be done by the patient or family, it may be inappropriate and inefficient in the long run to automate much beyond the use of couplers.

Good maps used by intelligent travelers should be our goal. The shape of each person's path will not be known until the input stops. All travelers will have their own input and generate their own path, choosing from the large number of options and combinations of options that the map offers. In the field of medicine, a central facility for coupler production that makes a subscription service and an 800 number available to all practitioners and institutions would make implementation of guidelines an immediate reality in everyone's practice. A fair audit of providers for responsible behaviors would then be possible. And patients would have more assurance that the best that is known in medicine is applied to their unique situations on every encounter.

Concluding Discussion of the Database

In the original description of the problem oriented system of medical care, there were relatively clear boundaries between the database, the problem list, the titled plans for each problem, and the titled progress notes on each problem. Much of the mystique of the medical professional has resided in the unexpressed logic that underlies the generation of these four phases and the connections among them.

The computer and knowledge coupling tools are beginning to surface the logic and smooth the flow and obliterate the boundaries. Abnormalities in the systems review and physical examination automatically go on a prioritized work list which is, in effect, the first problem list stated at the lowest level of abstraction. For some of the positive items in the database, a management scheme is immediately printed out (for example, an immunization program) so we have for that item leaped into plans without requiring the initiative of any provider. The provider may have to approve it, but no longer are we dependent on that provider's initiative or memory to elicit the basic facts and the options for action they should lead to. And finally the knowledge couplers ("Present Illnesses") on specific complaints lead directly to the synthesis of findings and the stating of problems at higher levels of abstraction. All the logic is visible because of the way the coupler results are presented and can be accessed. But it is the function of the medical provider working with the patient to make the final problem list at the highest level of synthesis possible. We shall now go on to discussing the creation and uses of the problem list.

```
        -- Possible Causes --                    Obs/Tot

    1: Cauda equina syndrome                        1:4
    2: Fracture - (any part of axial skeleton)      1:1

    3: Disc disruption - internal                   5:5
    4: Dis4c displacement (Herniated nuc. pulposus) 1:10
    5: Unexplained pain disorder or drug need       1:8

    6: RISK FACTORS FOR LUMBAGO                      1:5
```

Figure 26

```
Suggested Cause: Disc disruption - internal

-- Findings Present --

trauma or unexpected weight lifting or axial load. . . . . .
weakness in lower extremity(s) . . . . . . . . . . . . . . . . . .
difficulty in rising from sitting. . . . . . . . . . . . . . . . . . .
deep-seated dull ache in the low back region . . . . . . . .
severe aching in legs as opposed to radiating pain/sensation

-- Findings Not Present --
-<none>-

In the internal disc disruption syndrome, the back pain can be a deep seated,
dull ache accompanied by weakness and clumsiness complaints. Since muscle
spasm may be rare and severe headache may occur, pts. are often labeled as
functional.

The internal disc disruption syndrome often follows a sudden unexpected
weight load or axial load or high speed injury. L4-5 and L5-S1 most often
affected. Some patients lose weight and others gain.

        F: First              P: Print   O: Options   R: Return
----------------------------------------------------------------
Associated Options: Disc disruption - internal

            -- Option --             Risk   Cost

1. discography - essential for the Dx of int. disc disruption .
2. spinal fusion. . . . . . . . . . . . . . . . . . . . . . .

Myelography has no place in the investigation of the internal disc disruption
syndrome.
```

Figure 27

Suggested Cause: **Cauda equina syndrome**
-- Findings Present --

weakness in lower extremity(s) . . . .
-- Findings Not Present --

bowel and/or bladder function changed as problem developed .
pain or analgesia or numbness at anus, genitals, perineum. . . .
patellar reflex depressed or absent. . . . .

CONSIDER THE CAUDA EQUINA SYNDROME AN EMERGENCY. SPONTANEOUS RECOVERY NOT TO BE EXPECTED. The sensory loss is usually higher than the motor. Perianal numbness and loss of anal reflex occur in an advanced lesion. Walking may be difficult.

Possible bladder abnormalities are: 1. vesicular irritability 2. loss of desire to void and unaware of need to 3. partial or total urinary retention. In spinal stenosis, the problem may be intermittent; unlikely in monoradicular involvement.

In the cauda equina syndrome, recovery after surgery is hard to predict. After 3 months, usually no more sensory recovery; if motor recovery not complete by 6 months, do not expect it; may be some partial recovery in 6-18 months period.

F: First   P: Print   O: Options   R: Return

Figure 28

-- Possible Causes --	Obs/Tot
1: Osteomyelitis, Diskitis or Epidural Abscess	1:5
2: Cauda equina syndrome	1:4
3: Occlusion of the aorta or iliac arterery	1:2
4: Spinal stenosis or spinal claudication	6:6
5: Lumbar neoplasm (primary or metastatic)	1:6
6: Spinous process impingement syndrome	1:4
7: RISK FACTORS FOR LUMBAGO	1:5
8: RISK FACTORS FOR A DISK DISORDER	1:3

1..8: Display Cause information
    D: Change display mode -- [normal]

P: Print Results   F: Findings   R: Return

Figure 29

-- **Possible Causes** --   **Obs/Tot**

1: Cauda equina syndrome   2:4

2: Disc displacement (Herniated nuc. pulposus) 10:10
3: Tabes   3:6
4: Disc disruption - internal   1:5
5: Pelvic disease   1:4

6: 5th lumbar root lesion   2:5

Figure 30

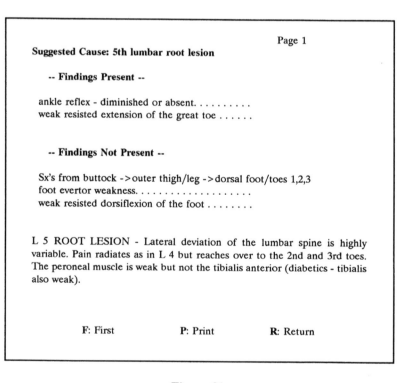

Figure 31

Chapter 2 Summary

The problem list is the second phase of the problem oriented system. In its initial most elementary form, it is a complete list of all the abnormalities found in the database. In its most fully developed form, it states problems at the highest level of synthesis of the abnormalities (diagnoses) that can be supported with evidence from the medical literature. Problem Knowledge Couplers are one of the principal new tools used to aid in this synthesis. The traditional device, the diagnostic *impression*, written by memory based, credentialed professionals, is discarded.

The problem list is the table of contents of the textbook on a unique individual, his or her medical record. It provides the basic structure for organizing all future efforts of individual practitioners and the patients themselves. It enables specialists to be aware at all times of the full context of their actions, and it enables the generalist and the patients to relate constructively and without *slip ups* to the specialists whose highly honed skills they require and deserve from time to time. Accordingly, the problem list has implications for the organization of the medical institutions.

For those medical personnel who have conceived of the medical care system as a hierarchy, particularly those who have thought of themselves as the top of the hierarchy, this honest confrontation with the need for a system of total care to unique individuals does not need to be just another threatening, unhappy experience. Rather, it can turn a forlorn, negative feeling—"Who wants to be a cog in a big heartless medical machine?"—into a clear vision of an architecture with logical and visible connections among the parts in which patients no longer need to fear being victims of an uncoordinated medical care system where efforts are not cumulative and where conscientious but provincial minds often work at cross purposes.

2
The Problem List

Lawrence L. Weed

The first page of the patient record should consist of a numbered problem list. It is, in a sense, a table of contents and an index combined, and the care with which it is constructed determines the quality of the whole record. Inherent in the problem oriented approach to data organization in the medical record is the necessity for completeness in the formulation of the problem list and careful analysis and follow through on each problem, as revealed in the titled progress notes. The precision of titled, problem oriented progress notes and conclusions is directly related to the precision and integrity with which the problems are initially defined.

The student or physician should list all the patient's problems, past as well as present, social and psychiatric as well as medical. The list should not contain diagnostic guesses; it should simply state the problems at a level of refinement consistent with the physician's understanding, running the gamut from the precise diagnosis to the isolated, unexplained finding. The teacher should demand that the student understand a problem and be honest in defining it, no matter how elementary the terms required. Only when both student and teacher are absolutely honest in clearly defining their level of understanding can they become intellectual colleagues, sharing thought and action in the solution of problems.

In proceeding to define a problem, the physician or student should first ask several key questions. Is the problem medical or social? If it is medical, it should be classified as one of the following:

- a diagnosis, e.g., ArterioSclerotic Heart Disease (ASHD), followed by the principal manifestation that requires management, e.g., heart failure
- a physiological finding, e.g., heart failure, followed by either the phrase "etiology unknown" or "2° to a diagnosis," e.g., ASHD
- a symptom or a physical finding, e.g., shortness of breath
- an abnormal laboratory finding, e.g., an abnormal EKG.

If a given diagnosis has several major manifestations, each of which requires individual management and separate, carefully delineated progress notes, then the second manifestation is presented as a second problem and designated as secondary to the major diagnosis, as follows:

Problem #1. ASHD with heart failure

Problem #2. Supraventricular tachycardia–2° to Problem #1

If the physician thinks in terms of the requirements of proper management and the later need for logical progress notes, there need be little difficulty in determining a satisfactory problem list. Indeed, such a system immediately identifies those difficulties that have assumed major management proportions. For example, the list for one patient with cirrhosis may consist of a single problem:

Problem #1. Cirrhosis manifest by jaundice and ascites (minimal)

In another patient with cirrhosis, the list may be better stated as

Problem #1. Cirrhosis manifest by jaundice

Problem #2. Ascites–2° to Problem #1

In the former case, management may involve treatment consistent with early stage disease. In the latter case, the ascites is a major problem that requires very careful diet regulation, paracentesis or diuretics, significant periods of hospitalization, even consultation for surgery. By these simple techniques, the magnitude of a problem is easily discerned, and we avoid the confusion that results when we are dealing with diagnostic entities that have different manifestations, which may or may not become major management situations in themselves.

If the problem is a social one, it should be defined no less honestly and precisely, for example, teenage pregnancy, bankruptcy, or severe delinquency in school. Precision in the progress notes follows from the precision with which the problems are initially defined.

As the problem is clarified, altered, or diagnosed, the original list should be modified accordingly. This modification is accomplished not by erasure but simply by the insertion of an arrow followed by the new diagnosis or by "dropped" or "resolved." Each change should be dated. In this manner, a record of the student's or physician's thought process is preserved. When several problems turn out to be separate manifestations of a single problem, such as a *pericarditis* and an *arthritis* becoming *lupus*, then the two may be grouped together and designated as *lupus*, using the number and position of the first of the two problems. The unused number then becomes inactive for all subsequent admissions and clinic visits. It may be preferable to choose to keep findings separate for purposes of good management and for satisfactory progress notes, as already recommended; but, in the case above, for instance, it should be clearly stated on the original problem list that each finding is secondary to lupus. When a new problem appears, it should be added to the list and dated accordingly.

Twenty-four hours should be allowed to reformulate the initial problem list where necessary. This interval enables attending physicians, chief residents, and consultants to provide maximal help in devising the best possible definitions of all the problems. (It may be remarked that procuring definitions of this kind should be a major goal of clinical teaching.) Deciding what is wrong with the patient and in what direction medical energies should be expended is of great value both to the patient and the physician, who is constantly reminded to be thorough and to act in context. After 24 hours have elapsed and the list has been reformulated, it or elements of it should not thereafter be obliterated or destroyed, but only modified as new evidence accumulates, so that a record of all revisions will be maintained. That is, the subsequent process is wholly supplementary to the original problem list, as it is finally revised.

In the course of a patient's illness, minor episodes arise which the physician may hesitate to define immediately as significant problems on a master problem list. In this situation, the progress note may be titled *temporary problem*, and the appropriate symptom or finding (e.g., *pain in the abdomen*) may follow the title. When the time comes for the second progress note to be written, it will be easy to determine whether the temporary problem should be transferred to the problem list or dropped as a transient episode of little significance, not to be referred to again. In organizations where coding of principal diagnoses is a ritual that can be easily disrupted by a problem list containing not only diagnoses but physiological and symptomatic findings, those doing the coding need only scan the problem list for the diagnoses. These are always readily apparent to experienced observers. That so many items on problem lists are not diagnoses may seem to be disturbing evidence of our failure to understand completely much of what we deal with, but lack of understanding does not justify omission or neglect in a final tabulation. Indeed, it is precisely on these points, not yet understood and still evolving, that we should continue to focus a critical analysis for the benefit of the patient. Our failure to include such problems in patients' records in the past is evidence of how thoroughly ingrained our episodic approach to medical care is and of how preoccupied we have been with performing medical *tours de force*, as we found solutions to major problems, many of which might have been prevented altogether by a more thoughtful and systematic approach. Physicians must actively develop a capacity and a tolerance for what Whitehead called "sustained muddleheadedness." We must learn to live with ambiguity in the pursuit of honest solutions to difficult problems.

The list of problems should include not only active but inactive or resolved problems (Figure 1). The latter category includes any previously significant difficulty which may recur or may lead to a complication. For example, removal of a breast, gall bladder surgery, or cholecystitis should always appear on the list. An arm fracture that occurred when the adult patient was a child can be left out completely if, in the opinion of the physician, healing has been complete and no significant future problems can rationally be attributed to it. Disorders such as diabetes or glaucoma should always be considered active problems, regardless of how well controlled they are at the present or how unrelated the current complaint of the patient may seem.

Even when their time is unavoidably limited, physicians should not abandon the idea of a complete problem list. Rather they should title the abbreviated list that they are able to formulate *problems not yet completely delineated* and specify the one or two problems they do recognize and propose to take action on. By labeling the list in this manner, physicians are being completely honest with themselves and with all those who depend upon the record. Later, there may be more time. New findings may be made, and the problem list will slowly grow. Honest, accurate notes make all our efforts cumulative, even when we lack time. The nature and extent of any incompleteness is immediately discernible in records containing an honest list of problems and accurately titled progress notes.

In a simple medical situation, such as an appendectomy in a well person, one problem labeled #1. *Appendectomy* and a series of progress notes and plans, each designated #1 and properly titled, will on brief examination tell any physician new to the case that there is a single problem with no complications in an otherwise well person. The student or physician who is the author of the record should immediately be corrected, however, if careful examination of the patient and laboratory data reveals that there are more problems, either not identified or simply neglected. The system is open ended and allows for the simple and the complex, the ill defined symptom and the well established diagnosis. All it requires is that the formulation of problems be explicit to a degree consistent with the current state of their identification and resolution at any point in time.

In those institutions where complete, current problem lists are available, they should be enlarged and displayed in the operating room, much as x-rays are, so that anesthetists and surgeons are continually reminded that the patient may have far more to contend with than the single difficulty that is monopolizing their attention at the moment. By such a simple technique, nodes that should have been cultured will not be carelessly dropped in formalin, and patients whose cardiovascular status is borderline will not be subjected to lengthy procedures that were hastily decided upon on the basis of a frozen section alone.

ACTIVE PROBLEMS	INACTIVE PROBLEMS
#1 Accelerated hypertension	
Retinopathy	
Renal disease	
#2 Hypokalemia–etiology to be determined	
#3 Vomiting–dehydration (central venous pressure–0, hematocrit 40)	
#4 Diarrhea–unknown etiology	
#5 Anemia, secondary to renal disease (Problem #1)	
#6	Remote peptic ulcer disease
#7	Cholecystectomy
#8 Exogenous obesity	
#9 (l) breast mass	
#10	History of chronic alcoholism
#11	History of gonorrhea Rx'd
#12	Personality disorder
#13 Decreased vision (r) eye possible central retinal artery occlusion	
#14 Cardiac murmur, continuous, Never before described → Chest wall flow murmur secondary to problem #9 (progress note 12/4)	

Figure 1. Problem list showing active and inactive
(or resolved) problems

In the audit or teaching process, the problem list should be the starting point. We begin with the question: Is every abnormality in the database represented on the problem list, either as a problem itself or as a part of the basis for a diagnosis (e.g., myocardial infarction accommodating the finding of chest pain) or a physiological finding (e.g., heart failure accommodating the finding of shortness of breath)? If all the abnormalities are accounted for, no matter how crudely, then the person being taught or audited has reached a minimal level of thoroughness. As we discussed in chapter 1, a serious mistake in the care of patients and in teaching medicine is to undertake discussions about diagnosis and management of one problem before establishing whether all the patient's problems have been identified and defined at the outset. Diagnostic or management actions that are rational in one context can be totally irrational in another context. (The exception to this total contextual approach is defined in chapter 1 when the issue of emergency physiological derangements is discussed.)

The approach recommended here teaches more than the technique of obtaining a good history and physical examination. It inculcates an analytical sense that formulates the data into precisely defined problems that may justly be taken as the foundation for explicitly defining further work. Such an approach emphasizes process and results, not initial diagnosis that contains elements of assumption and may as a consequence be poorly followed or left unresolved.

When the physician or student being audited lists as separate problems many findings that are manifestations of a single problem, then the auditor or teacher should immediately recognize this as reflecting the level of the student's understanding and the precise level at which constructive teaching and meaningful development can start. Rather than insisting on the premature resolution of the anomalies by ill advised guesswork, the physician teacher should systematically help the student to synthesize separate clinical symptoms into a valid single entity, just as the physician teacher, in his bedside teaching, helps the student to analyze a multiplicity of problems.

For the learning physician the problem list can be a source of considerable confusion and an index either to his or her lack of medical knowledge or of the ability to apply it with thoroughness and precision. The jumbled problem list must be recognized for what it is—a call for help and assistance—the student's clear statement of difficulties that should not be ignored. If it is so recognized, then the problem list may become, for instructor and student alike, the source of progress in knowledge and technique.

Psychiatric and Demographic Problems

By many physicians, nonorganic problems encountered in the practice of medicine are regarded as alien, baffling, and perhaps not even interesting. Consequently, personality and adjustment problems are usually ignored in summaries of patient problems, even though they could have been described easily using clearly understood nontechnical formulations ("cries easily," "family difficulties," etc.) if the physician is unfamiliar with sophisticated psychiatric terminology. Until all psychiatric, social/cultural, and medical problems are consistently objects of attention and have become titled elements of the problem list, it will not be possible for patients and providers to watch them evolve and thereby learn systematically from experience. By ignoring some of the problems, we fail to develop an appreciation of patterns of physical and emotional disturbances and their roots in the lives of the patients. In cross-cultural medical care, we develop in Putsch and Joyce's terms a biased *unilateral and ethnocentric view of "what's wrong."* (Putsch and Joyce 1990)

The computer is making a major contribution in this area. Much of the Wellness Coupler, described in the chapter on the database, deals with this aspect of people's lives and provides some guidance right at the outset. Also a vast amount of research on the Minnesota Multiphasic Personality Inventory (MMPI) and the computerization of the analyses of the MMPI have made it much more likely, where it is employed, that individual patients will gain from their physicians an immediate, sympathetic understanding of the forces with which they are struggling, and much inadvertent neglect and many inadequate analyses by the medical profession can be avoided. There are many physicians who reject the help of modern techniques on the basis that Osler for three hours followed by Freud for three hours could have done better. Even if this was true, modern techniques are not competing in that league, but rather they are competing with hasty, off the cuff, five minute analyses by untrained, impatient physicians who live from case to case and who have no systematic means of learning and improving from a highly organized and recorded database that is kept up to date.

First the Problem Oriented Medical Record, and now, the Problem Knowledge Couplers have done a great deal to overcome the false boundaries that have grown up among all of the specialties in medicine.

Indeed, whenever developing a coupler, whether for chest pain or headache or vomiting or whatever, it is strikingly apparent that a complete list of causes for the problem includes representatives from almost every specialty, and psychiatric diagnoses just about always have a place on the list. To quote a psychiatrist, Dr. Willie Yee, who has been involved in building knowledge couplers:

[N]ature does not respect the distinction between medical and psychiatric Causes, and neither do the Couplers. One recent study (Hall et al 1979) indicates that 9% of psychiatric patients have an underlying medical disorder. Another study (Farmer 1987), surveying chronically mentally ill patients found 53% of the subjects had undiagnosed medical problems. The use of the coupler system in diagnosis enables both the patient and the psychiatrist to consider all causes regardless of specialty and thereby extends their abilities in management. This integration of psychiatry with medicine has been recognized as a desirable trend and openly promoted by the American Psychiatric Association in recent years.

Health maintenance should appear on everyone's problem list. Under this heading are immunizations and other preventive medicine issues. It is important to review the results of the wellness and systems review couplers and the management options they produce directly. This is an example of where the computer leads us directly from the database to the plan. The single finding is the problem and a plan is automatically formulated, but the provider must take a moment to be sure the problem list is updated. When there is a one to one correspondence between the bit of information sought and the action to be taken, the user is led directly to the action. Any exceptions or modifying information that needs to be acquired is discussed in the comments under the management action to be taken.

In such a system, details are embedded in the computer that can allow actions to be more carefully tailored to a uniquely individual situation. In the past, we have either neglected a certain amount of preventive maintenance or have applied it in a broad demographic sense, insisting, for example, that all people over a certain age should have tonometry or sigmoidoscopy. We have expected a wide variety of practitioners representing many types and degrees of specialization to recall and process large amounts of this type of information. The literature is full of evidence of our failure to meet all these expectations. In a computerized system, appropriate action can not only be built in, but also be targeted to the individual's unique situation. For example, referral for visual fields evaluation by automated perimetry in someone with a family history for glaucoma may be warranted earlier than for someone without this risk factor. Likewise, for the patient with a family history of colon cancer, the same consideration would apply in the decision to do a colonoscopy.

In those situations in which the computer is routinely used as a tool, the provider reviews the recommended actions, identifies problems for the problem list (often under *Health Maintenance*), and places the recommended action under the appropriately numbered and titled plan. In this way, the problem list continues to be a complete picture of an individual's health status.

Physicians who seek to provide total care for their patients and who naturally integrate findings into well formulated problem lists should not, and usually do not, feel threatened by the challenge of creating a complete list. On the other hand, specialists who are annoyed or made anxious when health issues are raised that extend outside the limits of their experience may feel threatened by the strict accounting required by a rigorously constructed problem list. It is certainly true that such accounting demands precision and high standards; it is also true that we have compounded our problems by accepting a medical care system in which the efforts of individual practitioners and the patients themselves are uncoordinated.

A single problem oriented record available to everyone at every encounter, with a copy always in the patient's possession, will make the efforts of both providers and patients cumulative. Specialists will not be confronted with the impossible choice between

- dealing only with a specific problem relevant to their own specialty without regard for the total context, or

- trying to give total care to individuals while simultaneously keeping up with the demanding skills of their own specialties.

Either alternative is unacceptable to a busy, competent, and rational specialist. One of the reasons we have a malpractice crisis is that there are physicians who are accepting the dangerous risks of the first choice or trying to meet the impossible demands of the second choice. No single provider can do it all. But if everyone is part of a well defined and coordinated system, then a single database and a single problem list shared by all providers place everyone in the broadest possible context, and the efforts of everyone are cumulative. Furthermore, if the patient has a copy of the total record, he or she can help the providers avoid working at cross purposes.

The system described above could have a profound effect on the way larger medical institutions are run. There could be a single database section with highly skilled people keeping each patient's database up to date on a routine basis. These people could be trained to make sure that every abnormality in the database is accounted for on the problem list. Patients would be assigned to the place where there are specialists who are able to deal with the acute major problem of the moment (the cataract, the leukemia, broken hip, the heart failure). Those specialists could be brought up to speed and put into context promptly with one glance at a properly constructed problem list, instead of being forced to establish a broad context on their own.

For the other problems on the problem list that are less acute but still require ongoing attention, the appropriate providers could be made aware of the patient's whereabouts. For example, a patient may be on an orthopedic specialty ward for hip surgery but also has a glaucoma problem or a blood pressure problem that requires monitoring and informed attention, particularly under the new drugs and stresses of surgery. The orthopedic surgeon could elect to assume responsibility for the continuing care of this ongoing problem. Alternately, the surgeon could choose to have the system inform and mobilize the original providers for this problem or enlist the efforts of new providers if necessary. In this sense, the medical, urology, or orthopedic service of a hospital is not just some geographic area, but rather it is all the problems in that institution that belong to that specialty, irrespective of the physical location in the building.

This honest confrontation with what total care to an individual requires may be very unsettling to those of us who think of ourselves as physicians in charge of a patient's care, rather than as merely a cog in some medical care machine. The reality is, however, that we have always been just cogs in a big medical care machine. By not explicitly recognizing this reality and not rigorously defining an overall architecture with logical and visible connections among the parts, our joint efforts have not been coordinated and cumulative. Patients have been victims of the lack of a highly organized collaborative effort. Even in those institutions and group clinics where the stated goal was a disciplined collection of highly trained specialists, the information systems for coordination, guidance, and feedback have often not been commensurate with the stated goals.

Before focusing on two problem lists and reviewing some concrete rules for keeping them that facilitate coordination among providers, we should consider the importance of rules and discipline in any large system. The more parts there are in a living organism or dynamic organization, the fewer degrees of freedom for any one of the parts and the more controlled the environment has to be. It is the price we have to pay for the higher level of sophistication that multicellular organisms or multi-individual organizations provide. Change the pH of the human body a few tenths of a point or the temperature a few degrees and the whole organism will die; have the musicians of a great symphony "out of synch" by a single beat and we go from music to noise. For those who are oppressed by rules and who feel that they somehow take the art out of medicine, the words of Stravinsky remind us of how misguided is such a notion:

> A mode of composition that does not assign itself limits becomes pure fantasy. The effect it produces may accidentally amuse, but is not capable of being repeated. The creator's function is to sift the elements he receives, for human activity must impose limits upon itself. The more art is controlled, limited, worked over, the more it is free.
>
> As for myself, I experience a sort of terror when, at the moment of setting to work and finding myself before the infinitude of possibilities that present themselves, I have the feeling that everything is permissible to me....
>
> I have no use for a theoretic freedom. Let me have something finite, something definite—matter that lends itself to my operation only insofar as it is commensurate with my possibilities. And matter presents itself to me together with its limitations. I must in turn impose mine upon it. So here we are, whether we like it or not, in the realm of necessity. And yet which of us has ever heard talk of art as other than a realm of freedom? This sort of heresy is uniformly widespread because it is imagined that art is outside the bounds of ordinary activity. And in art, as in everything else, we can only build on a resisting foundation: whatever constantly gives way to pressure constantly renders movement impossible.
>
> My freedom thus consists in my moving about within the narrow frame that I have assigned myself for each one of my undertakings (1947).

Three Problem Lists

Problem List 1. The first problem list is of a patient who was worked up in an academic institution that was in the early stages of implementing the problem oriented medical record. It illustrates some of the difficulties a subspecialist has in coming to terms with some of its requirements and some of the consequences to the patient when a specialist takes too narrow a view. The patient came in on the 17th of the month and on that day a database was acquired, but no complete problem list was developed from it. Only the impression *bladder tumor* written at the end of it.

The initial plans related to only this one problem. By the 11th day of the next month, there was a problem list with seven problems on it. The problem list appeared as follows (the single initial impression having been written on 3/17 on the history and physical examination sheet).

3/19	Bladder tumor
3/19	Colonic (sigmoid) tumor
3/31	S/P Sigmoid colon resection and partial bladder resection
4/2	DTs, Alcoholic
4/3	Pulmonary edema
4/11	UTI

The following points can be made about this particular problem list:

- Two days should not have been allowed to elapse before a problem list was created.

- In the initial workup (database) done by this particular physician, there were abnormalities that should have been represented on the initial problem list on 3/17, the first day the patient was seen. Instead, the patient's course was allowed to evolve haphazardly, incurring dangerous risks and needless expense. At a minimum, the problem list should have included the following three items (the comments are for the reader, not the problem list):

  - Alcohol abuse
    (A history of drinking two fifths of liquor a day was in the database and no problem identified until the patient went into the DTs.)

  - Blood in stool and altered bowel habits
    (A history of blood in the stools and intermittent constipation and diarrhea were in the database, but no problem was identified and worked up until surgery was undertaken for the single impression

of bladder tumor and they found the tumor went beyond the bladder into the colon. They had to withdraw from that surgery, study the patient further, and then go back in again—a great deal of unnecessary risk and expense.)

- Dyspnea, cough, and wheezing—unexplained
(These findings were in the original history but were never accounted for on the problem list. They should have appeared on the problem list on the first day followed by an adequate plan. Perhaps if this had been done, the problem of congestive failure would never have developed.)

There were many other deficiencies in this patient's care that grew out of a disorganized approach. There was no flow sheet whereby effective monitoring of many variables could have taken place and some of the difficulties anticipated and even prevented. But many of these additional deficiencies have their roots in the absence of a complete initial problem list. As we shall see when we get to the section on plans for each problem, it is not possible to develop a good plan for one problem without knowing the other problems. Good management is contextual, and it is the completeness and the reliability of the problem list that determines the breadth and meaning of that context. In the case just described, the status of the heart and the alcoholism had as much to do with the ultimate outcome of surgery as the details of the surgical lesion and the surgery itself. We may specialize, but the patients do not.

Often specialists will say they have neither the time nor the skills to get a complete list of problems every time. But the case just described illustrates how dangerous is the illusion that it is more efficient to proceed without all the facts. The manhours spent by all types of medical providers in dealing with the messes in this one case would have been enough to develop complete databases and problem lists on many patients. A stitch in time really does save nine.

Cases like the one above happen every day in almost every medical institution. Indeed, they are so pervasive that we have come to accept them as the inevitable price of modern, highly specialized medical care. What we have here is not like an oil spill or a plane crash in which many victims suddenly appear and spark a detailed investigation into the system itself, often resulting in major changes in the way business is done. Rather it is more like the continuous underground pollution of a water supply in which the victims are not even conscious of the faulty system until it is too late for many of them. In the field of medicine, the patients themselves are not provided with the means of understanding how much better things might have been. Sick people are in no position to analyze and fight a bad system. Well people have no immediate incentive to study and change the system.

Undoubtedly, organized public scrutiny would come about if the innumerable victims of our misguided system—patients in major medical mishaps that occur daily—could be seen as the shuttle astronauts were after the Challenger disaster. For the public to watch thousands of patients entrusting themselves to physicians' care and then sickening further or dying at their hands would be a staggering perception. The result would be demand for change going far beyond our present piecemeal measures.

Problem List 2. The following problem list, from a general medical ward, is presented here for purposes of study and comment.

#1 Acute encephalopathy
    Probably secondary to uremia
    Transient anisocoria
#2 Uremia
    ?Dehydration
#3 Fever
    Pyuria without bacteriuria
    Leukocytosis
#4 Biventricular congestive failure
    Mild
#5 Moth-eaten skull
#6 History adult onset diabetes
#7 Hypertension
#8 Obesity
#9 Dental caries
#10 Abnormal chest x-ray
#11 Varicose veins

Our first question should be, Is this list complete? A quick review of the initial database suggests that it is not. The first few sentences of the description of the present illness that accompanies this problem list read as follow:

> 60-year-old white female who (according to her son) was well until 4 AM yesterday when she apparently awoke and was confused, muttering religious phrases, refusing to acknowledge her son's presence. Son denies any fever, chills, seizures, paresis. However, allegedly patient has been vomiting for 2 days.

The vomiting is not represented on the list and either should be recorded as a separate problem or should be represented as the first item in problem #2, followed by the presently listed dehydration and uremia, depending upon whether the physician thinks it is possible at the outset to attribute the uremia to this history of vomiting.

The next question that should be asked is, "Is each problem expressed properly?" The first five problems are reviewed one by one below. Each is followed by specific comments relevant to that question.

#1 Acute encephalopathy
    Probably secondary to uremia
    Transient anisocoria

Would acute encephalopathy best be expressed by omitting "probably secondary to uremia"? Unless there is no doubt that the encephalopathy results from uremia, a complete analysis of the problem is in order. Ascribing the encephalopathy to uremia, even "probably," may mislead colleagues and prevent a thorough attack on the problem.

#2 Uremia
    ?Dehydration

Question marks should not appear in the problem list. Uremia should simply be worked up and dehydration ruled out (or verified as one of the causes).

#3 Fever
    Pyuria without bacteriuria
    Leukocytosis

If the physician thinks that the fever is secondary to pyuria, then the problem is simply pyuria, and fever need not be listed. If, on the other hand, the physician is trying to record the probability that the fever is an independent problem since no bacteriuria exists, then fever should be listed and worked up separately. The plan for a fever of unknown origin is of course quite different from the approach to a fever which is merely secondary to a urinary tract difficulty.

#4 Biventricular congestive failure
    Mild

It should be indicated whether the etiology is unknown or is secondary to problem #7 or some other cause which the physician understands but has failed to mention.

#5 Moth-eaten skull

After reviewing the film, the radiologist objected to this expression, asserting that the film was consistent with hyperparathyroidism.

The attention of an experienced physician studying the amended problem list would no doubt be drawn to acute encephalopathy, vomiting, uremia, and "pepper and salt" appearance of skull in x-ray. In ascertaining the patient's serum calcium, the physician would not be surprised if it was markedly elevated and would, most likely, expect this patient at autopsy to have a parathyroid tumor. What of the inexperienced individual? If he or she rapidly reviewed the differential for each of the problems in a reference text, he or she would identify the diagnosis or finding that is a common denominator for several of the problems and would arrive at the same conclusion as the senior physician. Thus a disciplined, thorough approach to a set of problems may not only substitute for experience (or intuition) but may be superior to it, because the methodology does not depend on the necessarily limited reach of the mind of one man but permits the mobilization of the experience, and the accurate memory of it, of many experts through the ordinary coupling of a complete list of problems and readily available standard books and articles. *Experience* and *intuition* are words used by many as if their invocation leads to nothing but good. Experience can be incomplete and misleading; intuition can be wrong as well as right, directly relying as it does upon how accurately one interprets the accumulated range of experiences upon which all intuition is based.

The formulation of a problem list like that above, it may be argued, has already been recommended to every clinician and taught to every student. However, auditing of problem lists reveals that many physicians, regardless of intent, do not in practice create or demand thorough and complete problem lists. Nor can it realistically be said that they teach directly from the intern's own problem lists. Frequently teachers deal casually with an eccentric element of the findings, performing feats of synthesis in their own minds of which the house officer or student may be quite unaware. The obvious results may be confusion in patient care and student learning. The intern or house officer should be able to rely on the problem list as the complete superstructure of good patient care. Instructional pyrotechnics, improvisation, and ellipsis are revealed to be defective when the whole transaction between student and teacher is examined. The breadth and detail of the properly prepared problem list leave no gaps for the accidents of ignorance or error, in practice and learning, that irregular approaches inevitably allow.

Our second problem list is also from a general medical ward.

#1   Confusion, etiology unknown
#2   Hypertension, etiology unknown
#3   Psychosomatic abdominal complaints
#4   Urinary tract infection?
#5   Osteo. of spine
#6   Chronic alcoholism
#7   Fever of unknown origin
#8   Metabolic abnormality
        Hyperbilirubinemia
#9   Urinary obstruction, partial
#10   Probable pulmonary edema (see progress note 2/19)*
#11   Hyperkalemia

Comments on all but three of the above problems follow.

#1   Confusion, etiology unknown
#2   Hypertension, etiology unknown

The first two problems are concisely and clearly defined, and the experienced physician will quickly be in a position to evaluate the plan for the resolution of these not unusual problems.

#3   Psychosomatic abdominal complaints

This entry stimulates a careful scrutiny of the initial database. Has the physician mobilized enough symptomatic and objective data to justify defining the problem at this level? If the problem is accepted as it is, the plan will be quite different from the plan that would be developed, for instance, in the case of "abdominal pain, etiology unknown."

Question marks do not belong on a problem list. Either a urinary tract infection clearly exists or the problems that may suggest that it does should be stated, e.g., specific findings in the sediment, a specific change on an IVP, or a symptom such as dysuria. A logical approach to working up any of the latter can be taught; working up a question mark cannot. No scientist should be in the position of guessing what the problem is when exercising his or her science. When the problem is originally stated as above, the tendency is to do several urine cultures, to find them negative, and to conclude that the problem is thereby solved, leaving the original complaint, dysuria or frequency, forgotten and unresolved.

The expression *rule out* in a problem list can also trap the physician. For example, if the problem is expressed as *rule out diabetes*, the physician will do a glucose tolerance test, find it normal, and thereby dispose of a difficulty that never existed, leaving the vaginitis or neuropathy buried in some narrative history or physical exam, never to be identified again.

#5   Metabolic abnormality
        Hyperbilirubinemia

"Metabolic abnormality" is meaningless. What is the problem? Is the hyperbilirubinemia the abnormality? If so, the first phrase is redundant. If not, the specific finding should be stated. Also as the hyperbilirubinemia is encountered, the database must immediately be examined to see why the physician separates the jaundice problem from the chronic alcoholism and how in the face of both of them the physician can establish with conviction problem #3 as psychosomatic abdominal complaints. By carefully interrelating a problem list with a database and progress notes, the teacher can in very specific ways improve the care of the patient and the abstract quality of the performance of the physician.

#9   Urinary obstruction, partial

If problem #4 had been more explicitly stated, it would be much more
apparent whether problem #9 should be combined with it into a single, better
defined problem.

#10   Probable pulmonary edema (see progress note 2/19)

The word "probable" should not be used in a problem list. The student (or
physician) knows the patient is suffering from pulmonary edema and should
either so state the problem, or state it in terms of a symptom, or a sign, or an
abnormal x-ray finding.

Before leaving the problem list, let us mention three aspects of each
problem that should be immediately available to anyone proceeding to develop
the next section of the problem oriented record—the plans for each problem.
Indeed, it may be the practice of some to have these three aspects appear
under each problem before going to formulate the plan in the microcomputer
version of the problem oriented medical record.

- The *basis* for the problem statement:
  If the problem is hypertension, the basis may be simply three diastolics
  greater than 100 on three visits; or if the problem is pernicious anemia,
  the basis may be a B12 level or a set of clinical findings. Whatever it
  is, there should be no ambiguity in the statement as to which of the
  abnormalities in the database have been extracted and combined to
  drive the problem to a higher level of abstraction in the mind of the
  physician or other medical personnel. When knowledge couplers are in
  standard use, we shall all have a common language and it will be the
  positive findings under the cause we choose that will form the basis of
  our problem statement.

- The *status* of the problem:
  Is the problem getting worse, better, or staying the same? It should be
  possible to enter any medical environment at any time and to identify
  not only which patients are getting worse but precisely which problems
  are getting worse. Later we shall discuss how one further sets priorities
  among this group.

- The *disability* from the problem:
  A problem that might totally disable a manual worker might be a
  minor inconvenience to a radio broadcaster. The management of the
  disability is often as important to the patient as management of the
  problem itself, and the disability may be the most important issue to
  ancillary personnel who are helping to manage the ill person.

Chapter 3 Summary

It is the third phase of the problem oriented system, where every diagnostic effort and treatment is related unambiguously to a specific problem, that provides a record of not only *what* was done but *why* it was done. Since the context of every patient's life is unique, no single textbook approach can be applied to all people for solving and managing a specific problem. As providers embark on developing a plan for a problem, the system requires that they have clearly in mind the *status of the problem* (getting worse, better or staying the same), the *disability* from it, and the *basis* for stating it at the level of abstraction (diagnosis, symptom, etc.) on the problem list. Further guidance is then provided for constructing the plan in terms of the *goal*, the *parameters to follow*, the measures to take to *investigate the problem further*, the *treatments* to give, and the *complications to watch for*. As this framework is used over and over again in providing care, patients begin to develop a critical sense of their own as to whether their problems are receiving an organized and thorough approach. They soon learn that providers cannot set a goal for one problem without knowing the other problems. They also begin to realize that the choice of parameters and the frequency of observation is one of the most crucial activities in medicine. Management couplers can be very helpful in this regard.

Couplers are also essential to organizing and rationalizing additional investigative efforts to further understand the problem. The notion of knowing and systematically monitoring for the possible complications from each problem might do much to avoid some of the acute and emergency situations that are now routine byproducts of our present way of providing care.

3
The Initial Plan

Lawrence L. Weed

Plans for the possible diagnosis and management of each problem, keyed by number to the problem list, should be prepared as the next logical step after the problem list has been formulated. Each problem should have its own plan, numbered correspondingly, so that an experienced observer can see at a glance whether an anemia, or a urinary tract infection, for example, has a complete and reasonable plan. Too many serious omissions occur when sleeping pills, blood urea nitrogen orders, and side rails are all mixed up in a list of 20 items, which were spun off the top of the physician's head in a totally random fashion. As time goes on, detailed progressive plans for each problem will appear as a section of the succeeding progress notes. When a well conceived plan is written at the outset, all that is necessary for long periods in the progress notes is a record of the data as they are produced. The initial statement of plans is important because it establishes the character of the further data that are to be obtained and the treatment that is to be given.

Established headings under a problem are a useful guide to those developing the initial plan. In the microcomputer based problem oriented record, this set of headings is known as an element set; the software can bring up an element set under each problem, automatically providing guidance for the user.

Element Set for Developing the Plan

Basis
Status
Disability
Goal
Follow Course
     Parameters to be monitored
     Treatments to be instituted

Investigate further
>   Specific measures to be taken grouped under the specific hypothesis
>   being considered

Complications to watch for

The user is not necessarily required to develop entries under each heading
(in the computer based system an asterisk appears automatically in front of
each heading where entries have been made), but such a structure gives the
user an immediate appreciation of how and in what depth a problem is being
pursued.

Basis, Status, and Disability

This information, concisely stated, should be in front of the provider as he or
she develops the rest of the plan. For example, by reviewing the *basis* for the
problem statement, the physician may decide to substantiate it further or even
state the problem differently. The *status* helps set priorities and budget time.
For example, if the problem is "getting worse," prompt attention, adequate
time for assessment, and increased frequency for recording followup
parameters are indicated. Knowledge of the *disability* may affect the
parameters to be followed, the treatments, the goal, and the complications to
watch for.

Goal

The patient profile and the complete list of problems should be reviewed
before setting a goal for a problem. For example, if one problem is *terminal
carcinoma of the lung* and another is *hypertension*, then the goal for the latter
may be either to ignore it or use only the Hypertension Diagnostic Coupler
but not any expensive or invasive diagnostic procedures. At best, treatment
would only occur if it were necessary to keep the pressure within relatively
safe limits; it would not try to achieve normal values for the long term. In
another case, the goal might be stated in contingency terms, postponing any
action until the results of efforts on other problems are known. Also the goal
may be to defer any action until plans or drugs for another problem are
modified so that they do not interfere. When this careful interaction of
problems is not considered, investigative efforts often really tell more about
what is being done to the patient than about what is causing the problem to
be solved. For example, an x-ray dye needed in pursuing one problem may
produce information of minimal value and yet completely invalidate the
pursuit of another more urgent problem.

Patients must be involved when goals are set. If they know they will refuse surgery under any circumstance, then there may be little point in carrying out some textbook approach to a elaborate diagnostic workup that incurs expense and even risk to the patient. Also, an active role on the part of the patient is indispensable when setting priorities and discussing trade offs in the face of multiple problems. There are times when patients are defeated by the sheer number of things to be done if each problem were to be approached in the ideal manner. Wherever possible, the patient, after being fully informed, should decide what to tackle first and on what time scale. Morale is achievement, and achievement depends on reasonable goals set by the patient. Multiple specialists independently making demands on a multiproblem patient can all fail when each acts unilaterally and has no way of coordinating his or her efforts with others in the total context of the patient's life.

Follow Course and Treatments

It is here that the provider states the parameters that should be followed to reveal whether the problem is getting worse, staying the same, or getting better. For the purpose of always being aware of any problem that is taking a turn for the worse, it is better to have a few well chosen parameters reliably measured at regular intervals than a whole battery of things gotten at the beginning but then never systematically followed. Patients have been lost from rapidly advancing problems because no one was watching simple clinical parameters frequently, but instead relied on either a faulty diagnostic guess or a fancy diagnostic test whose results would either be equivocal or return long after the situation had gotten out of control. It is useful to think of parameters with the following points in mind:

- What is the most reliable and inexpensive parameter to keep track of the course of the disease?

- What is the threshold that should alert the observers of a parameter to notify the decision makers? (Major mishaps in medicine have occurred not because the right warning signals were not available, but because no one paid attention to them.)

- What level is the physician looking for to take what action? Not infrequently, physicians order tests and the acquisition of data way out of proportion to their capacity or their discipline in matters of interpretation and action.

- What parameter should be used to measure the response to therapy? The provider should have some idea about the criteria for success or failure and when to discontinue a therapy. If it is difficult to define such an endpoint, then the provider should question starting the treatment in the first place.

All too frequently in the practice of medicine, treatments are brought to a halt not by a conscious decision made judiciously at the proper time but by some crisis produced by a treatment that was allowed to go on too long.

• The frequency of measurement of various parameters should have some logical relationship to the expected rate of change. Also, all those who get data should recognize that when the rate of change increases, the frequency of monitoring may need to be increased and the decision maker alerted.

Choice of parameters and the frequency of observation is one of the most crucial activities in medicine. Management couplers can give much needed guidance in this area. If there are more than two or three parameters and treatments going on at any one time, there should always be a flow sheet; such a flow sheet should be organized and kept current right from the beginning, not several days after a hurricane of lab reports and other data have been scattered over the landscape. (See chapters on progress notes and flowsheets for further elaboration on this issue.)

Physicians have to be constantly on their guard that the parameters chosen for one problem are not invalidated by the treatment or course of another one of the problems on the list. Too much time and money are spent getting and discussing data which, with a little thought, never should have been ordered in the first place. It is not that the given test or procedure was not a logical step for the problem in a textbook sense, but when put in the context of a patient with several problems and multiple variables, the results would be uninterpretable since the original conditions of their use could not be met. Because of these issues, formulating plans in multiproblem patients deserves meticulous attention, and it is often efficient in the long run to do it in two steps: first think through what would be the ideal approach for each problem as if it were the only one present; then introduce the necessary changes based on an analysis of the contradictions and interactions that grow out of a multiproblem situation. Diagnostic and management couplers and the detailed guidance they provide facilitate this process.

In some instances, the provider would never reach this step in the plan because a quick perusal of the total list of problems would have resulted in the goal being set as "Defer any workup until Problems X and Y are resolved or stabilized."

Investigate Further

It is at this point that the provider states the hypotheses to be investigated and by what steps and in what order. As stated above in another context, before launching into investigations of all sorts, the physician should have a clear idea whether the sought after data will truly contribute to ruling something in or out and whether further action really depends upon the projected procedure or laboratory data. For the sake of the patient's health, comfort, and pocketbook, we should rigorously distinguish "nice to know" information from "need to know" information.

Before we had knowledge couplers to help us take advantage of the enormous power of simple findings in the aggregate, we were always looking for the powerful "one shot" deal that would make the diagnosis. And often without thinking, we would attribute more specific diagnostic power to a test or procedure that is highly technical, expensive, and sophisticated than to a single observation or a cluster of clinical observations. This tendency is perhaps exaggerated when the diagnostician is also the one who directly profits each time the expensive test or procedure is performed. An extreme case of this occurred recently in a leading medical center when a diagnosis of *hemochromatosis* was made by cardiac biopsy by a specialist when it could have been done earlier by eliciting and organizing a few clinical observations. Once a large number of diagnostic and management couplers are available, it will probably never be justified to generate a plan for further investigation from the memory of a single provider or even from a conference of experts extemporaneously working from their own memories.

Of course, there may be times that many simple findings in the aggregate do not differentiate causes well, whereas a single procedure may get straight to the heart of the matter and thereby be cost effective even though it might be invasive or expensive. However, until we start using couplers routinely, we will be unable to establish clearly when simple clinical methods fail in certain situations. For example, a recent study of arthroscopy in knee problems in children and adolescents found the clinical diagnosis to be in error in a large percentage of cases and therefore advised arthroscopy before arthrotomies or other corrective actions were taken on the basis of the clinical diagnosis. However, we often find that such articles do not state what the clinical criteria were used to make the clinical diagnosis, how consistently were they applied in all cases, and how competent were the examiners. When we build good couplers that take full advantage of all that is known clinically for a wide variety of options, we realize that unaided minds could not possibly equal them. Therefore, studies like the one just described may be drawing the wrong conclusions from their data. The arthroscopy findings may simply be revealing the need for couplers if we want to fully exploit the power of simple clinical observations in the aggregate. This is another example of where we have done *outcome* studies before we ever had control over the *inputs*. Persisting in such studies may be not only a waste of effort and money, but it may lead to the wrong conclusions.

The manner in which results of coupler usage are organized on the index of causes facilitates the development of a rational order for pursuing various diagnostic and management possibilities. Those possibilities for which the prognosis is bad, the course is rapid, and the effective treatment known should be investigated before time and resources are invested in self limiting disorders or those for which medical intervention offers little.

Complications to Watch For

In this section of the plan, as providers we can use effectively a great deal of known statistical information. For example, if it is known that patients with infectious mononucleosis can on occasion actually develop respiratory failure or rupture a spleen, then the physician does not fall into the trap of losing such a patient through inadequate monitoring, having dismissed the case as "just another case of mono". It was not just another case: it was a patient whose spleen was extremely large and tender or whose remarks about a breathing difficulty were completely ignored by the busy clinician.

On careful analysis, many cases in medicine never needed to reach the emergency stage. Many signals were being given by the patient for a long period of time before the crisis occurred—their significance was just not recognized and the "emergency" was allowed to develop because simple steps were not taken to anticipate and avoid it.

Obviously, the individual physician should not endanger an overall objective in order to pursue the "ideal" resolution or management of a single problem. Moreover, we must strive for a clear idea of what the norm is for a given patient in a given age group before plans are conceived, though it is unfortunately true that in many instances we cannot be provided with sharply defined standards when setting goals, either in diagnosis or management. All classification systems and programs for management are arbitrary. There is not a standard case of lupus or angina or emphysema or depression; nor is there an absolute amount of insulin or fluid or bicarbonate for a patient with diabetic acidosis. But there are variables prominently associated with each disorder and its management. If each variable is identified and restored to, or maintained in, a normal state, and as physicians we think more in terms of logical biochemistry, physiology, and psychology than in terms of artificially conceived syndromes and categories, then we are less likely to be frustrated and misled by what may be referred to as polemics in medicine.

In taking a physiological approach to a patient's difficulties, we must continually remind ourselves of how little of the total picture we are able to see, particularly in the first encounter with a patient. In general, if a patient has developed complicated difficulties over a course of weeks or months, we should not try to extricate the patient from those difficulties in minutes with an eccentric therapy that is directed only to the derangements readily apparent. Thoughtless, rapid readjustment of a few parameters, considered out of context, can be dangerous to the patient.

It is true that prognosis requires diagnosis, but diagnosis always leads to a degree of categorization that is never wholly justified. Physicians must learn for themselves, and teach their patients, a certain measure of planned ambiguity. Otherwise we will make absolute statements, draw premature conclusions, and neglect to follow carefully the progress of the patient, thereby failing in turn to introduce the critical control and continuing readjustment that good medicine always requires. The parameters to which we choose to pay continuing attention are the most important part of any plan, for such followup is the only protection the patient has against our misconceptions as we diagnose, treat, and prognosticate. Patients must come to think of a physician as a sophisticated guidance system and not as an oracle with absolute and immediate answers.

Many students find it difficult to separate diagnostic activities from those undertaken for immediate therapeutic action. For example, when a patient is in shock, the physician should first think physiologically; obtain information about volume, cardiac output, and peripheral resistance; and act immediately. Not until later is it time to systematically procure information to determine the cause. To say that in life threatening situations we must determine the cause before taking action is like saying that we must know why the child fell in the water before we will take steps to retrieve him or her. It is customary to take adaptive and contingency actions to satisfy immediate needs; therefore physicians are rarely justified in prematurely assigning causes before a reasonable body of facts is available.

When it is necessary to acquire diagnostic information over an extended period of time, it becomes difficult to think etiologically in a sustained and organized manner, especially after immediate physiological disturbances have been corrected. There is a great tendency to think vigorously about causes at the time of admission and then to fall into an uncritical attitude as day to day details are managed and the preponderance of the physician's energies are turned to new admissions. It is therefore essential that the initial plan be given much thought and that problem oriented progress notes, with supplemental plans, be so kept that overall execution can be judged and reassessments made without confusion. In complex cases, the emphasis should be on quick daily review of each active problem to ensure that a maximum effort is being exerted to resolve it, as opposed to an aimless collection of further information of questionable utility.

It is now generally recognized that our programs for educating patients in their own care have been woefully inadequate. Although teaching materials, such as medical magazines for laymen and audiovisual aids, have been employed and new personnel have been hired to overcome these deficiencies, it is not easy for patients to rigorously relate what they read and see to their unique situations. The "voltage drop" from all these materials and efforts to what actually goes on in a patient's day to day care can still be enormous. The best way to overcome this is to have the patient (or the family if the patient is not competent) be a full partner in the development and maintenance of the medical record. In this way, patients will know what data are being gotten and why. Everything they learn will be relevant to their needs or it would not be in their record. When they return home from the clinic or the hospital, there should be no confusion in their minds because they will have a copy of the plan and they will know exactly what parameters to follow. If, after such a system of care is implemented, a patient returns time after time without the proper data and with no evidence of having done his or her part, then the provider should at least give that patient a lower priority. Other patients should not suffer because the physician's time and intellectual and emotional resources have been exhausted by a patient who perpetrates crises out of delayed or neglected maintenance efforts. We should not be rebuilding engines for people who cannot be bothered to change their oil, and we certainly should not be doing it with the money of other taxpayers who are doing all they can to stay healthy. But these ideas cannot be implemented rationally and fairly without a well defined system of medical care and data management in place. We need a system to differentiate between those patients who are in difficulty through no fault of their own as opposed to those who indulged themselves and asked others to pay for the consequences. Our present system fosters delayed maintenance and crisis care. We pay specialists a fortune for rebuilding engines (coronary bypass surgery on an obese, sedentary smoker), whereas we pay nothing for teaching and demanding the oil be checked (a change in lifestyle).

In the past, to the extent that we have educated patients at all, we have focused on medical content relevant to their specific problems. There is another aspect of their education that must also be addressed. Each encounter they have with the medical care system should make them more sophisticated about problem solving in general. They will eventually absorb the underlying structure that supports the approach to anyone of their problems. They will think in terms of the steps described in this chapter: the goal, basis, status, disability, parameters to follow, the treatments, the investigation of further steps, and the complications to watch for. As they interact with various medical providers throughout their lives, they will not only be able to bring some rigor and discipline to that interaction, but they also will automatically get insight into how the provider thinks. In general, secure and competent nurses and physicians will welcome such understanding from the patient. When a provider resists these approaches, the patient may want to reconsider his or her choice of professional help.

Ideally in a hospital, the patients' medications should be in their bedside stands, and each four hours the nurse should come around and have each patient say which ones are due to be taken and then take them under the nurse's observation. Patients with multiple problems may be bewildered by all the treatments, but they need to get matters under their own control. Nothing is accomplished by doing it all for them if they eventually are going to have to go home and be in charge themselves. The goal should be to have a system of care operating as much as possible under the direction of the patient so at discharge there will be no doubt that it all can continue at home.

Physicians should keep in mind that their professional proficiency is the result of a repetition of basic concepts and principles through many years of medical school and residency training. They should not expect patients to grasp, after one exposure, all the implications and details of the management of their disorders. Indeed, if we dismissed students from medical school or physicians from training on the same standards of learning that some doctors apply to their patients ("they just don't understand"), I venture to say that there would be few doctors left in the system. As individual physicians learn best through their own work and their own progress notes, if carefully led and observed, so do individual patients learn best from their own experiences, when carefully led and observed by their physicians. Present patients and potential patients are the largest untapped resource in medical care today. Advantage can be taken of that resource through education of the patient and through clear formulation of the role that patients themselves can play as effective paramedical personnel.

Chapter 4 Summary

The uncertainties inherent in complex biologic systems make properly titled progress notes and up to date flow sheets crucial parts of a responsible medical care system. Any system without a feedback loop runs wild, and medical action can run wild if we do not monitor the progress of each problem and the results of the interventions for that problem. The defined steps of the problem oriented plans described in the previous chapter provide the basis for highly organized progress notes and flow sheets. There is not time in a busy practice to think in depth about every problem at every encounter. Without a good plan and conscientious efforts to follow it, progress notes can degenerate into random recordings of whatever parameter strikes the fancy of a given observer at the moment, and there is nothing cumulative about the overall effort.

By reading the progress notes, one should be able to quickly determine the progress of the problem from the patient's point of view (symptoms and disability), and from the point of view of reproducible objective measurements. The frequency of progress notes should be directly related to the rate of change of the parameters being followed—the more rapid the change, the more frequent the notes. If the patients understand this rule and are involved in their own care, they can make a major contribution to keeping potentially dangerous situations under control. They live with the situation at all times and are the first to be aware of significant change. The patients should be guided more in their thoughts and actions by what the data in their records actually show than by the statistical information they see in books or articles or hear from authoritarian providers.

4
The Progress Notes

Lawrence L. Weed

The uncertainties inherent in complex biologic systems make properly titled and numbered progress notes the most crucial part of the medical record. They are the mechanism of follow-up on each problem. Faulty understanding and defective decisions may be expected at the outset of a new case. Indeed, they are inevitable in the face of multiple variables. But failure to followup rigorously the results of those decisions is inexcusable. Action without followup is arrogance, especially where the objects of that action are living systems about which nothing is completely understood and in which conditions never remain fixed.

The progress notes should be written in a form which relates them unmistakably to the problem. Each note should be preceded by the title of the appropriate problem. This method immediately tells the reader that it is the progress of the anemia, for example (or the urinary tract infection, etc.), that is the subject under discussion. If a new problem is being discussed, it should be added to the original list and dated accordingly.

The physician should resist the temptation to write a single progress note and then say it covers four problems such as *renal failure, congestive failure, chronic obstructive lung disease,* and *hypertension* merely because they are interrelated and it seems inefficient to deal with each problem separately. The sets of parameters required to objectively assess the progress of each of those problems are not identical; and if each is not focused upon in an organized manner, crucial elements on one or more of the problems are frequently lost sight of and the whole exercise may even degenerate into general phrases like "doing well" or "situation not improving." There may be far less likelihood of yielding to this temptation when using the computerized problem oriented record and the guidance it provides in both plans and progress notes. (See Bartholomew's discussion of the use of the computerized problem oriented record in medical practice and Abbey's description of Problem Knowledge Couplers and their use in dentistry.)

Progress notes should be written with the original plan clearly in mind. There is not time in a busy practice to think in depth about every problem at every encounter. Without a good plan and conscientious efforts to follow it, progress notes can degenerate into random recordings of whatever parameter strikes the fancy of a given observer at the moment, and there is nothing cumulative about the overall effort. In this latter sense, progress notes should more accurately be called daily observations that are made with no real effort to measure progress against established goals with well defined parameters.

As can be seen from Figure 1, each problem oriented section of the progress note may consist of any or all of the following elements:

- Subjective data (headed "Subj"—or "Sx", for symptomatic data)

- Objective data (headed "Obj")

- Assessment (headed "Asses")

- Plan (Immediate plan)

Additional elements are sometimes added with self explanatory headings (see examples in chapter 2, e.g., Disc in Figure 7, Neg in Figure 4).

Moving within this framework immediately affects the physician's ability to choose the important parameters to be followed, standards of logic, and sense of responsibility in the attack upon and resolution of the patient's problems. In addition, the selection of certain problems to work on reveals which ones the physician thinks important and, conversely, what the physician chooses to ignore.

Each of the four elements listed above is commented on below.

Subjective Data

This element includes those parameters from the original plan that are subjective or symptomatic in nature. By putting them first, the provider ensures that progress is assessed from the patient's point of view. A physician should notice when data of this nature do not parallel objective measurements and should be alert to the possibility that there has been a misstatement of the problem or an error in a particular piece of data such as a cardiogram report or a laboratory value. Also, providers have to keep reminding themselves that patients come to have their symptoms explained and relieved —not just to have their x-rays reported as normal.

Progress Notes
1/5

#1. Failure to thrive

    <u>Subj</u>: Patient in no distress, feeding well

    <u>Obj</u>: PE: T = 37.3

                    HR = 140/min

                    RR = 28/min

                    Otherwise unchanged

                    CXR: no infiltrate, no cardiomegaly

                    Weight: up 150 gm after two days of formula #2

    <u>RX</u>: None

    <u>Ass</u>: Thriving well on present diet.

    <u>Plan</u>: 1.   observe and maintain on present formula.

#2. RUQ mass, questionable

    <u>Subj</u>: None

    <u>Obj</u>: PE: abd.-the RUQ mass can no longer be palpated with certainty.

          Flat plate and upright: no masses or fluid levels

          UA: negative, except s.g. = 1.007

          Urine culture: negative

          RFT: BUN = 26; Creatinine = 0.6

    <u>Rx</u>: None

    <u>Disc</u>: Although original RUQ mass not supported by any of the studies

              so far obtained, the possibility of a neuroblastoma or Wilm's

              tumor cannot be ruled out on flat plate. Thus will do IVP.

    <u>Ass</u>: Probably no RUQ mass

    <u>Plan</u>: 1. Schedule IVP

Figure 1

Objective Data

In the objective data section of the progress notes, physicians are frequently inclined to omit physical findings and emphasize laboratory data. For example, there may be a detailed discussion of an x-ray and no mention of how the patient coughs or of the character and quantity of the sputum.

In those problems that require the creation of a flow sheet (as described in the next chapter), the physician or nurse simply enters "see flowsheet." The same data should not be put in the prose progress notes as well as on the flowsheet.

Assessment

In the assessment section of the progress note, physicians should keep in mind the original plan and objectives. Also, when disagreements arise, for example on the subject of whether surgery should be employed in an elderly patient with a number of problems, the progress notes should contain written evidence that expert consultants, representing both sides of the issue, personally met, discussed the matter, and reached a conclusion. Unilateral action is practically never necessary if systematic approaches to difficult situations are formulated and followed.

Plan

A significant modification in therapy or diagnostic action should never be made without careful reference to previous progress notes on the same problem. Frequently, earlier evidence, however unassailable, is neither supported nor refuted; it is never interpreted or even appreciated. It is ignored. Often these data were obtained at great discomfort and expense to the patient and, if studied, may provide the evidence needed to solve the patient's current problems.

The plan section of the progress note, like the initial plan, should be prepared not only with respect to the specific problem but to other problems as well, so that therapy, which ordinarily would be satisfactory, will be withheld when contraindicated by other problems noted in the complete list. As soon as modifications or additions to the initial plans are indicated, the notes should state these clearly.

Organizing progress notes in the above manner continually reminds physicians to think systematically about each patient and provides evidence of whether they have actually done so. The younger physician will develop a pattern of ideation for each type of problem and will thereby create a framework upon which to build an individualized course of postgraduate self education.

Nurses' notes, social service notes, and physical medicine notes should not be separate parts of a medical record but should themselves be progress notes of the kind recommended here, properly titled with respect to specific problems and placed in sequence with all other data pertaining to a given problem. In this manner, the medical and paramedical professions assume an integrated and easily audited role in solving the patient's problems, and each avoids establishing the kind of identity that permits or encourages the possibility of dealing with problems out of context. It serves an educational function for every nurse and social worker to review constantly the total problem list and to enter all observations and actions under the appropriate heading; understanding (or the lack thereof) is immediately revealed when such entries are associated with the appropriate (or inappropriate) problem.

Occasionally we hear the complaint that nurses and doctors think differently about patients and that "Nursing care plans and notes" are necessary to deal with important aspects of care that doctors have traditionally neglected. There has been some truth to this in the past, but the way to deal with it is not by fragmenting the approach to solving a problem, but rather by having the original plan for a problem be complete from the patient's point of view. We believe that if all the aspects of a good plan mentioned in the previous chapter are conscientiously attended to, then the patient's full needs will be met. When the progress notes are written by various individuals, it may well be that one note by the nurse will go into more details on the progress of the disability or the nature of the pain, whereas another note by a physician may be principally on the interpretative aspects of one piece of objective data. But read in sequence and all under the same problem, the notes will give a complete picture of the progress on that particular problem. Too often, the first time crucial findings in a separate nursing part of the chart are ever fully discussed is in a courtroom, where even the physician is hearing the information for the first time. Also, as more and more patients have complete copies of their records and take more and more control of their own care, they should see all the data relevant to a given problem in one place, logically developed. In this way, everyone focuses on what is best for the patient and the patient does not become a victim of turf battles among providers.

When to Write Progress Notes: Setting Priorities

How often the provider writes a progress note on a problem is related to the goals that were set and the nature of the problem. A very slow moving problem or one that is completely under control may have a note once a month or once a year, e.g., a pernicious anemia problem that is well treated and that is producing no symptoms or positive findings. On the other hand, a patient with a recent coronary may need a progress note every few hours or entries on a flow sheet even more frequently than that. It is important that all medical personnel observing the patient and recording objective data realize that this is a process that cannot be done mindlessly, sticking blindly to the frequency orders of the original plan. It is the rate of change of a given parameter that should determine the frequency with which it is followed.

Although good clinicians can make some reasonable estimates when the original plans are written, they can never be sure. The provider should never look at the value of any finding without comparing it to the last value and noting the rate of change. The greater the rate of change, the more frequent should be the observation and the sooner the responsible provider should be notified. In this regard, patients should always think of themselves as the most important provider of their own care, and if they recognize the simple rule just stated, they will know when and when not to call the doctor. Too often they feel bound by someone's earlier and mistaken estimate of the course of a finding and then sit on a crucial piece of data too long. For example, a patient with a sore throat, fever, and malaise noted that what seemed like a small harmless rash suddenly started to spread—in other words, a parameter undergoing a rapid rate of change. She notified no one because a physician said she was doing fine and he would see her the next day. The next day never came for her, and a meningococcemia the physician did not foresee took over. It could have been treated earlier and probably successfully if she had been taught to understand the significance of rapidly changing parameters, no matter what they are.

A physician with a very large load of patients and problems should first attend to those where medical care can still make a significant difference—to individuals whose lives are still meaningful to themselves an ˙ to others. Then having identified such patients, the physician zeros in on those problems that are undiagnosed and that are getting worse. It is far better to have no note on an arthritis problem that has been smoldering along for years and an excellent note on an abdominal pain that is unexplained than it is to have incomplete, perfunctory notes on both of the problems. Unexplained problems in the head (psychiatric and neurological complaints) and in the abdomen require special vigilance. They can get out of hand very quickly, and valuable opportunities can be lost.

No audit of an individual physician's performance can be complete and fair if the auditor is not aware of the physician's total load and methods for setting priorities. We must not drive providers to wealthy environments where help is abundant or to patients with easy problems by refusing to take into account the total clinical load and the total amount of good care contributed to an environment over a long period of time.

Resident Notes

The approaches to the medical record described here can do much to define the role and the responsibilities of the resident physician. The conventional extended note of the resident is no longer recommended. Instead, after "working up" the patient, the resident should review and correct where necessary the list of problems as defined by the intern. Residents must first ascertain whether all the problems have been identified, critically examining the historical, physical, and laboratory evidence that bears on each. They should then insert after each problem an entry that consists of either "agree" or of a specific amendment.

Residents should use the problem list as the focus for work rounds and the implementation of complete day to day care. They should insist that the list of problems be complete and current and that the level of resolution of each problem be apparent. A good resident rapidly learns what problems should be given priority and naturally refrains from casual discussion of complex issues without carefully reading the appropriate problem oriented progress notes and flow sheets.

Residents can measure their own progress as teachers and leaders, not by how extensive their notes of amendment, are but by how brief, and by how infrequently it is necessary for them to reformulate the list of problems. If an intern fails to develop under a given resident, then documentation of this failure, explicit in the medical record, and particularly in the resident's notes, should be made available to the faculty, preferably by the resident. When house officers, students, and practicing physicians are evaluated in any other manner, interpersonal factors irrelevant to their capacity to care effectively for patients may intrude. The more tightly coupled care and education become by means of the medical record, the more secure are the welfare of the patient and the rights of the physician in charge of patient care.

Operative Notes

Operative notes are elements in the record of the patient's progress and should always appear as numbered and titled entries in the progress notes. If operative findings throw new light on the definition of problems, the problem list should be modified accordingly.

#1. Abdominal Pain -> Carcinoma of the pancreas (Date of finding)

Complications following surgery should be stated as new problems, followed by the entry "secondary to problem # [the original problem]." Data on a series of complications, such as pneumonia, phlebitis, fistulas, and the like, should not be consolidated into a single note because of the confusion that would result.

At the time of writing the operative note, the surgeon should quickly review the complete problem list, stating under the appropriate number in a titled progress note whether additional useful information about a kidney or a liver, for example, became available at surgery. No opportunity should ever be lost to add significant data to the medical record.

Consultant Notes

Consultants will of course examine the patient and the data in the customary manner. They will be expected, however, to enter their notes in a form that differs significantly from that usually observed in most medical records, in which known facts are intermingled with new information and conclusions are buried in pages of narrative.

Consultants should identify the problem for which they were consulted. They should employ its proper number and title and immediately state in not more than a line or two their conclusions and principal recommendations. They should then, under a separate subentry entitled *Discussion*, defend the position they have taken, repeating data already recorded in the chart only when employing them analytically to support any conclusions.

Having completed this annotation, the consultant should then review the problem list, adding any new problems that may have been revealed and recording under the appropriate problem number and title any new information or additional analysis that a specialized point of view contributes. When there is nothing significant to record with regard to a specific problem, the consultant of course omits mention of it. If this approach is taken and if all the data on any given problem are retrieved in sequence, all relevant contributions are immediately available in context to the primary physician and others. At the present time, many specialists either do not consider all the patient's problems and so provide a stereotyped analysis rather than one tailored to the patient's problems, or do not integrate their own analysis with the ongoing analysis by the physician in charge of the patient. If the specialist cannot use the existing list because it appears incomplete or inadequately expressed, the first order of business should be to discuss it with the physician in charge; otherwise any notes the specialist makes may be ignored as fragments never fully integrated into the ongoing appraisal of patient needs.

Critique of a Progress Note

The progress note that follows relates to the second of the two problem lists that were discussed in detail at the end of Chapter 3. The complete problem list will be found there. We are concerned here only with problems #1, #7, and #10.

Progress Note 2/9*

#7 Fever of unknown origin
    Sx: None (specific)
    Obj: This AM the patient spiked a T of 41°
            RR = 36-48 min BP 200/160 -
            ↑ 130/80

Lung rales at bases-rhonchi diffusely throughout
Chest x-ray—no localized infiltrate
Gm stain sputum: gm + cocci
Gm stain urine: gm - encap. rods. Probable
Klebsiella

Asses: Prob. gm-sepsis
Plan: 1. Cultures blood, urine
         2. Ice blanket
         3. Rx pen. kana + colistin

#1 Confusion
Sx: Completely obtunded today—unresponsive
Obj: Neck rigid
         Neuro exam unchanged
Asses: ?Secondary to intracranial bleeding
Plan: Will not do spinal tap now
         Other problems more important

In any patient with single or multiple unexplained findings or problems, each should be pursued to its logical conclusion. Often when this is done, synthesis of several problems into a single entity occurs as a natural consequence of thoroughness of exploration and application of simple logic. For example, had a lumbar puncture been done and pus found, problem #7 as well as #1 might have been far less obscure. Accurate, complete information is the foundation of good management, and it is ultimately economical of time to obtain it rather than to attempt to improvise without it.

#10   Probable pulmonary edema
       Sx: As above
       Obj:BP falling → 160/90
       Hr 160/min
       RR 36-48/min
       Patient suddenly developed acute SOB + frothing at mouth.?Pulm.
       edema
Asses: Pulm. edema
Plan: Rx dig., morph. + phlebotomy 150 cc
       CXR-did not confirm
       No diuretics because of possible gm neg. sepsis

Many elements of these progress notes suggest the physician is inexperienced and unsure of the entry, but this useful observation could not so readily be made if the notes had not been titled and facts and interpretations grouped accordingly. Without the titles, the incongruity, incompleteness, and faulty analysis might well have been overlooked in the review of the notes.

When the progress note is read by the resident or attending physician for the purpose of guiding the intern, the critique should be presented in an orderly manner. First the title: If "probable" indicates that the intern was not sure of the entry, why did not the title reflect what the intern was sure of— in this case the findings? The resident or teacher should sit down with the intern and actually prepare a note that is more appropriate under the circumstances. Such a note should not be entered into the record but is intended instead as an example from which the intern may learn. For instance,

> #10   Acute fall in BP, tachypnea, and tachycardia
>   Sx: Unresponsive
>   Obj: See #7—particularly chest findings and chest film
>   (should make time relationship to physical
>   findings clear).
>   BP now 160/90
>   H.R. 160/min
>   "Frothing at mouth"
>   Chest exam—see above
>   Imp: Except for "frothing" not picture of
>   pulmonary edema (if rales only at bases)
>   BP fall, tachypnea and tachycardia consistent
>   with pulmonary embolism or with septicemia
>   as discussed under #7, or infarct
>   Plan: a. R.O. pulmonary embolus; EKG for typical
>   change, enzymes, *call resident* about
>   further emergency studies.
>   R.O. pulmonary edema suggested by "frothing."
>   R.O. myocardial infarct-EKG
>   b. Consult resident about instituting morphine.
>   phlebotomy and digitalis, even though Dx
>   much in doubt.
>   c. No entry for patient education.

Titled progress notes should be consulted at autopsy so that the findings may be correlated as precisely as possible with the perceptions of the physician in the progressive identification and analysis of problems. (This patient underwent another episode in which the blood pressure fell to 90 and at autopsy showed massive pulmonary emboli.) The original physician should be asked to discuss exactly what was meant by "frothing at the mouth," since that factor played a major role in the conclusion.

With regard to patients such as the one described here, the teacher can be very explicit about the occasions on which the intern should request assistance. Whenever uncertain and able to define the problem merely in terms of findings that suggest that the patient is in danger, the physician should get help. That help was obtained should be reflected in the patient's record, either as a note by the resident or teacher or a direct quote of his or her advice. A call for the right help at the right time is often the most intelligent part of a good plan.

New house officers rotating into difficult general medical services from specialty services are suddenly confronted with enormous responsibilities that are well beyond their experience and that require more time for careful consideration than is likely to be available. If they will cooperate in revealing the structure of their thinking to the extent that this house officer did, they will be guided in a manner that is sufficiently relevant for intellectual growth to occur. Naturally, to be intelligible may mean to be found out, and the physician may sometimes wonder whether it is prudent to be explicit and thus become vulnerable to rigorous analysis. But it is this explicitness and vulnerability that lead to sound education, and that, above all, is what the student physician is after.

Progress Notes in the Microcomputer Based Problem Oriented Record

The microcomputer based problem oriented record gives the physician immediate availability to the original plan which provides the structure and guidance for providing highly organized and disciplined progress notes. As discussed in chapter 3, the following headings (or element set) form the basis for such guidance.

Basis
Status
Disability
Goal

| *Follow Course:* | Parameters to be monitored |
| | Treatments to be instituted |

| *Investigate further:* | Specific measures to taken are grouped under specific |
| | hypothesis being considered |

Complications to watch for

The user is not necessarily required to develop entries under each heading at every encounter (in the computer based system an asterisk appears in front of each heading where entries have been made), but such a structure gives the user of such a record an immediate appreciation of how and in what depth a problem has or should have been pursued. Furthermore, the user can select any one of these headings and a display will appear on the computer screen that contains the specific elements of the plan such as a parameter to follow or a cause to be investigated. The user can then select one of these elements and enter values of the parameter as they appear or the results of the particular investigation of the cause. This continuous electronic flow of the data from the problem to the plan and on through the progress notes means that there is no separate section of the record for progress notes. Also such a system facilitates immediate review of the plan and of the last note when the user goes to update the situation on a given problem. It is also possible to retrieve data in flow sheet form regardless of the problem for which the data were originally ordered.

5
Flowsheets

Lawrence L. Weed

In either a problem oriented or source oriented medical record, data can be entered in narrative (prose), graphic, or flowsheet (tabular) form. In all records each entry is dated, that is, the data are time oriented. In a paper record, the data for all retrieval purposes are of necessity in the same form as the entry. Computerized records, on the other hand, may allow retrieval in many forms. Indeed, flowsheets with almost any number and arrangement of variables have become an expected feature of any computerized medical record system. The emphasis, therefore, from the point of view of good care and good education must be on how to choose the correct variables for the flowsheet and how to interpret the relationships among them. But it is also important for those who do not yet have computers to recognize that a useful mixture of problem oriented flowsheets and narrative progress notes can easily be generated at the time of data entry if the original planning is done with the desirable number and arrangement of variables in mind for a given problem.

To emphasize this point, we have reproduced the entire chapter on flowsheets from the 1969 book on problem oriented records. Although the medicine represented in the flowsheets may be somewhat out of date, both the flowsheets and the discussion of them show what can be routinely accomplished in a large city hospital where the pressures of time and load were often extreme. Indeed, the one whose job it is to steadily and methodically enter the data onto the flowsheets is often the one who makes the most astute observations about trends, hitherto unrecognized correlations, and data gaps, that need to be filled in in the care of the patient. Such people not only serve the individual patient well, but also they may contribute to the development of medical science since every unique patient may be the source of new and useful insights in complex biological situations.

For certain problems, progress notes are not an adequate means of relating multiple variables. Data involving physical findings, vital signs, laboratory values, medications, and intakes and outputs can lead to sound interpretations and decisions only if they are organized to reveal temporal relationships clearly. Too often younger physicians may observe that the senior physician is likely to scan a patient record, expound on a single laboratory value, call at random for others in an expressionistic way, and finish by reaching doubtful conclusions, prefaced perhaps by the phrase, "in my experience." Time relations are ignored, crucial data are never brought to light, and wrong decisions forever go unrecognized because no logical tracks are discernible in the randomly recorded data.

Flowsheets like those reproduced at the end of this chapter can be used to facilitate the comprehension and interpretation of interrelated and changing variables. On certain fast moving problems, the flowsheet may constitute the only progress note. The time required initally in setting up a proper flowsheet is small compared to that lost in unraveling and reassembling disorganized and misplaced data.

In the construction of flowsheets, basic principles should be emphasized to the student at once. The teacher should spend more time helping the student decide what parameters to follow and how frequently to follow them and less time predicting conclusions. The data will tell young physicians what to do, but they need help in acquiring the discipline to keep their information orderly and to audit it systematically.

In choosing the appropriate parameters to follow for a given problem, physicians should keep in mind that they must strike a balance between an excessive number of variables and a compulsive preoccupation with the precision of a single variable, which, if interpreted by itself, could be very misleading. For example, the determination of four or five variables of a completely different type with speed and reasonable accuracy will solve an anemia problem faster than the investment of expensive time in procuring one determination of a single variable to an unreasonable precision or at a frequency that is physiologically absurd. This principle applies to narrative as well as numeric information. The limited time of the physician should not be spent disproportionately on qualifying and quantifying a single term like *hemoptysis*, if no time is left to resolve the problem by exploring other questions and obtaining and making use of physical findings and a chest x-ray.

The frequency of record keeping (or data collecting) depends upon how steep the curve is. A chart of a rapidly changing burn patient might show recordings every hour, whereas a chart on a patient with cirrhosis and persistent ascites might show recordings once a week or once a month. The frequency should be such that the configuration of the patient's course can be detected at a glance.

The bulk of the rapidly moving problems that require a flowsheet are fluid balance problems, and fortunately a few fundamental parameters common to all of them can be emphasized. For example, all patients being maintained on intravenous fluids and patients with renal failure, cardiac failure, shock, acute intestinal problems requiring fluids and drainage, and acidosis (either metabolic or respiratory) require the same careful consideration of the total volume of fluid in the body, of the circulating volume, of the tonicity of fluids, of the potassium level, and of the pH of the fluids. If told to follow the patient's blood pressure, pulse, respiration, venous pressure (by physical examination alone when indicated), hematocrit, and weight, the student will almost invariably mobilize common sense, make intelligent decisions about volume, and so prevent either the overloading or the "work-up" dehydration that occurs on medical and surgical services. Matters should of course not be allowed to proceed to the point that gross symptoms and physical findsings are necessary to alert the physician. If told to watch the serum sodium, the student will not create or ignore significant derangements in body tonicity. Carefully watching and maintaining flowsheets that record the serum potassium and the factors like pH that affect it, the student will gradually gain understanding and pursue the relevant literature as actual cases require it. The same is true where pH and blood urea nitrogen are the prime factors.

Having become disciplined about these few parameters common to many problems, the student will quickly learn to add the more specific ones, such as pCO_2 and minute ventilation in the respiratory problem or a series of EKG strips and medications in a patient with a hypertensive crisis or an arrhythmia.

The important point is always to keep from inundating students or interns with information when what they need, over and over again, is the opportunity to see principles operating naturally in their own patients as they line up, side by side and day by day, all the related parameters. If teachers looked more carefully at flowsheets with students, pointed out missing parameters, and directed reading to very specified points, they would misinform less and inculcate discipline more—and learn a great deal themselves.

Problem List

#1.   Arteriosclerotic heart disease

#2.   Seizure disorder etiology

#3.   Irreversible shock

#4.   Pernicious anemia—doubt

#5.   Diabetes mellitus

#6.   Status post cholecystectomy

#7.   Hepatomegaly

#8.   Azotemia

#9.   Mild dehydration

This single flowsheet offers an excellent opportunity to discuss many aspects of the shock problem. Parameters that deal with volume and cardiac output and indirectly with peripheral resistance are all present, and the quality of care can be assessed with respect to some of the finest details. If concerned that certain other parameters should have been followed, experienced observers should point them out so the student may add them to the next flowsheet and literally experience developing in the management of difficult problems such as this.

Name — W. Q.   Date

Date/Time	BP	P/RR	Wt	CVP	Hct	Arterial pH	pCO₂	O₂Sat	Na/K	pH	Venous pCO₂	O₂Sat	In	Out	Notes
6/12 9ᴾᴹ	109/90	80/90	52.7	—	48	1.34	53.1	91%	125/4.3				1675	↑40 Incont	1 mgm Isuprel in 1 L D₅W
6/12 2ᴾᴹ	°/₀	89/24	53.4	290	51	7.11	20.5	93%	125	0UN-49	6.3	34%	50cc NaHCO₃	Coma	Intubated - onto Bird
3ᴾᴹ	°/₀	88/24	—	226					7.6	1.02	O₂ Δ vol% 11		D₅W 450cc	50cc Blood	Isuprel - 1mg/250cc D₅W 12gtts
4ᴾᴹ	°/₀	—	—	270	44	7.15	26.5	97%		7.02	50	53%	50cc NaHCO₃	250cc Coma	S20 Isuprel 1mg/250cc 320 120cc/h 75mg Heparin
5ᴾᴹ	Intubated 80	80/32		166	39					O₂ Δ vol% 1.5			50cc NaHCO₃ 250	50cc Incont Blood	OFF Bird - IV Bird restarted
5ᴾᴹ	78	100/		158					125/4.8			53%	50cc NaHCO₃	135	Skin warm
6ᴾᴹ	88	110/24		190							O₂ Δ vol% 4.0		50cc Isuprel	885	
518	84	100/32		190		7.21	36	77%						95	Sleeping but arousable
8	78	109/32		180					125/5.7	BUN-42	12%	73%	50cc	990 45	Seizure - Dilantin 150mg IU
9	73	73/24		177	63	7.29	49	95%	125/5.0	O₂ Δ	3.5	4.0	50cc	1025	Isuprel 2mg/250 w.60cc/h
10ᴬᴹ	72	111/32		170	36	7.32	50		0UN-49	12L	44	75%	D₅W	7080	
10ᴬᴹ	80	100/24		181						O₂ Δ - 3.4	4.0			140	Sleeping but arousable
12ᴺ	70	105/24		146										1240	
2ᴬᴹ	95	122/96		143										12cc	OPNS EYES on Command
4ᴬᴹ	70	100/24		181										18cc	
7ᴬᴹ	72	111/		193									N/	12cc	Isuprel - 45cc/h, 12.5cc Mannitol - aliquoted
8ᴬᴹ	70			171	74	7.41	74	90%		7.39	44	99%	NSS		Isuprel to 100/h Mannitol - 100 (off) Isuprel off (cont)
5ᴾᴹ	90	108/30		183						Δ 7.39 - Δ 54.			50cc N₂		Isuprel - 40cc/h, Seizure - 5min
4ᴾᴹ	65	100/32													Seizure 5min - 10mg Blood

Problem List

#1.   Acute respiratory insufficiency
        —Acute CO_2 retention
        —Respiratory acidosis

#2.   Chronic restrictive and obstructive lung disease
        —(L) pneumonia

#3.   Tribolar pneumonia

#4.   Thyromegaly

#5.   Acute cor pulmonale with right ventricular failure

#6.   Pulmonary tuberculosis—inactive

It is apparent from this flowsheet and list of problems that this patient was desperately ill with pneumonia throughout her only lung, with a pH of 6.94, a pCO_2 of greater than 150, and an oxygen saturation of 85 %, when she was receiving oxygen before the intubation and subsequent tracheostomy. With all the parameters (including the minute ventilation), recorded at the time by the intern in a routine ward, there is no better vehicle than the flowsheet for the presentation of the principles of respiratory physiology and total care.

Date • Time	B.P.	P/R	T/V.P.	Wgt.	Hct/BUN	Na/K	CO2/Cl	pH/pCO2	pO2/O2-Sat	Min Vent	SH HCO3	I-V P/T	Input	Output Urine		Meds & Procedures
5-27 6 PM	170/120	112/36	/30		62/32	141/5.2	27.5/	6.94/150	/85%	4/min						① ↓ Sat O2 - intubation done with Bird respirator 65 psi ③ Venesection - Removed 600 cc.
6:30 PM	180/90	108						7.05/123	/96%							
7:00 PM										3.4						→ 10 mg. morphine SO4 no respirations without Bird unresponsive
8:00 PM	116/76	104	36.0/21							3.8		500/500	0.5			→ Aminophylline 250 mg I.V over 15 min
9:00 PM	120/70	104/9	/21					6.97/145	/94%	3.8						9 PM Given 176 meq Na+HCO3-
10 PM	130/70	96/9						7.11/140	/98%	3.8		500/1L	0.5	Hcont	Large amt	
11 PM	110/66	108/9	/15		50			7.21/106	210/	4.2						11 PM Ampicillin 2 grams I-V 11:30 Tracheostomy performed
5-28 12:30 AM	98/60	110/9						7.30/75	110/	3.8				Hcont	Large amt	
5-28 2 AM	130/80	120/9								3.3						Says Responding to multiple stimulations
4 AM	126/74	116/9	/16													
6 AM	148/84	106/14	/25		50/							150/1150	0.5	600/600+		Blood for lytes, CFS.
9 AM	147/80	108/14	/21	60.6	46/22	138/4.2	28/	7.18/98	/93%	4.0		550/1700	0.5			→ 230 cc of Blood removed venesection Digoxin 0.25 mg. I.V.
12 noon	138/82	104/				138/4.4										Propylthiouracil/200 mg. 1 PM 1% NaI given I.V.
5 PM	170/90	100/12	/20		46/14	↓	37/	7.24/97	/95	4.2		↓		60+/1700+		
12 noon	162/112	104/16	38.?/					7.33/99	/97							

Problem List

#1.   Paroxysmal atrial tachycardia

#2.   Acute pneumonitis—bacterial

#3.   Chronic obstructive lung disease—acute asthma

#4.   Hepatomegaly

#5.   Calcific pericarditis, status post-op pericardial stripping

#6.   Calcific pleuritis

#7.   Stasis dermatitis—legs

#8.   Acute myocardial infarction 11/17

#9.   Diabetes mellitus—adult onset 11/19

This flowsheet on an arrhythmia problem reveals to the student or house officer how difficult it is to draw conclusions about drugs when four or five agents are used in rapid succession. With data such as this available, it is not easy to fall in the trap of saying (and believing), "I had a patient yesterday with an interesting arrhythmia which we handled with Dilantin."

Although the problem list includes chronic lung disease, no pH, pCO_2, or O_2 saturation are on the flowsheets as appropriate parameters to be watched while the attempt is made to control the cardiac rhythm. Drugs such as Dilantin cannot overcome the wrong metabolic enviroment in which the heart is trying to function. Also there is no column in which the sedation can be carefully followed.

Date: 11-13-65
Name:

Date/Time	EKG Strip (II α AVF)	Medications	Comment
7/11 2 PM		E w 150 PM	On Maintenance Digitalis leaf 100 mg B.d. for 6 mos ?PAT ? Parasystolic Tachycardia
6 PM 730		3B 3:30 pm Cardiac Sinus Massage (Quinidine 200mg P.O @ 7pm)	To Response
55 PM 7		5 m notes later after 14mn Nasal O₂	Spontaneous Conversion to wandering Atrial Pacemaker
30 8 PM			Wandering Atrial Pacemaker
7/12 5 AM 30		Midnight Quinidine 200mgm P.O	N.S.R.
6 PM 30		@ 6th Quinidine 200 mg P.O	Sinus rhythm c̄ PAC
		8 PM Digitalis leaf - 100 mgm P.O Noon - Quinidine 200 mgm P.O	
2 PM			Wandering Atrial Pacemaker
10 3 PM		Dilantin 250mg I.V	? PAT ? Atrial Fibrillation ? Parasystolic Tachycardia
15 3 PM		Dilantin 100mg I.M	Sinus Rhythm c̄ PAC's
80 4 PM		Dilantin 250mgm I.V	No change in rhythm
80 4-6 PM		40 meq KCl I.V	No " "
6 PM		Nasal O₂ 3 L/min Cedilanid 0.8 mgm I.V	? Atrial Fibrillation
30 7 PM			N.S.R.

The EKG strips appearing above are not exact originals.
They have had to be retraced by hand due to difficulties
in reproduction of the originals.

Problem List

#1.   Organic heart disease
        a) rheumatic heart disease
        b) generalized cardiac enlargement; MI, AI, AS, M.S.
        c) *sinus mechanism—atrial fibrillation (now)*
        d) congestive heart failure—predominately right-sided
        e) class III *consider* AV malformation right-sided overload
           —doubt

#2.   Goiter with past history of thyrotoxicosis
        Benign vs. toxic—resolved (see PN 5/16/66)

#3.   *Doubt* diabetes mellitus
        Resolved (see PN 5/16/66)

#4.   Past history of duodenal ulcer

#5.   Azotemia ? etiology (discharge diagnosis—chronic renal disease)
                Consider prerenal (doubt with long standing nature)
                Consider chronic mercurials

#6.   *R/O-COPE* (see PN 5/16/66)

A flowsheet on a patient such as this, with multiple problems, each of which has a long, complicated history, is an invaluable aid to grasping what is essential in the history within a reasonable time. It is also necessary to prevent the provincialism in time that makes the physician overinterpret single events, types of therapy, and temporary change (e.g., in cardiac rhythm, hypertension, and diabetes) which in reality are merely ripples on the surface when viewed against the 20 year background of all the data. Off the cuff oral presentations and pages of narrative data are no substitute for a well planned flowsheet in the presentation and comprehension of a complicated case.

DATE	Wgt	V.P. (cm)	B.P.	Hct.	FBS 2hpc	ECG	NA / K	CO₂ / Cl	BUN	PBI / BMR	CHEST FILM	CHOL-ESTEROL	ANTI-THYROID	DIGITALIS	ORAL HB+ Thio	QUINI-DINE	REMARKS
12-46 Adm #1	159**		140	80		Atrial Fibrillation			14.7	Normal cardiac diameter							Right high saphenous Ligation / Bilateral low sapheno
2-47 Adm #2	145**					Atrial ECG Fibrillation			13.7	A55	cardiac hypertrophy ca 163		THIO URACIL				Adm for hyper thyroidism / placed on digitalis to control rate
3-47	157*					Atrial Fibrillation											Antithyroid MEDS followed by BMR's
4-48	185**					Atrial Fibrillation											
7-50	200**					Atrial ECG Fibrillation				+8							I-51 2629 yrs. / I-131 2629 yrs. / WNL: Dx antithyroid
10-51	190¾					Atrial ECG Fibrillation											
1-52						Atrial Fibrillation											
10-54	192					Atrial Fibrillation ECG											10-54: I-131 25% in 24 hrs. / I-131 25% in 24 hrs.
1-55 Adm #3						P.A.F. us? RSR ≡ ECG	131		33	moderate enlargement						½ss / I-131 40% / Adm for CoB +edema / after dc MICED ischemia
9-59	180*			48	112	R≡R ≡ 1 AV Block	4.8	100	264		cardiac enlargement I/020320						No Dx workup / Adm for ↑ Sx + / further Dx
4-59						R≡R CLINICALLY				7.4							
11-59						Atrial ECG Fibrillation											
1-27-60	173*					Atrial Fibrillation	140	25	32	25% ↑ above expected	174					3-10-60 PTS WNL / radiologist: DK: 6 / 7 MI 11 MS
Adm #4 3-7-60	167*				104,90	QUINIDINE	50	103	16	cardiac enlargement I/020320						I-131 4/47 in 48 hrs
to 3-21-60	160*		150	65	73,93	sinus Arrhythm			29 to 34/1.2	2/0							I-131 4/47 in 48 hrs
Adm #5 6-4-60						give ↑ check Hyperthyraphy + steroid											Adm for pleurisy"
6-28-60																	

DATE	WGT	VP Circ	B.P.	HCT	FBS	ECG	NA+ K+	CO2 CL	BUN Creat.	PBI Uric acid	CHEST FILM BMR	TRIAM-TERINE	DIGI-TALIS	NAQUA	QUINI-DINE	REMARKS
6-61	81 Kg				108											
8-62	182#					Atrial tachy cardia with variable A-V block										↑ 3x ↑ edema so Naqua begun
	225#					Sinus arrhyth.										T-rac of edema
11-62	173# 76.5					with rare PVB's										D/C Naqua
2-63	170#					Sinus Rhythm E.J° Block. occas. PVB's.										1 + edema Naqua resumed
5-63	172.5															Ran off of Quinidine in 4 hrs
5-63	80.0					RSR (Clinical)										D/C 4:45
10-63	78.2					Sinus arrhyth - variable A-V Block wandering pacemaker occas. PVC's				37	Gross cardio meg						
							139			2.0	General Mgt 2-13-7-63 Same 2-13-63					No pericardiodesy
3-66	73.1	26	150				43	97		4.8						
5-10-66	190# 82.0	26	154	90		Atrial fibrill.	139 138 141	24 25	36	1.9	Generalized cardiomegaly c pleural effusion Hyperexpanded RC					Amylase < 200
5-11-66	178#	9	150 90	09% 132	90	Atrial fibrill.	43 134	108	45		pleural effusion				added KCl↓	Hospital admission
5-23-66	150#	19	140		171	Fibrillation c runs of PVC & Bigeminy	41 138	95 35	37	—	Generalized cardiomegaly ...					Hospital discharge
6-17-66	185#	25	150	58		Atrial fibrillation	49 137	94 28	1.0	① pleural effusion by PEM				D/C	Biventricular failure c OR tde w/
6-27-66	190#	16	160	58			53	120	41	= 1 from SU3-					Compensating CHF Hospital admission

---

Problem List

#1.   Laennec's cirrhosis with hepatic failure

#2.   Acute renal failure

#3.   Gastrointestinal bleeding

#4.   Staphylococcus enteritis

#5.   Deceased

This flowsheet illustrates the value of having all the parameters immediately available in order to make quick and reliable decisions concerning volume, free water (tonicity), potassium, and acid base. On August 6, for example, the volume parameters show an increase in venous pressure, no fall in weight, no dramatic change in hematocrit, and yet a marked fall in blood pressure. What was done to evaluate cardiac output? It will be noted that the free water decisions may have led to a serum sodium of 119, whereas the patient was admitted with one of 138. Exactly why and how much free water was given? It will be noted that the potassium reached 6.6 before KCL was discontinued. Why was therapy handled in this way? Why is the calorie column so empty before August 1? What should be the management of the blood urea nitrogen in the face of all these difficulties? It is from data such as these, observed over and over again, that students slowly absorb the significant factors in managing difficult problems.

In such cases it should be pointed out to the student how rarely the course of any given parameter can be predicted with confidence. Any teacher or older physician who makes such statements as "the patient should have had three liters of fluid last night with that rising blood urea nitrogen," or "That patient obviously has classical ---, and there is no question about exactly what she needs," is a clinician whose experience has not included the detailed analysis and following up of the data on multiple, interacting problems. Even if the possibility of hyponatremia in the face of a given water load was recognized in this case, the clinician could not be assured of such a response. There are in complex cases so many forces operating which we do not fully understand, and so many forces unperceived and yet to be detected, that our whole system of management must be based on the assumption (and awareness) of possible error in all decisions coupled with data systems designed for feedback and corrective action. Flowsheets and titled progress notes are the most crucial portion of an effective feedback loop in medical care.

A rotated patient flow sheet (vital signs and laboratory data chart). Column headings read: B.P., P.R., Wgt. (LBS), CVP mm H₂O, HCT, NA⁺ K⁺, Cl⁻ CO₂ BUN, pCO₂ pH Creatinine, INPUT, OUTPUT, Daily, Cumulative, Evaluation, Remarks, E.W.

Date	B.P.	P.R.	Wgt.	CVP	HCT	NA⁺/K⁺	Cl⁻/CO₂	BUN	Input Daily	Input Cumul.	Output Daily	Output Cumul.	Remarks
7/27				34	155								
7/26			150		138/7.5	97/28	25	20	1440	1440	700	700	SAR estimate 7/27 was Patient 5% dehydrated
7/31			150%		130/3.4	97/3.5	29		3085	5500	700	3600	
7/28			148		136/3.5	100/3.50	40		3600	9100	250	2850	
2/0			151		133/3.9	109/3.5			3500	11600	95	5775	
7/31					132/3.5	98/3.5			2570	14170	90	4675	Paracentesis for distention (Relief) → 2 liters YA Leakage @ 250 cc aspirated
8/1	140/70	90			125/2.6	100/3.5	6.5/5.9	800	2500	16650	1400	6100	NGT placed in stomach to relieve gastric distention @ 9: gastric material Removed
8/2	120/70	110		31	129/3.3	/21	30.8/67/3.58		2500	19150	3000	9100	KCl D/c (oral) 1000 cc urine out
8/3	100/60	98		27	119/4.3	87/3.3	6.9/6.4		2700	21600	440	9540	24 hr urine 13 mg. NA+ 1.27 Mag K+ 25 gm Glucose given in 20 minutes
8/4			154	30	120/4.0	/20	76/2.6	1400	900	22500	130	9600	Many Tubular casts seen in spun sediment. Small Staph aureus Demade 2 Remnant
8/5	70/40		151%		125/5.6	93/20		→	2600	27100	260	9900	Blood — 1 unit given. BP Decreased 7% — co all day 2 branding pulse Loose
8/6	60/40 70/50		153		123/3.2	/17	8/1		3310	30000	200	10200	Begin maintenance 2 Bali Electrolyte solut in Lipechol Dawn No urine Round
8/7	82/50				124/3.2	/13	77		1220	31.2	350	10.5	Maintenance Fluids plus Lipanol + Alidex No urine Round
8/8	90/50		141/4		131/3.6	140/2.54	94	→	1110	32.3	100	106	Maintenance + Bifida Lipamal or Glucidex 4 Loose stools
8/9	80/50			25					1000	33.3	100	10.7	
8/10													Lavaged in (7mg m/500 cc) Run at 0.3L mgm/min HW A

Chapter 6 Summary

The discharge summary should be problem oriented. There should be a concise statement about the basis, the course, the present status of each problem; the specific parameters that should be followed (if any); and the action that should be taken when certain thresholds are reached. Since the inidividual completing the summary cannot anticipate what problems may confront future users of the summary, the amount of detail to be included is arbitrary. When electronic records are complete and easily available, the need for dicharge summaries as we have known them may disappear. With a complete problem list and the ability to extract, tabulate, and graph any parameters in any relationship, a provider can extract details as the need arises. What is relevant and useful to save in one context may be useless in another.

It is important in ongoing care to practice data reduction at regular intervals. Otherwise, users of the record cannot see the forest for the trees, and important signals get buried in masses of data.

No discharge summary, no matter how well conceived or implemented, can substitute for an informed patient who has a copy or his or her own record and has gained the ability to interpret the data to others.

6
The Discharge Summary and Data Reduction

Lawrence L. Weed

The discharge summary as it has been conceived and produced in the past may well have done more harm than good. It is natural for us all, when confronted with a patient for the first time or after a long interval, to want a quick summary of the case so we can get on with the problem at hand. But is it possible for anyone creating a discharge summary to have in mind the needs of all possible future users of that summary? Those needs should logically determine what should be extracted from the whole original record. If a patient is admitted with a recurrent pneumonia, we may want to know every detail on that problem from the day it began. For the quiescent *meniscus tear* problem, we may be content with no more than appears on a complete problem list. The reverse would be true if the same patient came in complaining of a painful knee. And not infrequently the patient comes in with the blossoming of a problem that had barely begun when the patient was last seen, and the writer of the discharge summary neglected to even mention it on the summary. This can be overcome by a problem oriented structure to the discharge summary in which every problem has at least a minimal statement about its basis and course. Ideally, the best summary for a given user would be created at the time of its need with the new problem situation clearly in mind. Such a focus could assure that no resource that the original data have to offer would be overlooked. With electronic problem oriented medical records and modern search techniques, we can begin to approach this ideal. Furthermore, once patients routinely are given copies of their records with an up to date problem list at every encounter, the need for the old fashioned inadequate summaries may disappear.

Outcome studies based on discharge summaries may be misleading. It is easy to draw the wrong conclusion from such studies because the full context of the inputs may not be known. It is true that two geographic areas may have different rates for a given surgical procedure, but unless we have a full problem oriented record with the same defined database in both places, we do not know whether some did too many, some did too few, or all were justified. To do studies merely to show a difference is insufficient. Every patient has known for years that different doctors and different clinics respond to the same complaint in very different ways.

The foregoing has focused on the traditional concept of a summary at discharge from some medical unit. This is not the only time (not even the most important time) in the course of caring for a patient that we should be concerned about keeping the data down to a manageable volume. It is in the day to day care that we should be able to see at a glance where we are and what we are trying to do, without being weighted down with data that have outlived their usefulness as the course evolved. For example, the record may contain the details of the preparation for a barium enema or a whole series of hourly findings the first postoperative day. Such details are really quite useless in our thinking after we have seen the results of the barium enema or a week after the patient has stabilized postoperatively. We would like to be able to have such data drop out of the sequence for day to day perusal of the course, but not be lost completely from the system. Of course, we can conceive of situations where, for legal reasons or research studies, we might some day want to know exactly what the preparation for the barium enema was or precisely to what was the lowest point the blood pressure fell postoperatively, although at the time the patient seemed to have returned to a completely normal state.

It is this sort of data reduction that is already in operation in one site where the computerized problem oriented medical record is now in use. The complete database as described earlier is acquired in the electronic form, but all of it may not be stored in the problem oriented medical record. After studying the prioritized initial list of problems and the results of all the couplers that were used, the provider and patient decide what problems it all boils down to and then put them on the problem list. Then under each problem, where the basis for the problem statement must be concisely stated, we can pull out of that database only those elements that are necessary to justify the conclusions reached. The complete database can always be accessed if necessary, but it does *not* need to be a working part of the current medical record. This sort of thoughtful, regular data reduction forces us to digest data, formulate problems, and pursue hypotheses in a steady and forward moving manner as opposed to spinning our wheels by getting data way out of proportion to our capacity to use those data effectively.

Also, the issues of data reduction and the patient's role in his or her own behalf are more closely related than may first appear. It is important for both patients and providers to have the essential elements for management in mind each time they deal with one of the patient's problems. This is not possible if we get lost among scattered bits of data on pages and pages of a disorganized record. It is possible if we are careful to keep the problem list up to date, if we can have immediate access to the original overall plan for each problem, if we can retrieve all the data on a single problem in sequence, and if we can generate at will a flowsheet with multiple parameters regardless of the problem for which the parameters were originally ordered. In other words, as stated above, data reduction can best be done if we have a specific problem in mind. What is relevant and useful to save in one context may be useless in another, and we can always conceive of a context that can be used to justify the saving of almost any piece of data. Since we cannot anticipate every future problem and do not have the time in the usual paper record to instantly arrange and retrieve data in multiple ways, we can only have the ideal data reduction when the record is in the electronic form and supported by a structure that is common to and used by us all.

Chapter 7 Summary

The coupler editor is a tool for building and editing of couplers and requires no computer training or background. The choices are presented to the user on a main working display; the user can simply make a choice, or refer to a simple manual, or listen to an audio tape that accompanies the software.

Difficulties, when they arise, are more likely to have their roots in the confusion and ambiguities in the medical literature from which specific information must be extracted. In making linkages from finding to cause, or finding to management option, or comment to cause or management option, the user is asked to reference each linkage to the overall knowledge network developed to support coupler building. The knowledge network is a knowledge *cache* whose contents are much better organized for the purposes of coupler building than the present medical literature is organized.

The knowledge network makes the whole effort of coupler building more cumulative—the efforts that go into building one coupler contribute to the building of other couplers. When new knowledge arises, it can be entered into the network; if it contradicts information in the network, the contradiction is apparent by making the proper traversals.

The combined information tools of the knowledge couplers and the knowledge network make the efforts of all medical workers coordinated and cumulative. They are the basis for corrective feedback loops, and they allow a much more precise linkage of the research community to those who practice medicine.

7
The Building and Editing of Problem Knowledge Couplers

Lawrence L. Weed

The Coupler Editor

The coupler editor is a tool for the building and editing of couplers that requires no computer training or background. The main working display is seen on Figure 1. The choices on this display provide the necessary framework for thinking about medical problem solving and knowledge coupling. In effect, the display says to the user:

1. State the topic of the coupler (the problem).

2. List all the causes for the problem (a diagnostic coupler) or all the management options (a management coupler).

3. List the findings to be sought in the patient that will include salient findings for each of the causes or for each of the management options.

4. Develop options which may be used to further delineate a cause if the cluster of simple findings from the history, physical, and routine laboratory work are strongly suggestive but insufficient as a basis for diagnosis and action.

5. Develop comments about causes or management options or findings or options that were culled from the literature when reading about the coupler topic.

With the above materials in hand, we can build a knowledge coupler by designating the proper linkages among the various parts. In this way we have electronically linked the literature of medicine to everyday practice and problem solving. All this can proceed without the inordinate dependence on the poorly defined memory based knowledge of costly credentialed experts. If we pick one of the choices on the display in Figure 1, the choice labeled "Causes," for example, we get the display shown in Figure 2.

Every choice on this display is intelligible to a user simply by making the choice or referring to a simple manual or by being guided a simple audio tape that accompanies the software. No computer training is necessary. Difficulties, when they arise, are more likely to have their roots in the confusion and the ambiguities in the medical literature from which specific information must be extracted. In this regard, the demands placed on the coupler builder at every step in the process often go beyond the demands placed on the average textbook writer who is free to use ambiguous prose, and free to leave many consequences and connections unstated (if indeed they were ever explicitly worked out in the first place).

As Whitehead says, we think in generalities but we live in detail. Knowledge couplers either help us rigorously match the details of our everyday actions with the details of authoritative sources available for the problem at hand, or rapidly confront us with the gaps in, and fallibility of, medical knowledge.

The coupler editor is useful in developing effective management tools. Routines can be established for emergency departments, the front desk in a busy practitioner's office, telephone answering services, and paramedical personnel. In these cases we are coupling daily actions of office personnel, not to just authoritative sources in the medical literature, but also to well thought out approaches to the activities of workers in a busy environment. This assures coordination of effort and a working situation less vulnerable to changes in and variability of personnel.

The steps above suggest how the tools we are describing can serve everyday workers in the medical field. If users are going to routinely depend upon couplers the way a traveler depends upon a map, then they must be confident that the work of the research establishment and the current literature are related to the couplers in a systematic manner. If couplers are up to date and complete, then the user of a coupler should not have to be concerned with keeping up with all the journals or using modern computerized search services of the vast literature at the time of problem solving in a busy clinic. Engineers use tables of logarithms and integrals (or their electronic equivalents) so that they will not have to derive them at the time of building the bridge. In medicine, all of the provider's energy needs to go into getting the right data to feed into the coupler and into helping the patient negotiate the coupler results and all the ambiguities that inevitably arise when real problems are honestly matched against what is known in the literature.

How can we maximize the efficiency of the efforts of those whose job it is to build couplers? We first of all should recognize that the field of medicine does not have an infinite number of building blocks, but there are almost an infinite number of relationships among the building blocks. Just as a good carpentry shop allows the woodworker to fashion a wide variety of useful ob-

```
- - - - - - - - -   KNOWLEDGE COUPLER DEVELOPMENT SYSTEM   - - - - - - - -

Coupler: Acute Low Back Pain and/or Leg Pain of not > 2 months durat. (9)
Revision date:  8/13/89

-Build/edit/review- lists of and links between:
_____

          Q: Questions (+ Sequences & Coupler info.)
          F: Findings
          C: Causes
          O: Options
          N: Comments
_____

  R: -RUN- Knowledge Coupler        I: -INITIALIZE- a Coupler
  G: -Get- different Coupler        U: Coupler Editing Utilities
          S: System Command Processor
```

Figure 1

```
          - - - - - - - - - - - - - - -  Edit Causes  - - - - - - - - - - - - - - - -
  Cause 1

  Text: Cauda equina syndrome
  Global entity number:  0
  Display weight:  10
  Prognosis: [ Unspecified ]  ....w/ Rx:  [ Unspecified ]

  Associated components:  FND   CMT   OPT   REF
_____

    T: -Edit- text                  K: Knowledge Network functions
    D: -Edit- disease prognosis     G: -Edit- global entity number
    W: -Edit- display weighting     E: -ERASE- this cause

    Add LINKAGE to = = = = = = = = = = = = = = = = >
                    1: Finding  3: Comment  5: Option  7: Ref

    Review/Edit/Delete LINKAGE = = = >
                    2: Finding  4: Comment  6: Option  8: Ref
_____

    PRINT = = = = = >              P: -Print- Causes

          Active: Rel = 126, CmLnk = 87, OpLnk = 21, Ref = 296

        X: Extend list     S: Specific Cause   R: Return   N: Next Cause
```

Figure 2

jects from a basic set of tools and materials, so does a good knowledge shop allow the knowledge worker to fashion a wide variety of diagnostic and management couplers from a basic set of medical facts, a *knowledge cache* whose contents are much better organized for the purposes of coupler building than the present medical literature is organized. The knowledge cache can make our whole effort more cumulative—the efforts that go into building one coupler contributing to the building of other couplers. The knowledge network has become this knowledge cache.

The *knowledge network* was organized so that the physician can start with a problem at the level a patient states it, such as dizziness or chest pain, and make multiple traversals of the network to find all the causes or all the treatments or all the findings for one of the causes, regardless of the original source of the information. Just as we found in hospitals that medical records were not problem oriented, we have found the literature is not problem oriented. The very title of a journal, for example, may refer to a sponsor or place of origin such as New England (*The New England Journal of Medicine*) or a specialty such as surgery (*The American Journal of Surgery*). Our present knowledge network, which contains thousands of entities and thousands of relationships among those entities was built by exploring the present literature with specific problems in mind, using a whole variety of search techniques, textbooks, and review articles. Traversals of that network and software tool known as the coupler builder are used to construct the couplers. When new knowledge arises, it can be entered into the network, and, if it contradicts information in the network, it is apparent by making the proper traversals. A linkage between the coupler and the network allows immediate update of the relevant coupler. We thereby use computers not to "learn medicine" or "teach medicine," but rather to practice medicine in an up to date manner—just as we use maps not to learn geography, but to get to a destination every time regardless of how unfamiliar the territory may be.

Different issues arise as we tackle different problems, and the introductions to the couplers suggest the flexibility that the coupler builder has in presenting results to the user.

A Methodology for Dealing with the Medical Literature

How do we go about digesting and excerpting the medical literature in order to load our knowledge cache which in turn is used to construct and update knowledge coupling tools? This knowledge cache is a network of relations among clinically significant entities of all sorts. These relations are searched for and extracted from the standard medical literature. Examples include relations among diagnostic entities, pathophysiological abnormalities, various categories of potential findings (symptoms, physical findings, health habits, social and demographic factors, laboratory results, radiology and history findings), drugs and treatment regimens, diagnostic and therapeutic procedures, environmental hazards, and more.

Associated with each relation between a pair of entities is a body of conditioning or qualifying information. One part of this information, which we may call here the relation type or class, allows selection of sets of entity relations for particular needs by an automated database retrieval operation. The other part is essentially a body of textual commentary, composed and entered by the database builders, which may explain or illuminate the significance of the relation. This latter information is useful in developing the *comments* of the couplers that will be used by the practitioners.

Linked with entity relations, and the associated commentary, are specific citations of the medical literature from which the information was extracted and put into the form of excerpts with a specific and standardized structure. Knowledge coupling tools are derived from and linked in detail to the knowledge network, and the knowledge network is derived from and linked in detail to the medical literature. Adherence to the rules governing this vital chain of documentation is absolutely fundamental to the mission of building well documented, up to date couplers.

The process of constructing a knowledge coupling tool from the knowledge network can be only partially automated. Much thought must go into the selection and editing of knowledge network content for use in a coupling tool in light of the point of view being adopted in the tool, and the detailed nature of the medical knowledge being captured. However, it makes perfect sense to develop and support the human expertise required for this process in a central facility, whose products can be easily reproduced and widely distributed.

The value of knowledge coupling is not mitigated by possible flaws in the knowledge being coupled. On the contrary, it is vitally important that medical knowledge be reliably coupled to everyday action, precisely so that we may get a clear view of its strengths and weaknesses in real applications. What is disparagingly referred to as anecdotal evidence could take on a whole new significance if it was derived from experience gathered on such a basis.

Insights Gained During Coupler Building

The very process of coupler building affords many insights that may otherwise not occur to us as we teach or practice in the traditional manner. Some of these insights are discussed below.

Efforts Are Cumulative

Couplers make the efforts of everyone in the medical care system cumulative. Once a coupler is built, we have the means of assuring that the same points are covered in every patient with a given problem; thereby, we have corrected one of the main flaws in all the outcome studies that have and are being done, i.e., the inputs to the system are now better defined, thereby making the outcomes more interpretable. The coupler builder's intellectual energy and understanding (which are extensive upon completion of a good coupler) are now available to every patient every time that coupler is used regardless of the location or time of day or night. One teacher or one lecturer formerly available at certain hours in certain courses in certain locations suddenly becomes a thousand teachers available at all times in many places.

Policy Implementation

When society as a whole determines how limited resources are to be applied in matters of health—what therapeutic options are to be made available to individuals vs. what resources are to be applied to cover public health issues for populations of individuals (schools, sanitation, prenatal clinics, etc.)—such policies can be immediately implemented by adding to and altering the specific content of the relevant diagnostic and management couplers to be used in a given community. Patients themselves and their families should be the principal force in choosing among options made available to them by society. By understanding the details in a universally used guidance system, an individual can deduce what the policy is. But in the absence of concrete guidance systems to implement policy, no one can deduce from a general policy statement what the actual care and application of resources will be.

Corrective Feedback Loops

Every user of couplers who finds an error, an omission, or a contradiction to known evidence can communicate that finding, along with a reference to support it, to a centralized coupler building facility. The central facility can make the necessary correction and immediately update the couplers of all other users. Unexplained differences from different reputable sites can be revealed to the users in the comments section of the coupler, so patients at all times have the broadest possible view about their own problems and the ambiguities in their individual situations, as well as the areas of dissonance among the experts. Once such guidance systems are in universal use and the inputs into the system are known in the broadest possible context, then outcomes will be an automatic byproduct of the use of the system in providing care and subject to rigorous interpretation. Use of the guidance system and analysis of its outputs will become one of the principal sources of knowledge for updating and correcting the system.

Economy of Knowledge Transmission from Source to Patient

Enormous sums are now invested in teachers, lecture halls, conferences, examinations, libraries and wide distribution of journals with virtually no means of overcoming the great voltage drop in the transmission across such systems. Malpractice suits may punish a physician or give money to a victim, but they in no way correct the basic flaws of the system. Knowledge couplers leapfrog over all those problems. It is feasible through their routine and reliable use not only to bypass many of the steps of transmission in the present system, but also to have the potential to do it without the voltage drops that are plaguing us now.

Precise Coupling of the Research Community to the Practice Community

Since the steps on the maps are well defined and universally available, each investigator, on the completion of a new piece of work, can traverse the knowledge network and review with experienced coupler builders if and exactly where in the care system the research knowledge can be placed so that it will immediately be applied in practice.

Library Size and Expense and Availability

At present, the size and expense of libraries grow a hundred times faster than the new knowledge within them. Each new article has 100 old facts for every new one because each author is obliged to create the context of his or her thought. Even at that, the context is limited and often the article available only to those in the author's specialty. The knowledge net and the couplers provide an almost infinite number of contexts across many specialties and fields. A new piece of knowledge added can be viewed in many contexts by altering the conditions of the traversals through the net or the choice of coupler.

Diminishing Patient Risk in Choosing a Provider

At the present time, perhaps the most important decision patients make is the medical door they first choose to walk through for their care. Providers see what their specialized training has taught them to see and what rationalizes the procedures and routines they charge for to make a living. Real problems cross specialty boundaries, so many patients may find out from a specialist what they *do not* have, but not necessarily what they *do* have. Couplers have no such bias and every coupler has causes from many specialized areas of medicine. At the present time, the patient with an abdominal aneurysm who goes to an orthopedic surgeon for presenting back pain may lose precious time. When a complete set of couplers is used at all sites, where and how the patient enters the system will not be as critical as it now is.

Emphasis on the Technical and Interpersonal Skills of Providers vs. Memory and Knowledge Retrieval Skills

A credential based system can be replaced by a performance based system since couplers define precisely what skills are needed to approach a given problem and only those with those skills will be allowed to pursue those problems. Many will be able to acquire those skills because there will be so much less time spent in the educational system on the memorizing, regurgitating, and forgetting of the facts themselves. Indeed, the reservoir of people from whom medical providers of all types are selected will change both qualitatively and quantitatively. People who were selected under the former premises and tools may be quite different people from those selected under the new system. The economic and educational implications of these shifts can be very great.

Chapter 8 Summary

Once the computerized problem oriented medical record and knowledge coupling tools are in place in the medical community, many benefits may flow from their routine use by all patients and providers.

- The interdependence of social and medical problems will be revealed by the complete problem list on the patient. It will be recognized that sophisticated understanding and management of one of the problems requires an awareness of all of them. The knowledge coupling tools will reveal, and enable action to be based upon, the interactions among problems.

- The efforts of providers of different skills working under a variety of conditions will be coordinated and cumulative. The patients themselves will become increasingly effective in organizing and doing much of the work required in their own care.

- Much of the defining and assuring of quality in the medical care system will reside in the new information tools and the rules of the problem oriented system. The quality of performance of the providers of care and the patients in their own behalf will be measured in terms of their capacity to be thorough and reliable in the use of the tools and their compliance with the rules. Safe travel depends upon a well developed system of roads, facilities, and rules combined with reliable compliance with and enforcement of the rules. Keeping the information tools and rules up to date will become a well defined quality control responsibility of society and the medical establishment as a whole.

- Providers can be classified and evaluated in terms of the specific tasks for which they assume responsibility in the well defined system of care. Terms like primary physicians, nurse practitioners, and specialists of endless names and varieties with their vague boundaries and ill defined division of responsibilities can be abandoned.

- The basic science training of providers can be defined in terms of how scientifically they behave (astute observations and logical analyses) in the performance of defined tasks within a system of care as opposed to what scientific knowledge they have been exposed to in formal courses, programs, and examinations. This shift in emphasis has broad implications. Our ideas about faculties and facilities will change, and the economics and distribution of medical care may change along with them.

- Standardization of medical terminology and disease definitions is a fundamental prerequisite to precise inputs and interpretable outputs of the medical care system. Such standardization can be pursued more fruitfully if it is driven by needs that arise in the development of knowledge coupling tools and their incorporation into the practice of medicine. By their very nature, such tools embody characterizations of disease entities. Furthermore, they define explicitly the uses, roles, and interrelations of medical entities of all sorts that occur in clinical medicine. The development and disciplined use of knowledge coupling tools define the agenda for standardization. (A consequence of this is that standardization should not be pursued in advance of tool development in order to facilitate that development. It should be considered an integral part of the ongoing development process.)

- As telescopes give us a view and understanding of the universe unachievable with the unaided human eye, so might the consistent use of modern information tools in the solving of medical problems give us a view and understanding of medicine that is unachievable by the unaided human mind.

8
Implications of the Computerized Problem Oriented Medical Record and Knowledge Coupling Tools

Lawrence L. Weed

The structured, computerized problem oriented medical record and the computerized knowledge coupling tools enable constructive action on a variety of difficulties now besetting medicine:

- Medical problems dealt with out of context

- The burdens on the physicians and other providers that are imposed by the requirement of dealing with all of an individual's problems in a broad context

- Lack of control over the inputs of the system and the consequent inability to interpret the outcomes upon which reasonable economic, social/ethical, and quality control decisions must depend

- The lack of a coherent, effective approach to the medical malpractice problem that deals with root causes and basic defects in the system of care

- The lack of coordination of the efforts of all providers in the total care of an individual over a lifetime and the inefficient use of human resources in the health care system

- The absence of a system of health insurance that covers all the people for at least a basic level of care

- The lack of a defined and consistently applied system of incorporating new knowledge (basic science and clinical knowledge) into daily efforts of all providers

- Inefficiency in education (resulting from faulty premises and inadequate tools)

- The lack of a consistent and organized approach with feedback loops to the evolving definitions and diagnostic classification systems in medicine.

Problems Out of Context

In the earlier chapters on the problem list and the database, it was emphasized that sophisticated understanding and management of one of the patient's problems requires at least an awareness of all of them. Where the findings, for instance, show heart failure and azotemia, it is apparent that the right treatment for one may be the wrong treatment for the other. In other situations the interaction may not be so obvious, for example, in paroxysmal hypertension, dehydration, and hypovolemia. In such cases, physicians always risk faulty interpretations by treating problems out of context. If our index of suspicion of possible interactions among problems is high, we are in a much better position to detect unusual and even identify new phenomena.

For example, the management of *dehydration,* one problem on a problem list, dramatically improved *accelerated hypertension*, another problem on the list. The volume indicators and other appropriate variables were followed, using a flowsheet, as intravenous volume expanders were given. Aggressive conventional drug therapy of the marked diastolic hypertension, employed out of context, could have had disastrous consequences.

The interdependence of social and medical problems is immediately revealed by a complete list of problems. An awareness of a social problem (for instance, lack of proper heating in the house) may be more fundamental to the management of a medical problem such as pneumonia, than the management of other associated medical problems (for example, a urinary tract infection). Common sense approaches to medical care are facilitated by a complete problem list. The medical literature is replete with papers on single entities from series of patients (for example, myocardial infarction, cancer of the colon, or pneumonia) in which no complete problem list from a defined database on each patient was systematically presented. A paper may talk about X % mortality for perforated ulcer, when it should be saying Y % if heart failure is also on the list, or Z % if another problem or no problems are on the list. Pneumococcal pneumonia alone may well be a different disease from pneumococcal pneumonia in the presence of azotemia. Potent drugs are administered, and major management decisions made for specific problems taken out of context. It is no wonder that controversies in medicine abound; the present premises and tools used in the care of patients with multiple problems almost guarantee contextual chaos.

Until well conceived problem lists, management and diagnostic couplers, and patients and/or their families working directly from their own records are the rule instead of the exception, we cannot seriously attack the fragmentation of care in todays's specialty clinics and wards, and the fragmentation of the survey of that care on rounds and in conferences. The physician must learn how to move easily from a single minded focus on one problem to attention to the total list and the interrelationships of many problems. The essential combination of the clarification of a single problem and the integration of multiple problems is greatly facilitated by a medical record that is structured upon a total problem list and titled progress notes. Since the human body is a complex group of systems, each of which can develop abnormalities that reverberate through the other systems in varying degrees, the specialist, as a responsible scientist, must know the variables in the total system as they affect his or her specialized judgment and action. A patient's intuitive demand for a *whole doctor* is completely consistent with the demands that good science and a sense of all the relevant factors in a patient's illness impose upon the specialist, quite apart from general considerations of the need for primary physicians, total care, and humanitarianism.

The listing of individual but related problems separately on a complete problem list has been perjoratively called by some the fragmentation of medical care. This is not a legitimate complaint. If a complete analysis is done on each item on the problem list, integration of related findings occurs with clarity and inevitability. Failure to integrate findings into a valid single entity can almost always be traced to incomplete understanding of all the implications of one or all of them. The beginner who enters cardiomegaly, edema, hepatomegaly, and shortness of breath as four separate problems may be conveying that he or she does not recognize the problem of cardiac failure and has yet to achieve that level of synthesis intellectually. But the important point is that nothing is lost. On the contrary, the interest of more experienced observers is immediately aroused. The patient's problems are combined as appropriate under a single heading on the original list, and they are carried one step closer to diagnosis and treatment. The system does not prevent analysis and integration; it merely reveals the extent to which they are performed and defines the level of sophistication at which the physician functions. It is in this matter of immediately bringing a large number of seemingly disparate findings to a high level of synthesis that the knowledge coupler can not only help a beginner, but also go beyond that of the unaided minds of more experienced clinicians. Indeed, a coupler on memory loss and/or confusion, for example, that has many more causes in it that even the experienced person can routinely consider, may improve the performance of the expert as much or more than the expert can improve the performance of the beginner.

Burdens on Physicians Imposed by Multiple Problems Requiring Consideration in Context

We discussed earlier how the problem solving conditions of the usual PhD scientist differ from those of the physician. The physician is trying to behave as a scientist when confronted with multiple problems chosen by others under time constraints that basic scientists would find intolerable. We must build a system of medical care that recognizes and deals with these constraints. Many of our present problems can be avoided by the use of a defined system of care that employs skilled paramedical personnel, modern knowledge coupling tools, complete problems lists, and the systematic following of problems from the earliest stages with titled progress notes in a record of which the patient or family always has a copy.

A physician should always deliberately examine the patient's complete problem list. If time is limited, the physician should establish priorities and direct attention to those problems having the greatest potential for moving into the acute phase. As obvious as such an admonition may be, it is frequently violated by specialists who never see a complete problem list and who go straight to dealing with the problems of their specialties. In this regard, the most crucial decision patients often make is their initial choice of medical provider. In any case, the rule should be: When under pressure, the physician should select the problem or problems requiring immediate action, be thorough in dealing with these problems, and never attempt to deal with all the problems superficially for the mere sake of having dealt with them. If this approach is followed, the work reflected in each titled progress note can become a precisely defined building block, all effort can be cumulative, and sharply increased efficiency can result. Lack of time is not a legitimate argument against keeping data in order. Good form leads to ultimate economy of time in almost all human endeavors.

Busy general practitioners and their associated personnel who have learned to use problem oriented records and knowledge coupling tools wisely have demonstrated that the excuse of lack of time cannot be regarded as tenable. Medical students and physicians can be taught to deal with heavy work loads, to set priorities, and to direct paramedical help wisely. The medical record is an ideal instrument for achieving these goals.

Quality of Care

Quality is the excellence with which a well defined function is fulfilled, meeting a goal and conforming to standards that everyone understands at the outset. (In the field of medicine, quality has often been defined as that which people with credentials do, and only other people with credentials have a right to judge it. Such a definition is rejected here.) A Honda Civic may not be the same quality car as a Mercedes, but it can still be a high quality car within the standards and goals it set for itself in terms of price, performance, durability, and availability to thousands who could never even consider a Mercedes. We should always be clear in our minds when discussing quality whether the issue is the goal and its attendant requirements, or whether it is the excellence with which a given goal and its requirements are met.

What is the well defined function we should have in mind when we talk about the quality of medical care? Our context could be as narrow as a single surgical procedure or as broad as all the medical actions over the lifetime of a single individual or the performance of a few functions for a whole population in the presence of limited resources. Whatever context or goal we set, we then have to

- Define the system and the rules of the system for reaching the goal

- Audit providers within the rules of the system and on the well defined task or tasks assigned to them

- Audit the system itself with outcomes.

The following principles should be kept in mind in implementing the above three steps:

- Outcomes are always due to more variables than any single provider in the medical care system has control over. If an outcome is bad, we have to ask, "Was it a flawed system with bad rules?" or "Did someone fail to follow the rules of the system?"

- We should never bother to look at outputs until we have control over the inputs; otherwise, the results of studies are uninterpretable. As we stated earlier, outcome studies in memory based systems with credential oriented performers have been done for years with little benefit except to suggest there may be something wrong. Laymen have known for years that they can go to three different providers or institutions with the same complaint and receive widely differing approaches to the problem.

- We should never audit performers within a system if they were not aware of the goals or rules of that system beforehand or if they did not agree with them or if they believed it was humanly impossible to follow them (e.g., using the unaided mind to recall all the 70 causes of chest pain and all the relevant variables in the patient for choosing among them).

- Bad performance by a provider is often an indicator of a design flaw in the system itself; for example, an intern is assigned more patients to workup than it is possible to do reliably according to the rules of the system in the time allotted. Large systems easily lead to intimidation of members of the system into trying to do things that they believe are beyond them. It is very easy to blame performers for bad outcomes (or for the performers to unreasonably blame themselves) when the root of the problem was a mismatch between the goals of the system and the rules and resources of the system.

- Patients must be aware of the goals, the rules, and their well defined role in their own behalf. Individual patients often have more knowledge of and more control over relevant variables in the system than anyone else, so their role in their own behalf is fundamental to good care. Every patient must have the right information tools to work with and the responsibility for and control over many of the variables.

The problem oriented medical record and the knowledge couplers provide the basis for a well defined system in which a universe of variables is considered and from which the inputs into the system are known to all. The quality of a practice should not be judged solely by the credentials of those in the practice or by the sophistication of the techniques they use in practice, but rather by the

- Completeness and accuracy of the database obtained on the patients in the practice

- Efficiency (time and cost) of acquiring and interpreting data

- Adequacy of the formulation of all the problems

- Defensibility of every component of the initial plan within the context of the medical literature and the patient's life

- Thoroughness and analytic sense demonstrated in titled progress notes on each problem as the initial plan is implemented

- Total quantity of care the practice is able to deliver.

In the above discussion we have laid the foundation for a system of quality control that has three major components.

1. *Auditing for a core of behavior among providers within a well defined system as opposed to examining for a core of knowledge in a credential oriented system.*
The behavioral traits of thoroughness, reliability, sound analytic sense, and efficiency take on a very precise meaning when applied within the rules of a well defined system. The details of such an approach are discussed by Nelson et al. (1976) in the article on "A performance-based method of student evaluation." In addition to the rules of the problem oriented system, both the examiner and examinee may now have available to them the same minimal set of variables and the same linkages and arrangements of those variables within the context of current medical knowledge as presented to all providers as they routinely use up to date diagnostic and management couplers in practice. High quality care is the sum of competently performed and logically linked steps within the well defined system. No two patients will ever progress through the same system in precisely the same ways and their uniqueness will thereby be recognized in a manner that neither compromises quality nor our capacity to assess it.

2. *Keeping the information tools of the medical care system up to date.*

3. *Auditing the role of individual patients in their own behalf and their compliance within the rules of a well defined system.*

Since new information gathering and processing tools such as knowledge couplers do much to define the language and logic of medical practice, they allow more precise communication between physicians and all other groups such as lawyers, nurses, and the business and government leaders who pay many of the medical bills. In the absence of such tools and with no control over the inputs to the system in the broad context of an individual's life, we have had to content ourselves with endless economic and medical analyses of fragments of the system. And, of course, an improved fragment here and there may be better than nothing at all if we have not gotten to the root of the problem. Indeed, the sense of triumph both patient and provider feel over single medical achievements—such as a hip replacement that transformed a person's life, a heart transplant that literally restored a life, or a miracle drug or new technique that made the impossible possible—all tend to stifle analysis and criticism of the system as a whole when it fails the average patient on the average encounter with an everyday problem. Nothing could be a more dramatic achievement than a landing on the moon, but we should not let it obscure analysis and necessary change in the system when something of the magnitude of the shuttle disaster or even minor misfortunes occur.

Malpractice

Having defined quality of care above as the conformance to standards to which everyone agrees at the outset, we can define malpractice as the failure to conform to those standards. Lawyers who have conceptualized malpractice law in terms of physician negligence and the patient's right to informed consent need an infrastructure for data gathering and presentation of options as the basis for standards of care. The problem-oriented medical record and the diagnostic and management couplers not only provide such an infrastructure to formulate such standards, but they do it in a manner that makes daily implementation and compliance a feasible goal for all practitioners. Without such information tools, it has not been reasonable to expect all practitioners to know and present to patients all the known diagnostic and management options for all the problems that confront them on a daily basis. Our failure to recognize this as a profession has led to serious ethical and legal consequences. Both patients and providers of care have suffered a great deal of injustice in the courts and less than optimal care in the hospitals and clinics.

Lack of Coordination Among Providers

Inefficient Use of Human Resources in the Health Care System

The word *providers* should not be interpreted to mean merely various types of physicians. Indeed, the group in our society that may be giving more care than any other is the nurses. For specific problems, the same diagnostic and management couplers should be used by all providers to avoid the bias that specialization always introduces. The knowledge needed to solve real problems always crosses specialty boundaries and in the early stages of a disorder, the patient often has no way of knowing which provider to go to. The system should protect patients from the wrong choice of provider, and protect the providers from getting trapped in areas outside of their own expertise. The main force for coordination will come from the patient or the family if the patient is not mentally competent. By definition, the patient is present at every encounter and is the focal point of every decision and interaction. There is no substitute for the patient's being in charge. A patient is in control of and aware of all the variables 24 hours a day seven days a week, whereas most providers are forced to deal with a few of the variables 20 minutes twice a month in a busy clinic. From earliest childhood, patients must be brought up to understand the role they must play and the communication tools that are used in their care.

The Status of the Primary Physician

It is legitimate to ask how much help the average layman will need in negotiating each step of a highly developed medical information system. Furthermore, when help is needed, the following questions arise:

- How much training does an individual need to provide help or guidance at a given step in the process?

- How many of the steps in the process that do require help can be assigned to a single individual whose job it is to provide the help or guidance?

Assuming a complete set of couplers and a computerized problem oriented record, the roles of patients and guiding personnel can be defined rather precisely, all adding up to total care for the individual, just as a well defined transportation system can add up to total successful trips under the control of the traveler using sophisticated professional help at the steps where such help is necessary (in piloting airliners, for example). Such a well defined system makes it possible to evaluate the performance of all personnel (both providers and patients) in very precise terms.

In the present system, run by credentialed personnel (doctors, nurses, etc.), we talk about primary care physicians and all types of specialists, but the boundaries of the activities and competencies among all the personnel are very poorly defined; each individual sets his own boundaries and the patient is often a passive object in the whole process. One primary care physician may have a much lower or higher threshold than another for performing procedures or for ordering drugs or for shifting the responsibility to the next level of care. Primary care physicians also vary enormously in how many personnel they have working for them making small decisions and how much autonomy those individuals have. A person has only to enter several offices or clinics with the same complaint and then note the variation in what transpires (the questions asked, the extent of the physical examination, the drugs and procedures ordered, the time spent in explaining and the clarity of the explaining, the charges made, and the timing and number of revisits requested). These differences raise the question of exactly what are the unique and essential elements that the credentialed *primary physician* brings to the medical care process and which, if any, of those elements are dependent upon long and expensive years of medical training and which elements are nothing more than manifestations of the power that has grown out of the physician's authority, experience, and control over his or her own environment. It is impressive how some of the physicians who declare the role of the primary physician to be essential are the same ones who assert that one of their main functions is to organize care and protect their patients from unnecessary surgery and procedures ordered by other physicians. All this suggests that primary physicians as they are now trained and as they now function are not a single well defined entity with known functions and defined boundaries that can be neatly plugged into a well defined and organized system of care. Such a well defined system, with properly trained guidance personnel at those steps where patients cannot act alone, may well add up to a better system of care with fewer dependency states and with much lower salaries than present credentialed physicians now require.

Concerning dependency states, it is often asserted that many patients do not want to take an active role and would prefer to leave the management of their health to others. The analogy is often used that many people could learn to take care of their own cars but choose not to because they have neither the time nor the interest in doing so. The analogy is so often used because it is true that people often do want to turn their health matters over to others while they live any life they choose. On the other hand, the analogy is a bad one because everyone can leave a car at a garage for repairs and come back when it is ready or even buy a new one if necessary. But patients do not leave their body and mind at the doctor's office to be picked up when repaired. They take the whole system home with them and are in complete charge of all the variables. They break medication schedules, they self prescribe, they persist in bad health habits, they go to multiple providers. The provider should say to such patients "I understand your wishes, and I would like to serve you, but in all honesty I must get you over the illusion that anyone other than yourself can be in charge of and manage your own health. Money cannot free you from the responsibility, nor can you buy a new body or mind when the current one wears out."

Health Insurance

Normally, we think of insurance as a group of people sharing risks with well defined endpoints in mind. The whole enterprise is dependent upon the availability of reliable data for assessing risks and assigning costs to each individual in the system. In life insurance, for example, the endpoint, death, is sharply defined; most people do not try to reach the endpoint prematurely and thereby avoid paying into the system over a long period of time; and the owners of the business have a reasonable assurance of a cash flow that is sufficient to maintain a profitable enterprise. Also, for the purposes of life insurance, enough information has been accumulated to enable the exclusion of high risk individuals that could bankrupt the system. And finally, those who never get life insurance may make it difficult for their survivors, but they themselves, after death, are no longer a burden that weighs heavily on the conscience of society.

In health insurance, the situation is far more difficult and frustrating for both individuals and society as a whole. The endpoints are not easy to define; people, through unhealthy lifestyles and clamor for maximal benefits (from hair transplants to new hearts), are more likely to extract benefits from the system far beyond their willingness and ability to pay into the system; and the owners of the business are more likely to run out of resources before they can get solidly established. Also the unavailability of reliable data (particularly on ambulatory and comprehensive care) and the social pressures to cover everyone make it more difficult to define and exclude high risk patients from the system to save it from bankruptcy. And finally, those excluded from the system do not just die and disappear from the view and the conscience of society as they do in life insurance; rather, they often slip into many costly illnesses which a civilized society cannot ignore.

Those leaders who unwisely fail to assure preventive and prenatal care could never be heartless enough to avoid the costly consequences of their neglect. And those families who refuse simple things like whooping cough immunizations even when they are free, are the same ones who demand costly care when the epidemic strikes. And those citizens irresponsible enough to indulge in a lifestyle that compromises their health are very unlikely to find a way to limit the impact of their self neglect to their lives alone. Other innocent people must also pay the price. In this sense, the fundamental issues in health care and health insurance are ethical, not economic. It is not endless analyses of outcomes by economists that we need, but more disciplined control over inputs and priorities by the community as a whole that will bring order to the system. This can only be accomplished through a defined system of care in which the management options are included or removed from a guidance system on the basis of society's overall priorities and not on the basis of maximizing the opportunities for all types of care for every individual that enters the system. A management coupler may not include a given option, not because it is not scientifically valid and medically desirable for a given individual, but because, on a relative basis, it is too high a price to pay in the health of the community as a whole.

Physicians and other providers should never be placed in the position of having to think of, and fight for, all options for individual patients at the time of the clinical encounter, anymore than pilots should be able to make individual and unilateral flight plan decisions in a complicated society. And we should not think of such an approach as unjustly limiting the freedom of either pilots or physicians; rather we should look upon it as relieving them both of an ethical burden that they should not have to shoulder alone. Indeed, our failure over the years to extricate physicians from their untenable position by changing the premises and tools of our medical education and care system, and our perseverating about many of the unfortunate outcomes of their actions have led to much unnecessary and unjust "doctor bashing", when in reality, physicians are victims, along with the patients, of a flawed medical care system.

How did we start off with a discussion of insurance and end up in a discussion of defining and controlling the inputs to the health care system? It happened because, if something cannot be defined, it cannot be priced, and if it cannot be priced, it cannot be insured. If in the process of defining and pricing the components of health care, the resources of society are easily exceeded if every option is made available to all, then choices must be made. And those choices must be made by society as a whole (as pioneered in the state of Oregon) and then placed in the guidance system. No longer can they be a burden placed on the unaided minds of providers who are the product of a memory based, credential oriented system.

Coupling New Knowledge to Practice: The Effects of Some Current Educational Approaches

Perhaps we have not taken enough time in the past to stand back and simply observe the overall panorama of medical information flowing from the sources where it is generated, to its final application in the lives of patients, both in the maintenance of their health and the management of their problems. This view would be much like the perspective of a person in an airplane looking down on a river winding its way to its destination in the valley below. If we are too close, the details along the course not only distract us from the larger view, but they also entangle us for years or even a lifetime, and so the larger view is never seen at all.

The larger view allows us to see fertile areas of growth, but it can also show us obstructions and diversions in the flow, flooded plains and desert areas that could be changed. The right engineers could recognize the bottlenecks and would concern themselves with alleviating obstructions and redirecting the flow.

In medicine, our first overall view of the source of information is a cluster of university laboratories, clinical investigators, and research institutes run by industry, government, and private foundations. Less conventional sources, including ancient and modern healers of all types, are also pouring forth large amounts of information. From these sources, new information flows into articles in innumerable journals and books in libraries and into conferences and symposia around the world. Each article contains one or two new ideas and hundreds or thousands of facts and ideas that are already in the library, so the physical size of libraries grows much faster than new knowledge. From the libraries, the information flows into the minds and courses of teachers of all sorts in medical educational establishments. And, from the latter, it flows into the heads of physicians, dentists, veterinarians, nurses, therapists, and a variety of technicians, who then transmit it to the patients they serve. The magnitude of this flood into human minds and administrative units in the name of education, credentials, and specialization is overwhelming; but the flow through those minds to patients is where a serious block appears.

As we focus down on the point where large amounts of the information are funneled into the human mind, it becomes apparent what the flooded, decompensated minds will do. They become totally preoccupied with their own circumscribed goals, often oblivious to the overall goals of the total system. A physician responsible for all the information in a clinical laboratory, for example, may establish as a goal for the service to receive and record every specimen and make a timely error free report on every laboratory result to the originator of the information request. That physician will also generate and maintain all the relevant financial accounts for that order, because that is fundamental to his or her own economic survival. But there may be no intention whatsoever to assure that the original order is appropriate for the problem at hand in the whole context of the patient's other problems, that the result was properly interpreted, that the correct action was taken, and the correct priorities were set in the face of limited resources and overwhelming demands. The field of medicine abounds with such individual computerized information systems—tumor registries, basic science departments, specialty services, consultation rounds, screening clinics, departments of medicine or surgery, research groups on artificial intelligence, problem solving, etc. We, in medicine, are like a group of musicians (some very talented), all with their own compositions playing on their own schedules, but all using the same concert hall, into which patients come naively expecting to hear a beautiful symphony rehearsed and conducted solely for their own individual benefit.

But the goals of individual parts of the medical establishment do not add up to the central and original goal of meeting the overall needs of an individual patient in an integrated and organized manner.

The development of knowledge couplers and the computerized problem oriented medical record and their routine use in the daily practice of medicine can do much to make the sophisticated parts of the present medical establishment add up to a system that meets the needs of the individual patient.

We no longer need to take brilliant pieces of medical and sociological knowledge generated in laboratories and clinical investigations all over the world and channel them to the patients through the unaided minds of providers. No longer do we need to allow terms such as *medical mystique, intuition,* and *clinical judgment* obscure the basic truth that the unaided mind is not capable of recalling and processing all the appropriate variables at the time of action no matter what the training program or how fancy the credentials. Furthermore, the time has come to examine critically our assumptions about exactly what should constitute medical school education.

What are the implications of the new premises and new tools for the basic science education of the physician? In the past, the premise has been that medical students should spend the first two years of their medical education studying the basic sciences of physiology, anatomy, biochemistry, pathology, etc. so that they would have the necessary knowledge and understanding to think and perform as scientists when confronted with clinical problems. Since the time of the Flexner report early in this century, this premise has been operative in American medical schools and has accounted for much of the curriculum and much of the expense of running a medical school. As stated above, it has been possible through the hiring of PhDs and through the expansion of basic medical knowledge to expose the students to a massive amount of basic science facts, but it has not been possible to create for them in clinical practice the conditions that foster the disciplined behaviors of a scientist—i.e., one or two problems, the necessary time, and a publication system with rigorous peer review. Whether the memorizing, regurgitating, and forgetting of massive amounts of material have made them better clinicians than they would otherwise have been has not been established by careful studies over the years. Some may have assumed that medical students are a fundamental link between basic science and medical practice because their clinical elders fall behind in basic science and technology and their PhD teachers do not know the clinical problems and thus correlations escape them. Others have said that if all this thinking is valid, then why did the basic sciences of psychology, sociology, ethics, and economics get left out of the curriculum since they involve clinical practice as much or more as the subjects now taught? Still others have noted that much clinical practice (in rescue squad activities, orthopedics, psychology, psychiatry, etc.) is being performed by people who have been highly trained for specific tasks and who have not had the *credentialed* basic science training of the physician. It also must be recognized that the fragmented and sloppy manner in which the medical establishment has managed medical data on patients may be indicating that medical students may have temporarily learned some of the facts of basic science, but they they do not think and act like true scientists much of the time. Furthermore, the malpractice crisis may be another indicator of false premises and inadequate tools; in reality we are dealing with educational malpractice in which the physicians are victims along with the patients.

With the appearance of new premises and new information tools, we simply *do not know* what the minimal background should be for personnel who are entrusted with the job of delivering large quantities of acceptable medical care at a low cost. But we *do know* that the more sharply we define the tasks of medicine, the more we make visible to all the logical connections among those tasks, and the more the patients are educated to act in their own behalf, the more focused can be the training of those who perform the tasks and the more precise the audit of that performance can be. Knowing these endpoints, we can work back to find the most efficient approach to developing reliable performers within the system. A reliable performer with the new information tools may consistently produce *higher quality with less training* than those who rely on old premises and old tools. An intelligent ten year old girl with a good set of maps and the ability to read them may be a far more helpful companion on a trip than a person with several years of geography courses but no maps. Both will learn from experience, but the girl with the maps will never be dependent upon her experience or her credentials—she only has to be sure she has a set of up to date maps.

We can see from the foregoing how the premises and methods of medical education and practice, the cost and the quality of medical care, and the role of patients in their own behalf all intersect. And it is by careful examination of these interdependencies that we begin to get some insight into why the product of medical science, medical care, has not become mass produced in high quality and made available to all at a much lower cost as has been the case with the products of many other branches of science. Indeed, if the personal computer had evolved the way many products of medical science have, each one would cost far more, current standards of reliability would probably not exist, and availability would be far more restricted. But the personal computer, and many other products, from washing machines to automobiles, did not evolve that way. No mystique surrounded what they were made of and how they are assembled, and no educational credentials were required to make a better component (a faster component in the computer) or to assemble the components or market the whole product in a more efficient manner. And that has been true because all the parts of the product were known and the precise requirements for assembly were clearly defined. Medical science, on the other hand, kept generating new bits of knowledge and technique, but left the organization and assembly of those bits into effective units of care up to the credentialed physician whose limited recall and associative powers were documented in the psychology literature but never generally acknowledged in the methods we have used to educate and license physicians. As a consequence, we have overestimated the precision and value of the intuitions and judgments that have been the product of these idiosyncratic recall and associative powers of the unaided mind of the practicing physician. And not only have the prices of the services of those minds been high, but those prices have not been subject to the disciplining and lowering effects of a competitive market place. A prerequisite to making something better and available at lower cost is a clearcut definition of what that something is and then not restricting its availability to patients by erecting credential barriers, which automatically create financial barriers. Similarly, a prerequisite to making our outcomes interpretable, our medical science more rigorous, the training of health care workers more efficient, the patients' role in their own behalf more effective, and the whole enterprise less expensive is defining and integrating the components of the medical care process for all to see. The profession can no longer excuse its lack of discipline and imagination in mass producing high quality care on the basis that medicine is a complex art. We have already witnessed what we can accomplish when we put our minds to it in the performance of rescue squads manned by nonphysician manpower. One of the principal issues of our time is how can we harvest far more high quality care from the billions spent each year. Much energy and time have gone into discussions of how medical care should be financed along with innumerable comparisons of British, Canadian and American approaches in this regard, but new premises and new tools can contribute significantly to the increasing focus on the economics and methods of the production of the care itself.

Can we realistically expect that the articulation of the above ideas will achieve anything? After all, long ago Codman (1918) wrote:

> The day of the general practitioner is passing; it has almost passed in thickly settled regions: but the day of the isolated specialist has also begun to pass. Economic conditions do not permit the average person to employ the latter. Combinations of experts will to a great extent take the place of both, except in the unusual instances when the individual can maintain himself by his actual superiority in his own field.
>
> Now the specialist sees few cases, and gets overpaid for each; the practitioner sees many cases, and gets underpaid for each.
>
> If an institution subdivides its work among many individuals, each, like the specialized laborer in industry, will do the same thing again and again. and become more and more skillful. The patient is like the buyer of a boot made by many workers. The general practitioner is the retailer. He fits the boot to the needs of the individual customer.

Since the above was written, we have not witnessed highly organized groups of specialists delivering large amounts of highly skilled but low priced care. Nor have we seen general practitioners organizing the delivery of the care of such specialists. The premises and tools under which the general practitioner operated could not then, and cannot now, enable the performance Codman expected. We can only hope that new premises and new tools will allow us to succeed where they failed in matters of integrating and delivering the components of efficient and specialized care. Specialists have profited too much from the present system, as Wendell Berry has said in other contexts, to expect them to lead us to the major changes and efficiencies that are now possible. Also the best intentioned and most dedicated specialists cannot do their job and change the basic system at the same time—anymore than individual members of a symphony can be expected to change the score or the manner in which it is presented.

The new tools do not bring to medicine some algorithmic "cookie cutter" mentality any more than a map constrains the choices of a traveler. It is the constraints of disorder and the lack of a highly disciplined communication system among providers and patients that we must fear. The physician's and patient's ignorance of all the options and their inability to weave the right options into the fabric of the patient's life is what has created the "cookie cut-ter" mentality of the credentialed specialist and expert. There is the story of the woman who finally after 12 weeks of waiting for an appointment got to see the famous specialist at a university medical center and exclaimed, "I am so glad I got in here—I understand you are the best physician in the country for what I have." In a moment of insight, the physician blurted out, "Lady, all I hope is you have what I treat." New tools not only open up to the provider and the patient all the options that no single specialist or generalist could ever remember, but also help the provider and patient get the best *match* to that option which best fits the patient's unique situation.

The Changing Roles and Expectations for Students in the Medical Sciences Educational Methods and Approaches

Basic Science Lectures and Laboratories in the First Two Years

When members of the population are empowered and given the tools and responsibility to be in charge of their own health care from childhood on, we will have students entering medical school with a much clearer idea of what medical practice is and which part of it they would like to devote their life to. They will recognize that medical information and guidance are embedded in the tools they use and will see how important it is to master the necessary hands on skills fundamental to practicing in their chosen part of the field of medicine. They will recognize from the start that no one can do it all and that the patient's long term welfare depends upon a well defined and highly coordinated system of care. They will be much like a person entering a professional team sport. From childhood on, they will have seen professionals perform in ways that are completely intelligible to them. They can see that different members of a football team, for example, bring different physical attributes and skills to the game and that all are subject to the same rules and that there is a referee at every game; although the rules and means of scoring outcomes are arbitrary, they are defined and performance is judged by all within the framework of the rules. Some of the arbitrary academic boundaries we have built up among physicians, dentists, nurses, librarians, other medical professionals, technicians, and paramedical workers will disappear. Providers will no longer be given credentials that suggest anyone can or should know and do it all and thereby have power and incomes far in excess of many of the other productive workers in the system. Much power and control will reside in the rules and tools of the system itself. Some entering the profession will gravitate toward updating the knowledge base of the system both through study of the medical literature and from analysis of the outputs of the system itself with its many potentially powerful corrective feedback loops.

With the above picture in mind, we can work backward from the tools of the system to the necessary training facilities. For example, knowledge couplers on the knee or shoulder problems will reside in anatomy laboratories where providers can go to understand in detail all the elements of the coupler, e.g., the cruciate ligament, etc. Those doing basic research can always be able to consider where the outputs of their work might fit into the ongoing system of medical care. They will start with the entities they are working on, traverse the knowledge network, study relevant portions, and then see exactly in what couplers are those portions used. All linkages in all couplers will be referenced to the network, and it will be known where in the coupler system all facts in the network are used. Throughout the system, the emphasis for every trainee and performer will be on making tasks and time the variables and achievement the constant. From the patients' point of view, how much of their care is provided by one individual will not be nearly as important as knowing that the part any individual provider does is done correctly and within the rules of the system. In other words, whether the oboe player can also play a violin or write music is not important to the listener of the symphony; what is important is that the oboe player plays every note for the oboe correctly and in time with all the other players. Patients will expect less and less to get everything from "their doctor" and will focus more and more on the quality of the total system and their own responsibility in using it effectively.

Once it is recognized that we should be teaching a core of scientific behavior rather than teaching and examining for a core of knowledge, then devices like lectures that were designed to do the latter will disappear. (Lectures to inspire, to interest, to give an overall view, or to entertain could continue, but should be recognized as such). Teaching a core of behavior is best accomplished in the context of the performance of specific, concrete tasks.

For the clinician, the knowledge couplers and other new tools described in this book do much to define precisely what those concrete tasks are and what hands on skills need to be mastered. For the basic science faculty, what should be the context and goals of their efforts if we want them to teach the behavior of a scientist as opposed to teaching and examining for an arbitrary collection of some of the facts of basic science? The modern clinical facility managed with modern information tools provides an incredibly rich resource and context for basic science faculty to inculcate into beginning students a rigorous way of thought and a capacity to confront and systematically analyze complex problems in medical science and practice. Basic science professors and their students can be charged with auditing the logic of orders and use of data on real patients in all types of settings without being under the pressure of time and the multiple tasks that plague the clinician in charge. Trying to understand why things were done and what the data actually reveal as the case unfolds will develop the student's analytic sense. Students will note the consequences of ignoring or not controlling variables or of collecting unreliable data (faulty laboratory tests or inadequate physical or radiological examinations, for example). They will have to learn to confront and understand new things (as opposed to memorizing what a professor thinks they should know) as they work together with the professor to unravel the logic of the clinician's actions.

An automatic byproduct for the student of such an endeavor will be a rapidly expanding vocabulary and understanding of the medical sciences. Following a transplant patient will expose students to more basic immunology that they might ever hear or understand in one of the current basic science immunology courses. Other cases will provide the vehicle for almost any content material included in current basic science training.

A byproduct of teaching rigorous analyses and thought on real problems will always be a great deal of medical content and understanding. Memorizing and regurgitating vast numbers of arbitrarily selected basic science facts will not result in rigorous and responsible thought processes when confronted with real problems. Students do not need months of lectures or courses to prepare them for such an approach anymore than new babies need a course in grammar and physics before they can learn to speak and interact with the physical world. It is the quality of the environment and the spirit of inquiry of the guiding professor that will determine the quality of the student. And from the point of view of medical care and the development of medical science, such an approach would provide an invaluable routine audit of medical care that could be afforded in no other way. Both the clinician and the basic science professor would be enriched by such an approach. But even more important, the diagnostic and management couplers and the computerized problem oriented record with its disease files and properties on all the medical entities would be the base on which all the interactions could take place and improvements in the information tools would continuously flow from the interactions of clinicians, basic scientists, and students. In this way, the combination of new approaches and powerful new information tools present an extraordinary opportunity for synergism and efficiency both in the medical care system and in the development of medical science. Our failure to link basic science education to the audit of clinical thought processes is perhaps one of the biggest wastes of intellectual and financial resources of which the medical schools and care system have been guilty.

Once students grasp the idea that from their own observations and their own analyses of real life situations they can go on to understand current concepts and theories and at times can even discover in real data the inadequacies of current theories, they will cease to fear the unknown. They will no longer think that they must have a core of knowledge in their own heads, and they will become proud of their capacity to tackle and solve new problems instead of proud of what they know. The novelty of the future and the growth of new knowledge are phenomena over which the faculty has no control; the confidence and intelligence with which students approach this novelty, however, are the faculty's obligation.

The faculty can keep problem lists on students as they perform, just like the problem lists kept on patients. The lists will show that some students are not thorough, while others are hardworking and thorough but not reliable. Others have great difficulty in seeking out and analyzing the logic in the cases they are auditing. Some listen but do not "hear" what they are listening to when they move from audit and thought to doing clinical activities themselves. Others do and write things that they cannot logically defend. Given a group of abnormalities they have reliably detected and recorded in the database, they then make a list of problems that cannot be logically defended in terms of the synthesis of those abnormalities. Or they write indefensible plans or progress notes. The reasons for such problems have to be found and the tasks repeated until the difficulties are overcome. In this regard, a distinct difference exists between the field of medicine and other areas of graduate studies. Not only do medical students work on many problems in many patients simultaneously, but often they do not do patient workups over and over until they understand. They just get criticism, make a few superficial changes, and then go on to the next task of a list of tasks that may be overwhelmingly long. This happens so often in years of clinical training because students (even though they are paying tuition) are often part of the workforce in a working environment that does not allow them to do a task over and over again until they do it correctly.

Once a problem list is established on a student, training and tasks are organized accordingly.

The Role of Computer Simulations and Computer Assisted Instruction

Any computer simulation that has as one of its goals the learning of content is in direct contradiction to the premises for education outlined in this book. It would be like a person going through simulations of various trips in preparation for traveling without a map. On the other hand, simulations as they use them for pilots in developing the right manual skills and reflexes may be very useful.

Medical Rounds and Conferences

In the past, rounds and conferences have been varying mixtures of efforts to present known data, check the reliability of data, get new data, discuss the possible meanings of the data (often off the cuff, with little thought and careful study of the full situation), teach patient interviewing skills and interpersonal relations, and present ideas unrelated to the specific patient under consideration. In many instances, the goals and content of such rounds and conferences are not systematically recorded, and there are no careful followup action and corrective feedback loops. As is often true in memory based, credential oriented systems, it is assumed that the educational efforts at such rounds and conferences will have a positive and cumulative effect on the future actions of those who attend them. Furthermore, those in the profession in need of the most help may frequently be the last ones to attend such events in the first place.

The introduction of new premises and the routine use of knowledge coupling tools in the practice of medicine could affect such rounds and conferences and the economics of medical education in the following ways:

- Rounds and conferences, in general, should no longer be conducted for the purposes of transmitting new information for the direct application to specific patients, or keeping people up to date as to what is going on either with the patients or in medicine in general, or informing or educating the patients about their illnesses. Rather, new information should be systematically incorporated into the information tools used routinely in the care of patients, thereby in one stroke getting to patients the best care and the best education as they manage more and more of their care through their own copies of their problem oriented records, while also keeping providers up to date in medicine as it applies to their patients.

- Conferences or rounds may from time to time be called to negotiate the ambiguities among various diagnostic and management options as revealed by the knowledge couplers and progress notes in particularly difficult problem situations. They may also be called to introduce new techniques and tools for getting data that have become required input for some of the knowledge couplers on specific problems. If, during these rounds or conferences, new knowledge comes up that was not in the information system or if an error in the system is detected, corrections to the system should be made so that all intellectual efforts are generalizable and cumulative.

- The large amounts of money and manpower now going into medical schools, lectures, conferences, and publications of all types could be used far more efficiently in the production of guidance systems used by all providers at the time of action. Such tools can be replicated, updated, and distributed at less cost than present efforts to inform, update, and distribute memory based, credentialed human minds. Furthermore, the former are more reliable than the latter in conducting knowledge from its source to the patients who need it.

Evaluation of the worthwhileness of changes must be against the values and goals we have set and not against the standards of the old system with its old premises and tools. Indeed, how we decide to evaluate a new effort is perhaps the most crucial decision of all.

Our new system frees us from the assumption that at the center of the medical care process is a physician who can, without aid, recall and synthesize isolated facts in the management of the health of another individual. Logically then it should free us from all those educational notions and activities that were designed to create such an individual. Our goal now is a medical care system in which the patient or family assumes a central and active role in the medical care process. It is a system in which the steps to be taken for keeping people well, for discovering problems at the earliest stages, and for solving diagnostic and management problems are well defined in easy to use knowledge coupling tools and medical records. Since much of the medical knowledge and logic can be available in the new communication tools themselves, anyone who demonstrates proficiency in the use of the new tools should be employed without having to present credentials based on memorized knowledge or a capacity to generate complete logic pathways extemporaneously as a result of courses in basic science and problem solving. No single provider needs to maintain the illusion of being a "total physician", nor does the educational system need to support that illusion by requiring students to be exposed to and examined on an enormous amount of material and memorization, at the expense of their developing a sense of responsibility and excellence in the activities that they actually perform for patients. Instead, training can be focused; a sense of the whole will be realized when providers are part of a system that actually achieves the whole for all to observe and for patients to experience. Moreover, the role of patients as their own providers must be emphasized and training given to them accordingly.

The key phrase in the previous paragraph may be, "demonstrates proficiency in the use of the new tools". The question becomes, How much preparation in the basic sciences of medicine should be required of one before he or she is allowed to demonstrate proficiency in one or several of the tasks and thereby become a working member of a team and system delivering medical care? In all fields, we are confronted with the question of how much background and basic understanding is necessary for an individual to function effectively at his or her chosen level.

How much mathematics training should a physicist have, how much organic chemistry should a biochemist have, how much knowledge and understanding of combustion engines does a good driver need? In the field of medicine, the question is particularly difficult because of the issue we discussed earlier, i.e., multiple problems selected by someone else to be managed under time constraints often beyond the physician's control. Even if we were to accept the notion that as much basic science as is now taught in medical schools (and for which board exams are given) is fundamental to performing well in medicine, have we not deceived ourselves in what constitutes understanding and what is needed to achieve it. Medical students may have learned and regurgitated the words of basic science through lectures and exams, etc., but the very volume of the material precluded any fundamental understanding. A great scientist develops the capacity to think of fundamental questions and is capable of the most astute observations of phenomena never recognized by others, whereas the so called basic science training in medical schools consists of learning about observations that the students never made and learning answers to questions which they never asked. Such an approach may have crippled them more than it prepared them. Many quotations from Bok, President of

Harvard, on what is wrong with the medical school curriculum and concrete responses to those criticisms in terms of new premises and new tools for care and education are presented in detail elsewhere. (Bok 1984, Weed 1987)

At this juncture, with a far better defined system of care and powerful new guidance tools, it may be wise to take people of minimal training and let them try to achieve proficiency in the tasks of medicine. Only then can we learn what the minimal preparation needs to be. After all, we do know that every traveler does not need to be a cartographer. Also, although there is a place for travel agents, bus drivers, and pilots, etc., none of those workers in the system have the controlling role over the traveler that the medical care system places in the hands of the physician.

It may be useful at this point to reread what C.C. Weed wrote about medical education at the conclusion of his paper on the philosophy, use, and interpretation of knowledge couplers:

We will cling to the assumption that practicing physicians can without aid synthesize and manage the use of isolated facts in an integrated fashion as long as that is what we require of them.

The reliance on human memory and ability to synthesize and manage knowledge at the time of action prejudices our efforts even if complete and well written records are kept and a system of continuing audit put in place. At best, such records and such a system of audit will only reveal the inability of the human mind to meet the demands we place on it.

A thoroughgoing and lasting change in the goals and methods of medical education can occur only when the use of well designed external means of coupling medical knowledge to everyday medical practice becomes widespread and the unaided human mind's ability to perform the knowledge-coupling function at the time of action can be regarded as superfluous. When this happens, both students and teachers can be released from the oppressive weight of accumulated knowledge, knowing that there is flexible and adaptable means for both preserving and gaining access to it that does not place an intolerable burden on their minds. Their attention can then turn to the dynamics of how knowledge is applied, critically examined and improved. In particular they can pay much closer attention to the uniqueness and novelty of each patient's situation, and to those anomalous cases that reveal the limits of present understanding and methods.

What goals should be moved to the forefront of medical education as knowledge becomes the function of the practitioner's tools rather than of his unaided mind? The key to answering this question lies in the observation that the relationship between correct memory and correct action is not direct, for correct action depends partly upon the proper discipline in approaching medical problems.

Some aspects of how medical problems are approached must be confronted in the design of knowledge coupling tools. The designers of those tools, not the practitioners who use them, must be directly responsible for those aspects. On the other hand, Problem-Knowledge Couplers do not actually gather data, make decisions, perform actions, or record the progress of care in the medical record.

In the same paper, C.C. Weed set forth what he believed to be the specific goals of medical education, as follows:

The first goal of medical education must then be a core of behavior consisting of thoroughness and reliability in the performance of a task. The second goal is the understanding of the scientific method as it applies to patient care. In the context of practice aided by knowledge-coupling tools, this means an understanding of how to use medical knowledge as selected and arranged by the tools, the limits of the tools' functions, and most importantly the fallibility of medical knowledge and how this fallibility will manifest itself when medical knowledge is coupled to the patient's unique situation.

More generally the second goal means an understanding that science generally and medicine particularly is a team effort that requires careful attention to the maintenance of a medium of communication with oneself and others over time. In medicine this medium is the medical record.

The third goal is a mastery of those aspects of observational and therapeutic technique ("hands-on skills") that cannot be executed by a machine or conveyed by a knowledge coupling tool at the time of action but must be carried to the scene by the provider. It is in achieving this goal that specialization continues to be essential. Human beings, if their learning is properly focused, improved and maintained through practice, can develop and maintain sensory skills that cannot be replaced by a computer or verbally conveyed to an untrained person on short notice.

We can all hope that medical education will at least select for and not against those people who care most deeply about alleviating the suffering of others. They should come to understand how essential the three goals of medical education are in enabling them to act properly on their concern. They should be inculcated with a willingness to recognize their own limitations and be receptive to those tools that help them do their work better.

In trying to reach these goals, with the availability of knowledge coupling tools and high standards of medical record keeping, participation in real practice combined with rigorous audit of performance can and must become central to medical education, in both initial training and later professional development of the provider of medical care.

Participation in real practice for students is a realistic goal right from the beginning wherever the tasks of medicine are precisely delineated. The time and tasks for the student should be the variables and achievement the constant. Where given students level off in the system will be a function of their own uniqueness: their drive and ingenuity, their manual, interpersonal, and intellectual skills. Students should be involved at every level, including coupler building and knowledge network development as well as coupler usage. Furthermore, they should have blocks of time to go to laboratories to explore cadavers and to examine details, e.g., to be able to dissect a knee at the time they are fully aware of the detailed results of knowledge coupler usage on a clinical knee problem in a real patient. In this way, cruciate ligaments, Lachman tests, and more come alive in very relevant ways. The creative student will go beyond what is there and suggest new connections, new questions, and new research. In this way, creativity and concern for the future of the system will be fostered but not legislated.

It will not be easy to find the proper environment to institute all the changes described above. The very environment that is the most sophisticated source of the new knowledge and techniques, that must be embedded in the new systems of care, is also the very environment where traditions are strong. It is where masters of the old paradigm of memorized knowledge and the extemporaneous verbal manipulation of it flourish; it is where the students were originally selected on their abilities to memorize, regurgitate, and emulate. It is not easy to start a symphony or a chorus in an institution full of talented and competitive prima donnas. But wherever we start, we should never underestimate the ability of the younger generation to assume responsibility for bringing about the necessary changes, once they understand and agree upon the goals. They can be enormously creative if given a free hand. Their vested interest in the past system is minimal; their vested interest in the future very great. And if they are caught early enough, it will be natural for them to design the system with the patient's point of view uppermost in their minds. Students must get a commitment from the highest authorities in the university that they can operate under the new educational premises. No faculty member in the system should be allowed to tyrannize them with the premises of the old paradigm. One of the main responsibilities of students will be to guarantee maximum agreement between what is taught and what goes on in the real world; the faculty should give maximum support to them as they try to fulfill that responsibility.

Above all, they should not be evaluated by the traditional instruments of the old paradigm, but in a manner consistent with the new premises and the new tools.

The guiding premises will be:

- Patients and providers will always work as partners in health care, both working from a complete medical record as the concrete basis for guiding medical care and assessing its quality.

- A core of behavior instead of a core of knowledge will be developed in students as they confront new problems in unique situations. Their tools will include electronic extensions of human memory and analytical capacity at the time of action. These tools will be kept up to date through the joint efforts of students, faculties, researchers, and practitioners.

- Acknowledgment of the limitations of all human minds in dealing with certain levels of complexity should be developed within all students. Decision making *tour de force* performances by experienced specialists on rounds in front of students should not be mistaken for the teaching of careful analytic thinking in the face of many variables at the time of action.

- Standards of good practice should be maintained by random audits of actual performance in the real world, and students should see by example how compliance is brought about. Students and practitioners alike should never be judged on what they know, but on how well they function in a medical care guidance system that has been designed to prevent, discover, define, and solve problems in a given population.

Within the above premises and guidelines, students will undoubtedly lead in the development of a whole new medical education system that will bear little resemblance to the medical schools of today.

Knowledge Couplers and Definition and Classification Problems in Medicine

At the present time, the memory based uncontrolled inputs and off the cuff processing of data by individuals has led to an epistemological *Alice in Wonderland* where words mean to each individual provider what he or she wants them to mean, no more and no less. Such a system makes feedback loops unreliable and scientific understanding and growth faulty and uncertain. But as we build and consistently use a Problem Knowledge Coupler System, we will achieve the defined inputs which enable meaningful interpretation of outcomes, which in turn can be the basis for constructive change. However, such a system does raise a new set of questions which we shall now deal with.

In the chapter on the database, we described physicians eliciting present illnesses in which facts were assembled about an illness, but which did not explicitly document how each bit of information was processed or interpreted by the physician eliciting the present illness. In the couplers, on the other hand, each finding that is elicited points to specific diagnostic or management options. In this latter situation, the significance of each finding is no longer the responsibility of the practitioner; it is the responsibility of the coupler builder.

Without rigorously kept problem oriented progress notes and the tools to work more precisely with our language, our options and our results have led most of us to live with all sorts of misconceptions. One is that there is a common understanding of the language of medicine and that all people think of diagnoses and medical entities in the same way. Another misconception is that thinking in medicine (rational and logical within a small number of known, stated variables) continues to be so when applied to a unique human being who embodies many more relevant variables (structures and processes) than were ever considered when the diagnosis or treatment was conceived.

Considered as a physical system, the human body is an enormously complex collection of interconnected structures and interacting processes. An important part of that complexity is the body's extraordinary capacity for self regulation (*homeostasis*) and self repair. These features make it far more difficult to trace abnormalities to their origin and to decide which abnormalities should be regarded as primary in a particular patient. They also play a central role in the way problems evolve over time. Furthermore, each member of the human species differs from every other member by virtue of his or her unique genetic heritage and unique developmental and environmental history. By virtue of the complexity and the uniqueness of each individual, we can expect that any illness will be a unique course of events, resulting from an evolving derangement of certain structures and processes that will never be precisely reproduced. Ideally, in medicine we would like to be able to say that our understanding of human beings and the special characteristics of individuals are such that, when encountering an illness in an individual which may be unlike anything seen before, we can pinpoint the abnormal structures and processes responsible. Ideally, we would also hope that we could develop from first principles an appropriate course of management for the derangements we have discovered.

In reality, we cannot reach this ideal. We do not understand all the structures and processes of the human body well enough, and the providers of medical care are not well enough informed about the unique situations of their patients. In fact, one of the things we have tended to do traditionally is look for clusters of findings which several patients have in common, regard each cluster as a disease, and assign it a name. Over the years, we have devised management strategies of varying effectiveness for the diseases we have identified. (Often we have been so focused on the few things a few patients with the same disease have in common, that we have not given sufficient attention to the thousands of things which they do not have in common and which may have a critical and predominant effect on the outcome of any given strategy. This reality is the Achilles heel of the specialist.) But also in many cases, we have also acquired considerable understanding of the derangements of the structures and processes that are causally associated with the originally observed clusters of findings and of the mechanisms of causation. This has put us in a better position to understand and manage patients who show clusters of findings similar, but not identical, to the defining clusters for the patients' presumed diseases. Moreover, it has allowed us to redefine known diseases, not as recurring clusters of certain findings but as specified derangements of certain structures and processes. As such they may produce very different manifestations in different people, thus freeing us from the requirement of clinical repeatability.

With all the above considerations in mind, we realize that it would be extremely unlikely for two individuals to have identical derangements and consequences; each individual is unique and has problems that are unique combinations of specifically identifiable derangements and other unknown factors. The more details one has on an individual, the more the uniqueness reveals itself.

Because of these facts, seemingly irrational ideas in medicine, could, from the total point of view, be more rational than the so called "scientific or rational" ones. For example, because of the breadth of the context in which actions are taken, the Indian medicine man could set into motion a series of complicated interactions, the basis for which has evolved over millions of years; these in turn could deal more effectively with the problem than the more parochial and superficial "diagnoses" and actions of the "scientific" specialist.

Indeed, we may be on the threshold of understanding many processes at the level of the body, mind, brain, and spirit that have heretofore escaped us. It is through this new understanding that we may see linkages among traditional Oriental medicine, Western medicine, American Indian medicine, and many of the new alternative approaches to healing. It is important for all those functioning within the medical sciences, from the patient to the specialist, to have a picture of how medical science has developed and how medical roles are developing and changing in the face of these difficulties.

Since dysfunction was seen and written about in medicine long before the rudiments of anatomy, physiology, and biochemistry (the structures and processes) were understood, the human mind and body and spirit were treated as a *black box* exhibiting all sorts of difficulties on the surface (symptoms and signs) for which all sorts of remedies were devised with varying amounts of logic and understanding. We would laugh at a person who put nickels in a vending machine and then wrote a paper on how candy bars are made of nickel; but much of our medical and biochemical literature has been just that naive as we have struggled to understand the human machine. As the medical literature has developed, there has been no rigorous method to keep the definitions of each disease entity precise and consistent among all users of and contributors to that literature; people using the same words have often been talking about different things. To the clinician, the diabetic may be someone with a high blood sugar and a retinopathy; to the immunologist with a new technique for measuring insulin in the blood, the patient is a particular type of diabetic with a high or low blood insulin; others may think in terms of the glucagon producers, or the high level of antibodies to insulin, or defective receptor mechanisms. The more we know, the more we realize that no two diabetics are exactly alike and so diagnostic tests and treatments will not have uniform effects on what we categorize as a single disease when looking on the outside of the black box.

Regardless of the past, we can now try to define all entities in medicine in in terms of structure and process and look for intersections among them (Weed 1982, Weed 1986). We must not lose sight of how Addison defined Addison's disease, but we must continue to enlarge that definition as knowledge grows. The same is true of all the genetic disorders as we progress from definitions based on morphology or a metabolic error alone to a much greater understanding of many interconnections and consequences of various primary defects. Also, what we were once content to classify morphologically and chemically at birth may now require a more sophisticated definition in biochemical and genetic analyses early in pregnancy if management is to be adequate. It is becoming ever clearer that practitioners of medicine must use up to date information tools right from the outset of every encounter with patients.

Rules that are invented on the fly in response to unique situations are inherently difficult to document in the sense that ordinary scientific conclusions are documented. The uniqueness of the situations makes testing of the rules through straightforward repetition impossible. (Clinicians can and should document what rules were applied—what decisions were made and why—in medical records, even if the rules were invented for one time use.) However, the knowledge on which these invented rules are based can and should be documented, as should the general principles and strategies for generating rules for action in specific situations. More modestly, we can acknowledge, document, and standardize the methods we use to couple knowledge to action—the methods of retrieval and presentation we use to provide a useful basis for generating approaches to decision making in specific situations.

This is what we have tried to do in the development of the Problem Knowledge Coupler System, and its supporting database of medical knowledge, the PKC Knowledge Network. The use of every one of the basic elements in the content of a coupler is referenced to the a general database (the knowledge network). The basic elements of the knowledge network are referenced in turn to the medical literature itself. This chain of documentation is maintained as couplers are built and updated. Much of the work involved in this is done automatically, as a consequence of design of the data structures of both systems and systems for updating and retrieval. A consequence of all this is that although no two patients ever take exactly the same path through a diagnostic or management coupler and no detailed path can be anticipated, we still have documented the path in that each logical connection within the system is documented.

In this connection, we should comment upon the recurring preoccupation with the need for standardization of medical terminology and disease definitions. As we see it, such a standardization can be pursued more fruitfully if it is driven by needs that arise in the development of knowledge coupling tools and their incorporation into the practice of medicine. By their very nature, such tools embody characterizations of disease entities. Furthermore, they explicitly define the uses, roles, and interrelations of medical entities of all sorts that occur in clinical medicine. The development and disciplined use of knowledge coupling tools defines the agenda for standardization. (A consequence of this is that standardization should not be pursued in advance of tool development in order to facilitate that development. It should be considered as an integral part of the ongoing development process.)

It has taken us years to articulate and accept the need for standardized and common vocabulary in the medical sciences. It is hoped that we will not take quite so long to accept the need for efforts to be organized and consistent in our inputs to a problem solving system so that outcomes will be interpretable and corrective feedback loops on a sound foundation. Such an approach will no more limit the diversity we value than a defined alphabet unduly limits the number of sentences we can create. The highly valued diversity should have its origins in the almost infinite numbers of combinations of choices made by unique individuals as they employ the problem solving tools—not in contextually ill defined and chaotic inputs that defy rigorous interpretation.

In summary, modern communication tools can help solve many of the problems of complexity and context, and it is our obligation to use them and then to communicate to patients exactly where the boundaries are between our knowledge and our ignorance. By getting command of these details, we can build a system in which problems can be more precisely defined. Students will not flounder so long before they help us solve problems because they too will be able to see clearly the frontiers of our knowledge. The emphasis should be on building and updating the information tools (knowledge couplers and knowledge network), and on computerized problem oriented records so that we can bootstrap our way to a better understanding. Medical education got too deeply into the business of telling students and patients answers before honestly revealing to both groups the boundaries of our knowledge and the massiveness of our ignorance. Expectations of patients as they seek help from medical providers must be shaped realistically. They, more than anyone in the system, must understand their own uniqueness, the complexity of the healing process, and the likelihood for manmade interventions to run the gamut from the superficial and irrelevant, to perfectly focused or lifesaving, to disastrously inappropriate and dangerous. Two principles are implicit in the above:

- Single classification systems are frequently not of universal utility. To group objects or diseases or indeed anything on the basis of one characteristic will never create groupings that are appropriate to another characteristic.

● It has always been accepted that groupings of characteristics under a single name are necessary for practical purposes of management of common *problems* and for organizing our knowledge about specific relationships among *problems*. Also by focusing on a few variables and assuming all others to be similar and constant, statistical studies can be done on large numbers of patients with similar problems. The price we pay for such statistical knowledge is a certain amount of fiction in our conclusions about individuals, because the *constants* assumed are not constant and can vary a great deal in any given individual. The necessity for groupings can be greatly decreased as we more carefully delineate structures and processes.

Chapter 9 Summary

Not only do knowledge coupling (the combinatorial process) and the Problem Oriented Medical Record demystify the elements of medical care and their interconnections, but they also emphasize the role of every individual in revealing and managing all the variables relevant to his or her own unique situation. Physicians and other medical personnel see a fragment of the total during a fragment of the time. It is a scientific necessity that patients and their families have their records and learn to understand and manage the variables in their own care. The best textbook on a patient is his or her own record. Patients are unique but they repeat their patterns of uniqueness.

Patients, as partners with providers in the health care process, must learn that in all their efforts to solve their problems they must make time and tasks the variables and achievement the constant. Since each patient is unique, the time necessary and the tasks required to achieve the desired level of care will vary from person to person. The whole medical effort must rest upon a highly disciplined communication system among patients and providers. Quality of total care to an individual will be the sum total of the quality of each logical step in his or her care. Up to date knowledge coupling tools can assure logical connections among the diagnostic and management options and the unique characteristics and goals of the individual patient. Societal goals and ethical standards will be implemented through the management options that are placed within the system, from which all patients will make the choices appropriate to their needs. Physicians can no longer keep their secrets locked in a language that their patients cannot understand. The history of major changes in medicine, as in all other fields, is one of resistance by those in power.

9
Interdependencies and Potential Synergies

Lawrence L. Weed

Empowerment of Patients in Their Own Health Care

The Economics and Distribution of Medical Care

Evaluation of New Approaches to Ethics and Quality in Medicine

In previous chapters, we emphasized the role of every individual in revealing and managing all the variables relevant to his or her own unique situation.

In maintaining health, in chronic disease, and in the events that lead to acute illness, the patients themselves know and control more of the relevant variables than anyone else. Patients live with the variables all the time. When the values of those variables change (when the situation changes), they can be the first to know.

Physicians often know only a few of the variables and usually have direct control over none. Physicians and other medical personnel see a fragment of the total during a fragment of the time. With examples of two common disorders, we are reminded of these simple truths (Figures 1 and 2).

Physicians go to medical school and try to learn textbook averages about many diseases. Patients know many things that their diseases do to them as individuals; the facts are theirs with no formal education at all.

At the earliest possible age, individuals must become aware of their central role in the understanding and management of the variables in their own life and health care. This is not just some starry eyed, humanitarian goal; it is an absolute scientific necessity if major problems are to be avoided and the best

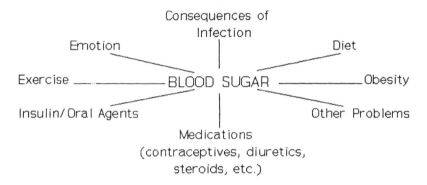

Figure 1. Diabetes management.

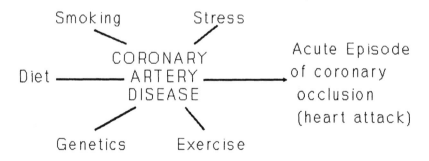

Figure 2. Coronary disease management.

possible care over time is to be achieved. A byproduct of this for every individual is an introduction to, and education in, the general principles of problem solving. Let us state some of the basic principles that all will learn, and under each principle we can emphasize those particulars that apply to medical care specifically. It is recognized that any professional knows the principles that follow, but most professionals have not accepted the obligation to articulate them for the purpose of communicating this common framework of thought to patients. What follows is such an effort. It is hoped that this formulation can be used by both patients and providers as the basis for a sound partnership in health care.

Variables

The more variables an individual knows and considers in a situation, the wiser he or she becomes in that situation. The more continuous the observation of the variables, the smoother the necessary adjustments can be.

In medicine, the patient needs the responsibility involved in knowing and managing the variables; otherwise a dependency state is created, self respect is lost, motivation diminishes, and the patient withdraws, leaving the situation to professional providers who cannot control or even know many of the variables.

Variables and Records

Keeping track of variables over time and examining for crucial interrelationships are beyond the capacity of the unaided human mind. Records are necessary.

By learning to keep and read their own records (including graphs and flowsheets), patients can discern their own unique patterns of response and be the first to see what works and what does not work. Real data can protect them from their own unfounded notions and from the misconceptions and generalizations of those who treat them.

Furthermore, if patients always have a copy of their total record, accessibility and retrieval problems will be avoided. They will not have to always be repeating their story or wondering whether professionals know all the facts. The efforts of multiple providers in many locations automatically become coordinated and cumulative. Without a single system that keeps everyone informed of all the variables, some physicians are trying to solve problems by extreme dedication and overwork, but they frequently end up disillusioned and dissatisfied. Many just give up on the whole issue of total care and select a specialty with a good income and reasonable lifestyle. But the specialist is always at risk, because the patients do not specialize—a uterus does not come into the office or hospital all alone.

House officers in training particularly are victims of a bad system. They may admit as many as five patients in one evening, and since providers do not simply add to a single, complete, organized, cumulative record, the residents stay up all night to do their own workups, and even then cannot get the work done properly in the absence of the right tools and support systems. Often there is tradition to "face it all alone" when it is the house officer's night on. To call others for help or to condemn the system is not what the "best doctor" is supposed to do; after all, it is a period of training and discipline that all must go through.

Under such a system, the patient admitted as the only patient on a slow evening in the presence of a skilled physician gets different care from a patient admitted with five other patients in the presence of a less skilled physician. Patients and families must be aware of these realities so that they can begin to mobilize cumulative accounts of their own situations and actively help the providers bring the information under control. And of course, as we said earlier, outcome studies in such systems are uninterpretable and continue to neglect the fundamental issues of inputs and a rationalized system.

It is true that some people who live to a ripe, old age have rarely been sick and have handled any medical problems they have with natural body defenses, sporadic visits to physicians, and no medical records. Compulsive thinking about health and medical record keeping may seem harmful or a waste of time to them. But others are not always healthy and have not found personal approaches that work for them. Such people continuously turn to the medical profession for guidance, where actions are taken and records kept (good and bad); these individuals must get involved, must understand the actions and the records, and must study the results of the interventions. Otherwise they may be victims of some of the bad effects that disorganized, uncoordinated medical activity can generate.

Relationships Among Variables

Scientists record and observe the course of variables to look for trends and associations among them. To separate coincidence from cause and effect, they have to make repeated observations. Some relationships are easy to see; every time the temperature reaches 32°F, pure water freezes; others are more subtle.

Scientists hypothesize and manipulate variables to bring out relationships, but they try to change one at a time so they will know what is causing what. They do not draw conclusions beyond what the data will support.

Patients without access to all the data and the physicians' thought processes may develop unfounded expectations and exaggerated ideas of the physician's power; they may demand diagnostic conclusions and specific therapies when none are possible. In an honest medical setting, simple conclusions are not possible much of the time. Patients need to be taught a tolerance of ambiguity; it can be tolerated when they have access to the data and the physician's logic concerning that data.

Physicians and other providers are away from the patients and the variables most of the time. Very frequently, the physician who will not take the time to organize data and interpret them carefully is the very one who introduces too many new and uncontrolled variables (excessive ordering of laboratory tests, drugs, and procedures of all types) and then draws unwarranted conclusions from uncontrolled situations. The pressure from uninformed patients for diagnoses and predictions increases these tendencies among providers. And of course, if the records are incomplete enough and not shared with the patients, the unjustified confidence of providers in their own handiwork can go unchallenged and undisturbed. Sometimes the only thing that interrupts this complacency and lack of insight is a crisis and a malpractice suit.

The medical schools are the worst offenders in these matters. They teach and examine for facts out of all proportion to teaching and examining for the capacity to collect and organize data effectively, control variables, and draw conclusions rigorously. The transmission of the medical school faculty's facts often overwhelms—even precludes—the transmission of scientific behavior to students. The failures in medical school education, in their own way, are every bit as bad as the failures in grade school education that are so widely discussed. The simple principles taught in a sixth grade general science course are violated day after day in patient care.

The scientific principles are simple, and patients can apply them to their own care immediately. Patients must stop expecting the impossible from the medical profession and start doing the possible for themselves.

Uniqueness

Multiple variables, constantly changing, lead continuously to unique combinations of variables.

A road map of the United States shows all the towns and many of the roads connecting them. The map facilitates travel, while the unique requirements of the traveler determine which paths are chosen. Every patient is a unique traveler through the medical landscape. There are no two patients, even with the same disease, who have the same manifestations, the same course, and the same qualitative and quantitative constellation of accompanying problems. Nor do they have the same goals and resources to reach those goals. But just as the map may be given to and used by many travelers, so the best medical options can be given to each patient who, along with the provider, will slowly work, step by step, through a medical or social problem.

People repeat their patterns of uniqueness.

The best textbook on a patient is that patient's own record. Unfortunately the medical knowledge about a patient kept in his or her record is often ignored in favor of textbook averages that really do not describe any real individual. Medical care is too often not tailored to an individual's unique needs as defined by his previously recorded unique patterns.

Time, Tasks, and Level of Achievement

No two people can ever do the same number of tasks in the same amount of time to the same level of achievement.

In the best educational institutions, we make time and tasks the constants and achievement the variable. All students start school in September; all take five courses; all stop in June; one gets A, one B, and one C. This is not written in the Constitution or the Bible: we could have made time and/or tasks the variables and achievement the constant. Society does not care whether we can do ten things or a hundred just so long as what we do is done right, and as long as we refrain from doing those things that we cannot do well. Because educational institutions have not acted on these principles, we have poured mediocrity at all levels into the streets. And often the public does not know how mediocre it is until it is too late. Most people in our society have had nothing but Bs or Cs or Ds or Fs in 12 to 16 years of schooling, never getting anything exactly right, or done to perfection, or simply complete.

Future historians may write that we were the generation enthralled by the precision, the discipline, the incredible regulatory systems, and feedback loops in the transfer of information among cells and molecules, but we were also curiously oblivious or callously indifferent to the lack of precision, the lack of discipline, the lack of regulation and feedback loops in the transfer of the information among the human beings who ran the medical care system.

It is true that we try to bring discipline to parts of the system but not to the whole architecture. There is no denying the triumphs of modern medical research and practice, but it is beneath us to ever use them as excuses for our failures to make every trip a safe one for every patient every time. We will always need research and new knowledge, but some of the most important new knowledge we need now is how to use knowledge effectively as members of a highly disciplined medical care system.

What the public expects from us now is for us to work together to produce a lot of high quality care at a very low price. For us not to think quantitatively about patients and resources has qualitative implications for most of the patients. The medical education and the medical care systems have been operating under flawed premises and inadequate tools, chains that hold us down and prevent us from building a better system. But as Rousseau said, "It is better to know your chains than to bedeck them with flowers." We have stated the new premises and we have the new tools. What we are confronted with now is a massive political problem as we try to restructure the medical care industry.

The Impact of Empowerment

Empowered patients operating under *new premises* and with *new tools* can have an impact on the medical care system in the following ways:

Decreased Dependence on Expensive Personnel

Empowered patients and their families can perform more reliably and more consistently many of the functions within the system that were formerly assigned to expensive personnel. The new knowledge coupling tools demystify the medical care process by making explicit all the components and the interconnections among them. This allows precise assignment of various functions of the system to people qualified by performance analysis to carry out those functions. Credentials or the lack of them are irrelevant in personnel choices in such a system. Random audits of the quality of performance of various personnel within the system and random audit of individuals' efforts in their own behalf will replace present credential oriented examinations of all types. Good human resource planning by governments and educational institutions must take these new realities into account.

Quality

Quality of total care to an individual will be the sum total of the quality of the functions used in that individual's care and the assurance of adherence to the logical connections among the diagnostic and management options and unique characteristics and goals of the individual patient. A single disease or procedure oriented *outcome* study is not an appropriate means for evaluating the quality of care of a unique individual. On the other hand, such studies rigorously interpreted in the broadest possible context of known *inputs* may be appropriate for adding or removing diagnostic and management options from the guidance tools from which choices are made in the care of individuals.

Distribution of and Access to Medical Care

Empowered patients in possession of their own problem oriented records and with a much clearer idea of what total care consists of will be able to solve many of the distribution problems of medical care on their own. They can seek in the marketplace the individual pieces at the best possible price and quality until their total care is complete. They can enforce a coordination of care among multiple providers that the providers themselves may never achieve if left free to pursue their own specialized objectives in a world of passive and uninformed patients. Each unique patient will generate the own appropriate mix of home based, community based, and tertiary care center based medical care. The correct balance of services will emerge as society implements its values by the options it makes available in the guidance systems used by all, and as individuals then make the choices appropriate to their needs.

Corrective Feedback Loops

The computerized record and guidance system that each patient uses for his or her care will be part of the total information system that will be subject to random populational analyses. The output of such analyses will be used to detect and correct any flaws found in the guidance system.

Ethics, Priorities, and Resources

Society's goals and resources will be reflected in the management options that are placed within the system. An individual's care will be reflected in the choices made by and for that individual from the options. In a very concrete way, society will be required to articulate its ethical standards, and individuals, through the use of the information tools, will be able to operate within those standards, protected from the biases, or whims, or self serving interests of any individual provider of health care. Ethical issues above all other things are contextual. The amputation of a leg under one set of circumstances is correct and lifesaving; under another set it is an unfair use of limited resources; and yet under another set it is wrong, even criminal. No human mind at the time of action can provide this context; a system of care must provide it and all providers and patients must be held accountable under the guidance provided by that system.

When resources are limited in a given region, society may have to remove certain options, not because they are not scientifically valid, but because on a relative basis they are ethically unsound. We should, wherever possible, avoid making absolute statements in ethical matters. Ideally, we would like to do everything for everyone, but we know we cannot. Setting priorities fairly requires a well conceived information system that is used by all.

Having stated how society as a whole can serve the common good through well defined information tools, it is important to single out for discussion one group in society that has had a large influence on how medical practice and medical research are perceived by most people. That group is the media. The lack of a well defined, highly coordinated system of care familiar to all and in which each person has a defined role and knows where to search for relevant options has allowed the mass media to create unwarranted expectations or raise unwarranted fears among the sick and the "worried well" by dramatically dropping fragments of medical knowledge into minds that up until now have not had any organized context whereby they could assimilate the bits of knowledge into their own unique situation. No one ignores the ideas of context and follow through more than the media, and there is no place where these ideas are more important than in the art and science of medicine. It may well be that those in the media, relating to the public in general, have no way of dealing with the issues of context and follow through. Now we have built into the very tools we use to provide care the guidance and currency of information that can serve the patient in the broadest possible context. No longer can isolated fragments of noncontextual pieces of dramatic journalism mislead unprepared and uncritical minds.

Medical Research

The results of medical research will be incorporated appropriately into specific diagnostic and management options in the system. The outputs of the total system can act as a guide to highlight further research needs.

Problems Associated with Change in a Large System

Having said all of the above, we must recognize that change from above and change from below within a given organization are often so difficult that real change must come from without. Stern, in his book, *Social Factors on Medical Progress* (Stern 1927), points out with multiple examples that "authority" is always in a struggle with basic change. He reminds us that in the middle of the last century when Oliver Wendell Holmes suggested new ideas about the origins of the death of mothers from childbed fever, he was attacked by the prestigious professors in Philadelphia who denied vigorously that they could ever be the vehicle of transmission of the disease. And Holmes answered their attack with a long vehement response which stated, "There is no quarrel here between men, but there is a deadly incompatibility and exterminating warfare between doctrines." Later in his statement, Holmes said,

> Let the men who mould opinions look to it; if there is any voluntary blindness, any interested oversight, any culpable negligence, even, in such a matter, and the facts shall reach the public ear; the pestilence carrier of the lying-in chamber must look to God for pardon for men will never forgive him.

At the same time in Europe, Semmelweiss was having similar difficulties with authority on the same issue. In 1909 William Sinclair wrote in his *Life of Semmelweiss*,

> It had to be confessed that all that had been taught for years about which thick-bellied books full of learning had been written, was error throughout; that a small piece of chloride of lime was sufficient to throw upon the scrap heap the whole learned apparatus, which so many distinguished men of science had been collecting and elaborating for centuries, with the industry and perseverance of bees; that the application of chloride of lime was sufficient to arrest the outbreak of the disease against which all efforts had hitherto been put forth in vain. All that appeared to be too simple to be seriously accepted.

If the professors and authorities resisted the notion that their "contaminated" hands doing pelvic examinations were the source of a single major problem and cause of death, how much more might they resist the notion that their unaided minds and *educational malpractice* are the source of many major problems in the whole field of medicine?

We should make some effort to understand how and why certain groups in the present establishment will feel threatened. Professors teaching the basic and clinical sciences and deans in medical schools are often judged on how well their students do on national Board examinations. Many of them feel that they were hired to organize medical knowledge and stuff arbitrarily selected portions of it into the heads of the medical students on a strict and fixed schedule with practically no feedback on the halflife of that knowledge in the mind of the student or on how it was used and integrated into the actual care of patients. New premises and new tools do away with this whole memory based paradigm and thereby may threaten those who have presided over it. Those who do welcome the change can turn their abilities to helping construct the new information tools, helping students to learn the hands on skills needed in caring for patients, and doing research to generate the new knowledge that feeds the new tools.

Many practicing physicians may demand evidence that quality of care will improve if they switch from the present system to a new one. They may demand evidence that change is justified even though they may not be able to produce evidence that much of what we do now is justified—that the hours of education, licenses, credentials, and costs are justified in terms of outcomes for patients. The first order of business is to define the functions and roles of all in the medical care system and build the proper information tools so that the system has corrective feedback loops and quality can be assessed. Until we do these things, Boorstin, the historian, will be able to write about presentday physicians exactly what he wrote about physicians of an earlier era:

> Physicians kept their secrets locked in a language that their patients could not understand; it is not surprising they enjoyed the prestige of learning and the awe of the occult. Aristocrats of the academic world, they were custodians of the means of life and death. They remained invulnerable to the attacks of laymen.
>
> The world of science was a world of separations—of books from bodies of knowledge of experience—and learned healers from those who most needed healing. But it is these separations that made the dignity of an awesome profession (1983).

Concerning the contention that physicians have an "abiding commitment to altruistic service and the protection it provides to patients," Katz (1984) has incisively discussed why this contention is flawed. He states, "Identity of interest (of patients and physicians) cannot be assumed and consensus on goals, let alone on which paths to follow, can only be accomplished through conversation." In the interest of such "conversation" being in as broad a context as possible and under control in terms of details and options, knowledge couplers and patient records in patient hands and new premises must be in operation. Otherwise, the authority and mystique of the physician will dominate the dialogue between the physician and the sick and often frightened and weary patient.

The goal and the basis for the dialogue are crucial. The goal should be not only that all diagnostic and management options are made known to the patient, but also that meticulous attention is paid to using the details of the patient's unique situation as the basis for choosing among the options. These details are often ignored as patients are told statistical information about a procedure or are told anecdotes about or shown videotapes of a few people who have had the procedure or the disorder, without regard for how well the example matches the situation of the patient. In a profession focused on single diseases and procedures, there is a great tendency when evaluating outcomes to look at only a single procedure or the four or five characteristics a group of patients with the same disease have in common, when in reality it is the hundreds of things that they do not have in common that may have the most effect on the outcome for a single individual. For example, a physician might say to a patient that a study on a given procedure on 100 patients has a 5% mortality rate without any effort to match the patient against each member of the series. Such a patient might get a very different idea of what is in store if it were pointed out that the patients who died had histories, physical findings, and other problems that match that patient's far more closely than the survivors. For that patient, in other words, the procedure may hold a far greater risk than the 5% figure suggests. Furthermore, if a patient observes other individuals discussing their personal experiences with a procedure without any detailed knowledge of how he or she resembles or differs from those individuals, then the procedure may be accepted or rejected for reasons that have nothing to do with how appropriate that procedure is for him or her as a unique individual. Patients must be far more focused on the details of the process of matching themselves as individuals to the options and the skilled execution of those options than to statistical or anecdotal data on the outcomes for large numbers of patients.

In medicine, those detailed steps and options are often hidden from the patient. We fail to point out that there was a bad outcome not because there was anything wrong with a given procedure but because some critical detail along the way was ignored. A well defined system of care is not only essential to achieving the best for each unique patient, but it is also essential if we are ever to judge with fairness among the options we are placing in the system. We should think of quality and good outcomes as the result of a calculus of many elegantly executed steps along a pathway unique to each person's needs. What is good for one patient is not necessarily good for another. Outcome studies, if not both carefully performed and critically interpreted, may end up throwing the baby out with the bath water. When properly performed in a broad and consistent context, we will be better able to determine whether a bad outcome is due to a bad procedure that should be removed as an option in the system, or a good procedure that was executed in an inappropriate fashion on the right person, or a good procedure executed properly but on a person for whom the procedure was inappropriate. Our failure to clearly articulate these issues and then build a system that deals with them has led to many of the unreasonable expectations of patients and much of the malpractice litigation against providers.

Such a tailoring of options to individuals cannot be done without modern information tools such as couplers. But even when we do the best we can, the public will come to realize that we will never be in command of all the variables and that providers of care and the procedures they use cannot always be held responsible for every bad outcome. They can only be held responsible for operating with integrity and discipline within the rules of a system that society as a whole understands and in which options and inputs are known to all. A memory based, credential oriented system can never meet such standards. Routine use of a fundamentally different system is required.

Administrators, deans, and third party payers may react to change in terms of the operational rules of the moment in the world in which they find themselves—per capita funding from government sources, national Board scores, voting tendencies of the faculty, payment mechanisms, etc. They often see their lives as being good managers and bookkeepers within the rules of the system they entered, not as philosophers who must use the power of their authority over purse strings to introduce new ideas that will correct the basic flaws in the system that they are trying to lead or manage. Boorstin (1983) said in this context, "To attack this citadel demanded a willingness to defy the canons of respectability, to uproot oneself from the academic community and from the guild—needed more passion than knowledge—more daring than prudence."

More than half a century ago, John Dewey emphasized the inseparable relationships between knowledge and action, research and consequences, science and ethics, and the natural world and human values. Contemplating all the ways that resistance and inertia may operate, we should not be surprised at George Kelly's observation, in *Daedalus* (1963), that "never have the unifying principles of knowledge and action been more obscure," making it difficult to draw conclusions from a fragmented knowledge system. For many an "expert," pride in "pure science" is giving way to a sense of being out of context, irrelevant, and irresponsibly unconscious of the importance of feedback loops on everything we set into motion in the real world. And the student in medicine feels stranded between two worlds, in Matthew Arnold's phrase, "the world already dead and a world powerless to be born."

Chapter 10 Summary

There are implications for all of education in what has been expressed about new premises and new tools for medical education. If we are going to switch to teaching a core of behavior instead of a core of knowledge in one part of the educational system, then we should consider the value of doing it in all parts of the system.

The quality of the work products in this country are more related to the work habits of our people than what knowledge children have been exposed to over a 12 to 16 year period of schooling. Society is not interested in a full set of credit hours from a university at the B, C, or D level. Society wants, and needs for survival in a competitive world, A+ work on every task for which a worker is responsible. It is hard for any individual to suddenly start meeting that expectation if for 12 to 16 years he or she never or rarely did.

Knowledge can be embedded in guidance systems, and children from the earliest age should, at a minimum, become highly disciplined in the use of such systems to do real work. Those students with the aptitude and interest can gravitate to the creation and production of new guidance systems for the solution of all types of problems. Athletics and the arts can continue as they always have among serious athletes and artists—i.e., tasks and time can be the variables and achievement the constant. The latter two groups of people have never been measured by what they were exposed to; rather they have been judged by how well they perform.

10
General Implications for Education

Lawrence L. Weed

There are implications for all of education in what we have been saying about new premises and new tools in medical education. To change part of an overall system without changing the total (particularly the early years of schooling), puts students into a double bind since their careers traverse the whole system and they run head on into the discontinuities we have created. For example, one group of educators may view the development of a core of behavior (thoroughness, reliability, sound analytic sense, and efficiency) as the cornerstone upon which all other educational goals and activities should be built; another group views the cornerstone to be a core of factual knowledge to be covered in a fixed time and credentials to show for it. For the student subjected to both groups, a double bind is inevitable since all of a group of unique individuals cannot be expected to cover a fixed amount of material in a fixed time to fixed standards of thoroughness, reliability, logic, and efficiency.

The double bind may be less obvious and less destructive to individuals in societies in which there is a long tradition of a given body of discipline and in which the members of the society are very homogeneous (for example, Japan or Germany), but it is particularly obvious in the United States, where there is great heterogeneity among those who enter the educational system and the marketplace. In heterogeneous groups, a choice has to be made—either sacrifice coverage of prescribed amounts of content to the goal of reaching standards of behavior (mastery), or sacrifice high levels of behavior to reach the goal of covering a fixed amount of material (*jack of all trades, master of none*).

If we look around us, we will see that society has already made its choice, if not in the schools it pays for, at least in the matters that are central in their lives—the cars they drive, the planes they fly in, the food they eat, the artists they listen to, and the athletes they idolize. For them, as Wittrock, Professor at the Virginia Commonwealth University School of Dentistry, likes to point out, the days of the percentage grading system are gone, even if some of their academic friends are not even aware of its disappearance. Who wants a pilot who is incredibly knowledgeable about aerodynamics and very good at most of the maneuvers of flying and got an A (90%) in his courses but failed to be a master of the 10% of the material which included the skill of landing the plane? Who wants, as Wittrock asks, canned food that is free of botulism only 90% of the time? But for the pilot to be master of everything he is expected to do and for the canning factory to be 100% free of botulism, there must be checklists, radar systems, detailed maps, and guidance systems for the pilot, and rigorous systems of production in the canning factory.

How did the schools get so out of synchronization with what society needs and expects? Most of us in today's society do not care about what individuals were exposed to or how much they know or have done; most of us care only that they are thorough and reliable in the things they do with and for us. Schools do not prepare students for this expectation. The result is schools plagued with dropouts—and graduates of our professional schools plagued by the malpractice crises.

If our premises are wrong and our tools inadequate, how did it happen? In "The Case Against Credentials," Fallows (1985) gives us some insights. He points out that credentials are usually based on an arbitrary coverage of a core of knowledge; anyone who has the right credentials and could pass the entry test is certified from that point on and is shielded from further tests of competence. He states,

> The rise of credentialed professions reflected the greater precision of scientific knowledge, and the greater complexity of modern business operations, but it also arose from a social choice. When it came to determining professional status, the trial and error of the market place would not suffice. Objective standards must be found.

He quotes President Eliot of Harvard as saying shortly after the Civil War that "There is a national danger in the vulgar conceit that the Yankee can turn his hand to anything....can leap from farm or shop to courtroom or pulpit, and we half believe that common men can safely use the seven-league boots of genius." Such thinking was followed, as Fallows says, by the idea that meeting objective standards meant getting an academic degree. Have we then, as this book suggests, exchanged Eliot's "vulgar conceit" for yet another—that we can equate performance on a credentialing examination with performance under all sorts of conditions for many years to come? We know that we cannot reliably interpret outputs in terms of optimum inputs in the memory based, credential oriented systems that are the hallmark of most professions. For professionals in sports and music and the arts, the situation is different; they are judged on actual performance in the real world and not on what they once knew at the time they were awarded their credentials.

Eliot was correct in believing that many human endeavors must be based on an extensive and complex knowledge base that is not a given in any interested Yankee who wanted to turn his hand to something. It is also true that the trial and error of the marketplace did not yield the objective standards that a fair assessment of outputs requires. But also it has turned out to be totally unrealistic to believe that an extensive and complex knowledge base can or needs to be stored in and retrieved from the human mind at the time of action in any field. Up to date computerized knowledge coupling tools used with thoroughness and reliability cannot only extend the mind of that interested Yankee, but they can also provide the objective standards that enable meaningful interpretation of outputs and corrective feedback of the knowledge built into the tools.

For those who repeatedly use the tools, much of the knowledge will gradually be retained by osmosis, just as a traveler learns geography from the repeated use of maps. But the important point is that the range of travel is not limited by the knowledge or previous experience of the traveler. It is limited only by the availability of the maps and the reliable use of the maps by the traveler.

In all fields, and particularly in medicine, there will be those who staunchly maintain that a basic core of knowledge must be memorized and examined for before an individual can even begin to discuss the field, let alone wisely use a guidance system to function. Elaborate structures of coursework, facilities, and expensive faculty have been developed on the basis of such convictions. These structures have then become embedded in the legal system in the form of credentials and licenses to practice, making it difficult for anyone to function outside of the system and without the formal preparation. Basic premises thereby go unquestioned for years, even generations. The simple fact is that we cannot know what the minimum preparation should be for performing specific tasks in any field or for fulfilling various roles in practice until we define more explicitly what those roles should be in a well defined structure of practice and guidelines. Without that well defined structure and explicit relationships among its parts, we have relied too heavily on the improvisations of individuals with professional degrees who sought or were given leadership roles because of those degrees. Observation in many areas of everyday life should have made us wary that such leaders, perpetuating the present system, tend to overestimate the amount of memorized knowledge needed for performance in their chosen fields; furthermore, they also tend to overestimate the meaningful retention and value of the knowledge preparation that we do demand. After all, children learn a whole language with a large vocabulary and how to negotiate the physical world with no formal preparation at all. The quality of what they develop is directly related to the quality of the environment they find themselves in. People of all ages travel extensively without any formal knowledge of geography, and the system and rules and guidance systems are so pervasive and easy to use that we rarely hear of anyone being lost on the basis of no formal preparation. We have also perhaps overestimated what is necessary in the way of resources and time to create good knowledge coupling and guidance systems in all fields. Indeed, the tiniest fraction of resources that are now going into our present system of coupling knowledge to action (long years of preparation, memory based credentials, expensive faculties relying on expensive educational resources) would create and maintain extensive guidance systems available to all. As we stated earlier, trying to make every traveler a cartographer capable of improvising maps along the way, has not only been disastrously expensive but singularly unsuccessful as indicated by the malpractice crises and the markedly uneven distribution of quality care to all the people.

The reason our vast investment of resources has not yielded what we had hoped for is, as Dawes (1988) states, "so much of what passes for education consists of memorizing connections between words, phrases, and images. These words, phrases, and images may or may not, in turn, have any mental link to external reality." People so educated are then allowed, even expected, to make global judgments extemporaneously when confronted with complex problems in the real world. But if we construct couplers and other guidance systems to be used routinely in all cases, our linkage to reality is assured right at the outset. Furthermore, the finding that such linear combination is superior to global judgment is strong: "it has been replicated in diverse contexts, and no exception has been discovered." Only with the use of such tools can we assure patients in medicine and clients in all other fields that they no longer need to be so dependent upon the inadequate memories or flawed experience of individual practitioners. As Dawes (1988) points out,

> while memory from our experience is introspectively a process of "dredging up" *what actually happened*, it is to a large extent determined by our present beliefs and feelings. We overlearn from experience. By viewing consequences as inevitable results of choice, we create a phony coherence in our experience, and if we believe in that coherence too much, it offers a poor basis for making decisions about the future.

And as Dawes is fond of reminding us, we do Ben Franklin a great injustice when we quote him as saying "experience is the best teacher." What he actually said was, "Experience is a dear (expensive) teacher, yet fools will learn in no other school." But in the field of medicine, as in many other fields, the educational system with its wrong premises and inadequate tools has made "fools" of many conscientious providers who could "learn in no other way" because up to date guidance systems and corrective feedback loops have not been created and then required for routine use in the provision of care.

The development and use of guidance systems for solving real problems at the earliest possible ages in the educational system would not only accomplish a more rigorous coupling of the best current thinking to everyday actions, but it would also yield other benefits.

- Ethical standards for a society would be built into the systems and thereby incorporated into society's everyday acts. Standards would not be something in specialty journals to be routinely ignored as individuals act "off the top of their heads" in their own self interest as problems are confronted on a daily basis.

- Since real problems always cross specialty and academic boundaries, the power of the credentialed "experts" and "specialists" could no longer be wielded in a biased, parochial manner. Allowing that bias to develop in the first place has only led to, in a field such as medicine, our present need for conferences on wellness, holistic health, environmental issues, etc.—efforts to "put Humpty Dumpty back together again."

- Real problems (practical or theoretical), the solutions of which have value to someone, can mobilize in students their collaborative instincts and can make their efforts, and those of their successors, cumulative. Everyone's energy goes into getting something worthwhile done and not into competing with one another and developing odious and destructive comparisons. By definition, if real problems are involved, no one knows the answer at the outset and therefore teachers and experts are not in a position to tyrannize others with what they know. Children would be spared the stultifying hours, even years, in schools that hold so little meaning for so many of them. The wall between the "real world" and the world of education would disappear, and fewer students would lose their footing as they try to move from one world to the other. School for all children should be an exciting place to go, and truly a haven for those from broken homes where real problems seem endless and nothing seems to get solved. The challenge to the teachers is to find a way through real problems to help the students realize the value of improving the way they use their minds. With our present system, the one thing the streets have over the schools is they offer the excitement of real problems and real payoffs. The reactions of children to schools may be considered analogous to the reactions of canaries to conditions in mines. They are highly sensitive indicators. And when they refuse to accept and assimilate what we are feeding them, we should begin to question what it is we are doing, and not merely hope that it might stay down if we pay higher wages to those doing the feeding.
  Furthermore, it is in school, at an early age, that children should develop a positive philosophy and understanding of productive work. We have recognized in the fields of music, athletics, social development, learning, etc., that a good foundation must be laid at an early age or risk its full development later on. In this regard, we have neglected the capacity of children to do productive high quality work and to truly enjoy it and find it an uncommon source of satisfaction and a restorer of balance in difficult times. And as we cannot learn basketball without

playing it, we cannot learn work without doing it. Have we been so fearful of returning to the unreasonable exploitation of Charles Dickens' times, so fearful of denying our children playtime, that we have forgotten how to be creative about turning work into pleasure and satisfaction? For some children, the job at McDonald's is the only place they have a chance to learn to do a thing right if they want to be needed to do it at all—and the better they do it, the happier they are. A disorganized and chaotic medical care system is the last place that students should begin their experience with real work, if we want to assure them of rewarding and happy feelings. The chances of negative feelings about medicine and about work in general are too great in our present medical care system. We should not be surprised that we see so many medical students clamoring for a few high paying "9 to 5" medical specialties that provide the lifestyle to which they have been or want to become accustomed.

- We must change our views about the relationships among education, the knowledge industry, and productive work in our society. Not only do real problems and productive work shatter false boundaries between bodies of knowledge, but they also offer us a means to harness the vast amounts of intellectual energy that young people are now expending in unproductive schools. We can no longer afford to waste that energy and some of the most vigorous years of their lives. After all, we respect workers who get worthwhile things accomplished and thinkers who make new observations, ask new and penetrating questions, and then seek and find the answers. As we said earlier in this text, too much of present education is memorizing observations that the students never made and regurgitating answers to questions that they never asked. This may actually inhibit, not develop, creative and productive minds. Our best people may have developed in spite of the educational system, not because of it. As Margaret Mead said, her grandmother wanted her to get an education so she took her out of school.

- We must abandon the idea that technical schools are somehow lower class than schools where students are passive receptacles of knowledge. The former are much closer to real work, and it is real problems honestly confronted that are the only immunization the students have against the misconceptions and generalizations of those who teach.

- Literature and the arts should be made available to those who have an interest in pursuing them for their own sake; they should not be allowed to become some busywork dreamed up by others. By force-feeding these subjects, we not only may not open up new worlds to students, but we may close their minds to them for the rest of their lives. They should come to believe that knowledge is something to be used, not collected, or something to be enjoyed, not something to be endured.

- The economic implications of changing the way we use and distribute knowledge can be considerable. Not only have our present methods failed us, but they have been based on the most extravagantly expensive resources in terms of personnel and the educational structures that house them. If we convert both students and patients from passive dependents to active contributors to their own development and health, then we may make a real dent in the two largest items of the federal and state budgets. Indeed, we may even affect the welfare budget as well, because it may be little more than a reflection of our false premises in education.

The number and types of skills that will be required to use the guidance systems reliably will vary from field to field and from specialty to specialty within a field. More of the energy that is now going into the teaching and examining for knowledge can be directed into devising the best possible means for helping people acquire hands on skills. The remainder of the time can go into helping people learn to accept and to skillfully negotiate the ambiguities that inevitably occur when such guidance systems are used in the solution of real problems. A map enables many trips; choices are determined by values and goals. Such training will help protect people not only from their own biases, but from the experts who are prone to tyrannize others with their knowledge as well as confuse everyone with disagreements that are so frequent among the experts themselves.

With the above principles and realities in mind, could we not introduce into early education the following assertions?

- Never judge people, from earliest childhood on, on what they know. Judge them on how thoroughly and reliably they accomplish the tasks assigned to them. Wherever possible, assign tasks that the student is interested in doing and tasks for which up to date guidance tools exist. It is almost inevitable that the skills necessary for one set of guidance tools will be transferable to many others. Universal use of such tools to solve problems will generate a demand for their production and an almost infinite variety of them will appear in many fields.

- Emphasize to each student that he or she is a unique individual and that no two individuals bring to any task the same level of skills, interest, and background; therefore, no two will ever accomplish the same number of tasks to the same level of achievement in the same amount of time. Students and faculty should never compare students, but rather judge them only against the goals of thoroughness and reliability in using the tools and completing the tasks they have embarked upon. After they are thorough and reliable, they can learn to defend logically what they have done. Efficiency should be discussed only after the other behaviors have been achieved.

- Each new group of students will naturally yield a few who become interested in building and updating the knowledge tools themselves. Others will focus entirely on the use of such tools to either make a living or to enlarge their interests or to solve specific problems relevant to them. In either case, we will no longer have an educational system that systematically produces large numbers of people who have never experienced an achievement of which they can be proud and people who are not thorough, not reliable, and who cannot logically defend their actions and be efficient in what they do.

  And efficiency is a matter of great importance in a society that is trying to get the highest standard to the most people at the lowest cost. When training an individual working under the new premises and with the new tools, we should make time and tasks the variables and achievement the constant. But individuals who remain unable to achieve mastery of particular tasks in an efficient manner, despite abundant training time, must accept that society cannot be expected to entrust them with those particular tasks. The school's job is to find the right tasks for the right people. The school's job should not be to become accredited on the basis of what they expose people to, without any responsibility for what their students actually do with their knowledge and skills after they graduate from the "accredited" institution. If schools had been held responsible for the latter, they would have long since come to the conclusion that they must build and teach the use of guidance systems for extending minds that are confronted with complexity.

With this simple outline, we have the beginnings of a new system that will enable us to escape from many of the traps set by a credentialing system based on a core of past knowledge. The new system will require, of course, that all who work in it are thorough and reliable, but that is a reasonable goal if the focus of the whole educational system is directed toward inculcating those behaviors. And those behaviors can be achieved by everyone if we do not defeat students right at the outset with too many tasks to be done in too little time. People will vary in the number and variety of their achievements, but the quality of the output of everyone shall be excellent. We may hope for not only a more productive society that produces high quality products but also a society of high morale, since morale is often related to one's capacity to do high quality work that is appreciated by others.

Chapter 11 Summary

Much of the present infrastructure of the medical care system, particularly that of medical education, must be abandoned if we want to adopt new premises and introduce new tools to achieve efficiency and quality in the medical care process. If, in the field of transportation, we wanted to shift from railroads to airplanes, we would recognize instantly that a whole new infrastructure must be built. No one would waste time trying to land planes in Grand Central Station.

In a new system of medicine, a whole industry of producing guidance systems must develop, providers must be randomly audited throughout their careers as they use the guidance systems in the care of patients, all the present facilities for inculcating and storing knowledge into human minds (lecture halls, Board exams, etc.) can be replaced by having the tools that all providers use to do their daily work having built into them the parameters of guidance and currency of information for doing that work correctly.

Since the knowledge couplers and other guidance tools do much to define the language and logic of medical practice, they form a sound basis for more precise communication among not only providers, but also other groups such as lawyers, nurses, and business and government leaders.

11
Can the Present Infrastructure of Medicine Support Radical Change in Premises and Tools?

Lawrence L. Weed

When we look over what has been written here concerning new premises and new tools and their implications at every level of medical education and medical practice, we wonder whether the present infrastructure of medicine can support or even allow such major change. Are we in the position of someone contemplating major changes in the mode of transportation, where it would be totally unreasonable to use the infrastructure of the railroads as the basis for air travel? How should we go about creating a new and satisfactory infrastructure for medicine?

To begin with, certain physical structures could be entirely eliminated and new ones created. Lecture halls, classroom facilities, and the large salary base of teachers for transmitting knowledge could in large part be replaced by computer guidance systems present at all sites of medical action and by sites for the acquisition of hands on skills. The guidance systems would be updated from a national or international coupler building center. The results from the use of such electronic guidance systems would be sent to the national or international coupler building center for analysis and updating of the couplers. The physical laboratories of people doing medical research could be organized around critical masses of people working on the same problems. No longer would each practice/teaching facility need a stable of expensive, prestigious, credentialed experts to set the tone and provide the guidance on clinical cases. The results of research and expertise would be channeled to patients through the couplers built at the central facility. The economic implications of such changes would be very great indeed. Our present system for coupling the best knowledge to everyday action not only has great voltage drops across it, but also is extremely expensive. A system of credentials based on memorizing, regurgitating, and forgetting, and guaranteed financial rewards regardless of the quality of future performance is not only intellectually unsound, but is also wasteful of costly human and physical resources.

Transformation of the System

The nature of the student body will change, and this in turn will affect the facilities that are required for their development in the medical sciences. More and more providers of health care will be people who chose a defined part of the health care system and went about achieving proficiency in that area. Autonomous physicians, empowered by credentials to define their own boundaries of activity and to carve out their own niches without regard for the architecture and requirements of an overall system, will become less and less a factor. If, then, a core of behavior instead of a core of knowledge is taught from the earliest years of schooling, the students accepted into the medical care system will be those with a demonstrated capacity for thoroughness, reliability, and sound analytic sense. They will be capable of more independent learning in the presence of the right guidance systems, structured to maintain standards, control inputs, and analyze outputs. The combination of such students and a well established guidance system will enable the establishment of an apprentice system with the one on one development of master performers for well defined tasks within the total system, much like we have always had in the arts. The apprentice system so prevalent in medicine in the last century failed because the preceptors for those apprentices were not supported by a system that provided standards and helped them negotiate the knowledge explosion and establish a coordinated system of medical care. They did not have the tools we now have to couple thought to action, and in the absence of such tools they elaborated a system of education that has become massive and expensive but not reliable in getting the right knowledge to each everyday action. Some of medicine's greatest present achievements have occurred in spite of the present system and not because of it. Indeed, in many instances, they are the result of islands of an apprentice-like environment that have sprung up in the midst of the present and pervasive memory based, credentialed oriented system.

In other realms, the apprentice system was not abandoned or stifled by licensing laws, because it continued to produce great artists and athletes—the goal of everyone. It continued to succeed because it made time and tasks the variables and achievement the constant, and the marketplace supported those who achieved excellence and simply ignored those who did not. What artist could reach present standards if forced to develop and perform under the conditions that confront a physician—playing anything that others might assign, with something different every 20 minutes in a busy concert hall, reading the music for the first time in the front of a highly critical audience who could sue for every missed note, for infinitely more than the price of the ticket, if they had the right lawyer?

If it is true that the present infrastructure cannot support the new premises and tools anymore than railroad stations could become airports, then how do we create a new infrastructure and where do we start? Frequently, major change starts in the laws and in the courts. Congress can change payment mechanisms and state legislatures can replace the credentialing examinations under present medical practice acts with the requirement that all practitioners and patients use guidance systems. The law should require all practitioners to limit their activities to well defined sections of the guidance system, sections for which random audits have demonstrated a core of behavior adequate to the tasks at hand. The law should also require that all patients be in possession of their problem oriented medical records and that continued audits take place within the rules of the new guidance system. A whole series of major changes will naturally follow.

- The coupler building industry will grow in every field that has to have them in order to function.

- Educators will have to switch their focus from the tyranny of memory and the development of experts, to making people thorough, reliable, and capable of defending everything they do within the boundaries of and rules of their chosen part of the well defined system. The more clearly the components of the medical care system and other systems are defined, the easier it will be to judge competence within in performing assigned tasks within the system. When random audits of competence in performing assigned tasks, not credentials, become the basis for deciding who can do what, then a large reservoir of competent personnel will emerge who charge far less than credentialed experts in various fields now charge. Furthermore, like volunteer rescue squads, volunteer efforts may emerge in many areas and co-op arrangements will be possible.

- The citizenry will become masters of the new tools through continuous exposure and usage and could be more in charge of their own health care, just as travelers with a good set of maps have many options open to them.

- The more the care system is defined and the more the public is informed, the more likely that creative efforts from many quarters will be directed toward technological and productivity advances that will enable better quality at lower cost. At the present time, new techniques and drugs make the system more expensive and on occasion more dangerous when their use is controlled by credentialed experts rather than by guidance systems available to all. Also at the present time, the incomes of specialists may be proportional to the use of the new tools and techniques, thereby predisposing to overutilization.

- As individuals, especially consumers, become more knowledgeable about the health care process, they will realize where, how, and why resources are limited and why priorities must be set. They will recognize the need to do far more for themselves, and they will understand why it is reasonable to give lower priority to those who ignore the guidance systems and fail to maintain health and prevent problems by reasonable measures.

- The diagnostic and management guidance that systems such as couplers provide will prevent individual practitioners working in the system from creating their own demand, as credential based physicians can now do. An informed public will no longer be in a dependency state. The focus will no longer be on the physicians creating a niche for themselves; within a well defined system, the focus will be on personnel of all types seeking roles that best suit their talents.

- Arguments among primary physicians and specialists about the distribution of income from various tasks will diminish. The highest income will go to those individuals who have developed skills that very few other people or machines can match and whose skills can be clearly assessed on the basis of ongoing performance. Credentials based on examinations for knowledge will be abandoned; there will be no financial reward for memorizing, regurgitating, and forgetting.

- Since knowledge couplers do much to define the language and logic of medical practice, they form a sound basis for more precise communication among not only physicians but also other groups such as lawyers, nurses, and the business and government leaders who pay many of the medical bills. The more clearly medical logic is revealed, the more apparent it will become to all concerned that there is much ambiguity to be seen and tolerated when we match the details on unique individuals to the arbitrary and statistically derived diagnostic classifications and management options that biased and credentialed experts and specialists have promulgated over the years. Not only will patients come to see how important it is that they assume a far more active role in asserting their uniqueness and choosing among options, but also their expectations will more realistically match what the medical profession can actually deliver.

Chapter 12 Summary

Those presently in the practice of medicine who have been educated under the old premises and who have never had any opportunity to expand their minds with the new tools deserve a great deal of thought and attention. In even the smallest shift of emphasis from the science of disease to the science of medical practice, we must be careful to do it in a way that does not deprive patients of the continued commitment and dedication of those who are now the custodians of so much specialized understanding and technical skill. It is our hope that many will feel that unreasonable burdens are being lifted from their minds, and that they can now give their full attention to helping the patients negotiate the difficult choices and ambiguities that the new tools present. Also providers can focus on collaborating in a manner that assures each patient that the best technical skills will be brought to bear on their problems. No provider should have to face the unreasonable expectations (and their associated legal liabilities) that our present credential oriented system places on their shoulders. Neither patients nor providers will have to make so many decisions on life and death matters off the "tops of their heads." The new approaches can also alleviate the growing frustration that so many now feel with the bureaucracy of the medical care system. Adherence to necessary rules and regulations can be an automatic byproduct of the use of the guidance tools used by medical personnel to do their work. Society's expectations of providers and patients can be built into the guidance tools through the options they offer and the codes they automatically place on the choices that are made. The computerized Problem Oriented Medical Record (POMR) can automatically provide many administrative byproducts such as auditing, billing and the documenting of how valuable resources are allocated.

Through the new premises and new tools, we can come to terms with modern medicine, and we do not need to be left with a sense of disillusionment. Expectations have not been met, because they have been unrealistic. Many professionals were too paternalistic with patients and too unrealistic about their own limitations. The new approaches can enhance, not detract from, a romantic and happy view of medical practice and medical science.

12
Conclusion

Lawrence L. Weed

It is not surprising that so much of our nation's intellectual power has been directed out into space or into the double helix, where rewards are well defined and the frustrations of dealing with a society that often seems essentially irrational and uncontrollable are largely absent. It is true that failures occur at the sophisticated levels, but they are made in tolerable obscurity and rarely under conditions of frustration and social unrest.

All of us would like to correct the imbalance, to see the organization of medicine well studied and well ordered, without at the same time shifting the weight of research and planning so far that the undeniable benefits of concentration on specialized subject areas are lost (Weed 1969).

In the last 20 years, since I wrote these words, we have continued to gain a great deal of knowledge at the analytical and biological level. And indeed, with three billion dollars planned for the genome project at the National Institutes of Health, we are poised to get a great deal more. But has a good balance yet been struck? As said earlier in this book, not only must we develop a much more rigorous science of medical practice in which our knowledge of how information moves among individuals is as good as our knowledge of nature's information system (from DNA throughout the system), but also we must develop much more discipline in the way we ourselves move information among and for individuals. It is worthy of equal resources and our best minds. It has been too easy to assume that, if we go on collecting new highly focused bits of specialized knowledge, richly rewarding the discoverers in prestige and money, such new knowledge will automatically be used effectively for all of society. There is much already known about the present genome and indeed much known in all of biology and medicine that is not being utilized effectively. There will always be a "voltage drop" from what is known to what is actually done for all the people, but must it always be so great and affairs so out of balance? The new knowledge we need now is the knowledge of how to use knowledge more efficiently and effectively. That we understand the significance of emphasizing such a type of knowledge will eventually be reflected in our educational and reward systems. Presently, as Lipp (1980) states in his book, *The Bitter Pill: Doctors, Patients and Failed Expectations*,

> [B]eing an artful clinician has gradually become a less prestigious and often less desirable goal for talented medical students than being a laboratory scientist....Medical school faculty members remain predominantly research-oriented scientists—and administrators—rather than clinicians with sustained experience with individual patients.

Students in our educational system cannot help but notice that people working in comfortable laboratories at regular hours enjoy the excitement of the research and even the possibility of recognition for understanding a single biochemical mechanism, whereas they never see such comfort, excitement, and recognition in medicine go to a creative and dedicated worker or leader in a big clinic or hospital in the poor and overcrowded inner city. In such places, students are much more apt to see exhaustion, disillusionment, and retreat into laboratories, specialization, or administration.

Much has been written about what is wrong with the practice of medicine and the information systems that support it. Ever since Codman's (1918) trials and tribulations with the medical establishment in 1918, many have made specific suggestions for change, but as Lipp (1980) comments, "like many of us, they are more helpful in analyzing the present state of affairs than saying how it should be different." The premises and tools presented in the foregoing pages are a genuine attempt to outline a conceptual scaffolding upon which a better medical care and medical education system could be built.

Once such a paradigm shift has been established, we should be able to sort out from our current activities in informatics and study of problem solving those things that will be useful elaborations on the new structures, as opposed to those current activities that should be abandoned because they represent little more than analyses and corrections of the efforts of unaided human minds that never should have been allowed to function under false premises and in such a sea of confusion and uncertainty in the first place.

We must acknowledge that simply stating new premises and describing new tools can by themselves assure nothing. In the field of psychology, Robyn Dawes, in his book *Rational Choice in an Uncertain World* (Dawes 1988), reviews in great detail all the evidence that has accumulated over many years that our unaided human minds are far more limited in their ability to recall accurately and to process variables systematically than we care to admit. He shows how little effect this detailed knowledge has had on the daily *practice* of *expert* judgment:

States license psychologists, physicians, and psychiatrists to make lucrative global judgments of the form, "It is my opinion that - " --- People have a misplaced confidence in their global judgments, a confidence that is strong enough to dismiss an impressive body of research findings and to find its way into the legal system.

This confidence grows as experts refuse external aids to their minds and then keep better track of their successes than they do of their failures. As Dawes reasons,

> The greatest obstacle to using external aids may be the difficulty of convincing ourselves that we should take precautions against ourselves. The idea that self-imposed external constraints on action can actually enhance our freedom by releasing us from predictable and undesirable internal constraints is not a popular one.

But it just may be that the problems and unpopularity of the present medical care system and the power and availability of microcomputers have finally reached a point where the necessary changes will be accepted.

Lipp catalogs, in a most articulate, personal, and devastating manner, many of the problems in the present system. He does it through vignettes of practitioners and the frustrations and agonies that haunt them. No one understands these better than Kenneth Bartholomew after his years in general practice in a small town in South Dakota. The sections that now follow were written by Bartholomew to convey how he has used the new premises and new tools to meet the responsibilities and frustrations that confront all busy practitioners. Three years ago, he volunteered to lead an effort to make his small community a health care laboratory. There the problem oriented medical record and the new information tools provided the basis for a system that would not only serve individuals but do so in the context of the health of the whole community. Once we have established in a small community that the electronic problem oriented medical record and its associated couplers can be the basis for an organized approach to the health of a community, we can then use the principles and tools in larger areas where vested interests and turf battles might obscure the value of a new and overall approach.

The efforts of Zelda Gebhard and Kenneth Bartholomew, in Faulkton, South Dakota, may establish from both medical and technical points of view that the principles enunciated in this book can be applied in a busy single physician practice on a multi-user microcomputer system in which all the medical records are in electronic form. It has already been established in other practices that knowledge couplers can be used on standalone microcomputers with printed results being integrated into an overall paper medical record system. Going to much larger institutions may introduce another whole series of technical problems. But it is important to have a model of the total system and what is best for the patient overall, so that, in larger environments with both technical and medical vested interests, we do not get trapped in all sorts of compromises of patient care just because we have made massive technical investments. Most of these technical problems can be solved, but it is essential that our efforts are well organized and deliberate and not just hasty automation of pieces with the belief that they all can be integrated easily at some later date. Until we have a center for coupler building and a full set of diagnostic and management couplers and complete and up to date disease and "property" files in the automated record, available to all physicians on a yearly subscription basis, we will not be able to assess the full impact of Bartholomew's pioneering efforts. However, he has already progressed far enough so that all of his actions and logic are intelligible, and a readily available basis for a fair audit and rigorous corrective feedback has now been established. Eventually many similar sites can become a useful source of feedback to the coupler building center itself.

Following the chapter by Bartholomew are the comments of three other physicians, namely, Burger, Cross, and Yee. Discussions of Problem Knowledge Couplers in other areas of health care are provided by Abbey, who looks at dentistry, and Nelson, who writes on veterinary practice. Zimny and Tandy (1989) have discussed in a separate publication the use of Problem Knowledge Couplers in the clinical practice of physical therapy.

In concluding this chapter, I shall paraphrase some of the thoughts of Lipp and others and comment on how the principles and tools described in this book may help.

Many physicians believe that their own feelings and reactions are among their most important therapeutic tools and that quality control devices do not measure such benefits. They believe they can provide the atmosphere that helps doctor and patient together "integrate information to form conclusions and develop helpful strategies for diagnosis and treatment" (Lipp 1980). There is a genuine belief in their own "idiosyncratic wisdom" and that somehow this will be lost in the midst of modern technology and arbitrary audits of their performance.

COMMENT. The knowledge couplers, when used together by the provider and the patient, assure both that the appropriate details will be elicited from the patient and that the significance of the positive findings will be known immediately to both. The physician can then use his or her skills to help the patient negotiate the results and the ambiguities that arise when the details on unique individuals are matched against the arbitrary groups of facts we place in books and journals. It is at this point that providers will use those "unmeasurable skills and wisdom" that patients seek. In the presence of modern information tools, the patients can select those physicians with whom they feel comfortable, without risking loss of the facts and integration of those facts upon which the personal interactions must depend.

Many physicians and nurses freely admit that when you haven't got the emotional energy and time to be both technically competent and humanely compassionate, something has to give. Both they and the patients have known for years that different people sacrifice different aspects of good care when placed under overwhelming pressures and demands that exceed their emotional and intellectual capacities—to say nothing of the financial temptations and pressures that surround them.

COMMENT. When the unaided human mind is expected to recall and process hundreds of relevant variables on a daily basis, fatigue will overtake it and some important variables will be neglected. Since the provider's credentials depend on examinations for facts about disease and not on a capacity for compassion or getting to know patients as human beings, these latter matters may be neglected by some. Others will just give up in the struggle for competence. The new tools and premises enable us to abandon such a system of credentials and begin to audit for the correct behavior in the use of new and powerful tools in the total care of the patient.

Many people still talk about "my doctor" as if somehow they can find a single individual to whom they can entrust their total care without any risk of significant mistakes.

COMMENT. There is no way to avoid multiple providers to a patient over a lifetime, if one wants the best care for all problems at multiple geographic locations. But the new guidance tools described can assure that the efforts will be cumulative and the diagnostic and management options up to date and properly related to the unique patient's situation. Those who prefer the science and technology of research and the epistemology of medical knowledge can keep the knowledge network and couplers up to date, can develop new knowledge, and can build the best possible hardware to move the knowledge. Those involved in direct patient care can use the new guidance tools, always being up to date since the very tools themselves will have built into them the parameters of guidance and the currency of information for solving clinical problems. After the patient and physician are done using the guidance tools together, they print out the diagnostic and management options they agreed upon along with the details on the unique patient that elicited those options. The doctor is no longer writing after the fact.

Having the patient in possession of his or her own record makes possible the understanding that can assure that the right hand always knows what the left hand is doing.

Many providers of medical care are concerned about the "ominous role of rules and guidelines" and the "breach between doctor and patient" that they may create. Every physician, sooner or later, has disillusioning collisions with the regulatory apparatus, resenting the loss of time that such encounters always involve.

COMMENT. Adherence to rules and regulations should be an automatic byproduct of the use of the guidance tools used by medical personnel to do their work. They are built into the guidance tools through the options they offer, the codes they automatically put on choices, etc. Also the computerized problem oriented medical record can provide many automatic administrative byproducts of the process of documenting medical care, contemporaneously with the use of the guidance tool itself.

Providers of all types are under increasing pressure to "find ways of limiting their emotional responsibility to patients, when the dimensions of their problems overwhelm not only our therapeutic skills but our constricted and enfeebled role on the production line." (Lipp 1980)

COMMENT. The more the total medical care system becomes defined, the clearer it is to the patient what can be expected from whom and at what points in the system. The content of knowledge couplers is interdisciplinary, and the combination of the computerized problem oriented medical record and the knowledge couplers provide: (1) a structure that allows one to see the context and dimensions of all the problems of a patient, and (2) the tools to zero in on any one of them and become informed at any level of depth appropriate to the situation at the time.

For a variety of reasons, many patients make demands for tests and x-rays and treatments beyond what the physician thinks are in the patient's best interests. This often leads to conflicts between physicians and patients that are harmful to both.

COMMENT. Neither physicians nor patients should be making decisions off the tops of their heads at the time of action. The human mind is prematurely biased and knowledge couplers are necessary. If a given problem should not have penicillin as a therapeutic option, it will not appear as an option and the patient will see this. He or she will also note that each option and linkage is referenced. A battle of wits between physician and patient is avoided.

In a mobile society such as ours, there are a large number of "worried well" seeking reassurance from new and ever changing physicians who have not had the benefit of a long standing relationship and all the understanding that implies. Such conditions of contextual ignorance may lead to frustration more than reassurance.

COMMENT. The patient's complete problem list, a copy of which is always in the patient's hands as well as the provider's, enables anyone at a glance to get an overall picture of the social, psychiatric, and medical problems that the patient is dealing with. The Wellness Coupler, Screening History, and Physical Couplers assure a minimal level of depth and breadth to the background data from which the problem list is assembled. Furthermore, the computer organizes all the abnormalities into prioritized work lists.

Evidence of thoroughness and a disciplined and organized approach to problem solving and an immediate printout for patients to take home with them make a major contribution to reassurance of the patient. Knowledge couplers and the patient having a copy of his or her own problem oriented record provide these things. One of the most compassionate things a person can do for another is to help him or her maintain a sense of control over a complex and changing situation. Just as the travel system and symphony orchestras can function smoothly with happy outcomes for the travelers and the listeners in spite of great complexity, so can the medical care system.

It is not easy for physicians and other professionals to find that perfect collection of patients who are just dependent enough to accept our paternalism, and just independent enough to assume responsibility for their health and much of their own care. As Lipp states, for many professionals trying to find their niche in this medical care system, "life is a process of retreat and the patching up of wounds. Retreat from aspirations and retreat from illusions. Wounds of the body and wounds of the spirit. Fortunate people retreat in an orderly fashion, tending to their wounds as they go; the unfortunate retreat blindly, erratically, agonizingly, the wounds open for all to see."

COMMENT. We can look upon the wealthy, organized specialist as one who retreated in an orderly fashion from the illusion of being a total physician under the conditions of the present system. Many general practitioners have been forced into an erratic and agonizing retreat. The specialists now need to understand their role in a new coordinated, non-memory based system based on new premises and tools. The general practitioner needs to shed illusions, carve out of a new well defined system the role best suited to his or her talents and energy and then with all others work contentedly and effectively within the new tools and premises, confident that total care for the patient will emerge. Crucial to the success of such a system is the family and patient being empowered with new tools as they become the central figures in their own behalf.

Through new premises and new tools we can come to terms with modern medicine, and we do not need to be left with a sense of disillusionment. There have been failed expectations because there have been unreasonable expectations. Many professionals were too paternalistic about the patients and too unrealistic about their own limitations. But new expectations do not need to mean loss of the possibility of a romantic and happy view of medical practice and medical science, anymore than discipline and order need to take away the romantic aspects of great music and great symphonies. Indeed, as Stravinsky (1947) has said, without order and discipline, we do not have great art and creativity, we have chaos.

By listening carefully to those on the frontlines as we discover new knowledge and develop new systems, we can slowly eliminate the *voltage drop* from the knowledge seekers to the knowledge users. By putting the right tools in the hands of those who do the everyday work of medicine, we may accomplish more than we will with endless studies by economists, think tanks, and lawyers who just keep telling them things they already know about their behaviors, the variations in their results, and their failures, without at the same time providing the changes in premises and tools that will help them in very concrete ways. It is recognized that new premises and new tools can by themselves assure nothing. They must be used with great discipline under strong leadership or the "clatter of the knowledge industry" and the frustrations of patients and providers will go on. As I look back on some of the things I myself wrote years ago and find myself saying many of the same things 20 to 25 years later, I understand more then ever the cynicism and frustration of many physicians and students.

In 1964, in an early article on the problem oriented medical record:

Conferences, research laboratories, and hierarchies of medical elite tend to obscure the haphazard and careless recording of the daily clinical data upon which all medical care, medical education, and clinical investigation depend....There is nothing wrong with the philosophy that what you do with your patients in a practical way should have relationship to what you know in a theoretical way. When such integration is not possible because the experimental approach and data collection process on the patient's problems are too sloppy and disorganized, then the display of unrelated erudition at the conference level or on rounds is pointless if not immoral (Weed 1964).

In 1969, in *Medical Records, Medical Education, and Patient Care*:

Medicine at its best can be generalized and made available by modern electronic means to each physician. And this aim can and should be achieved in such a way that, as the physician actually records his data and plans his treatments, the very communication tools he uses will have built into them the parameters of guidance and the currency of information he needs to define and solve problems (Weed 1969).

In 1975, in a book *Your Health Care and How to Manage It*:

Thousands of computer displays have been created and more will be. All require the framework of the POMR (Problem Oriented Medical Record) to meaningfully harness them to the pursuit and analysis of real problems....

The final pattern of care for any one person slowly emerges: the patient's uniqueness extracts the right choices at each step from the infinitude of possibilities offered, step by step, by the computer. At the end of the process that unique pattern is clear and complete, but no one could have predicted all its details at the outset (Weed 1975).

In 1981, in an article on "Physicians of the Future":

Corrective feedback loops in medical practice are essential. Growing wiser from outcomes in medical practice is impossible if inputs are undisciplined, poorly understood, or presented in too narrow a context or over too short a time (Weed 1981).

In 1991, here we are, proud of medicine's great technical achievements such as a heart transplant, "a *tour de force* of solitary expertise, which one may admire but not feel obliged to emulate," but still struggling to adopt a total system and new tools that "compel relationships and interdependencies as conditions of physician conduct" and result in "a system that is potent and feasible even in the practice of the average man" (Lawson 1974).

13
The Perspective of a Practitioner

Kenneth A. Bartholomew, M.D.

Couplers from a Patient's Perspective

Problem Knowledge Couplers have been explained in the previous chapters. I will now attempt to give perspectives as developed in my general practice of medicine from actual use and encounters with patients.

Prior to medical school training, I was taught in chemistry to analyze an unknown compound by using a gridlike approach. We would analyze the compound for a series of properties, place the positive findings on a grid, and overlay them on a grid of known compounds. We looked for a perfect match. Being close did not count. A failure to match meant a new compound, or at least one outside of the known compounds we were using for comparison. The gridlike approach allowed us to delineate what we knew and what we did not know about a given compound.

When I entered medical school, I remember very distinctly that I assumed this same approach would be taken in medicine. I remember how excited I was that I would soon know how to break down a problem into its components and arrive at a single diagnosis. However, that is not the way it is—huge volumes of data are memorized and the physician is expected to recall from memory the salient features. The task overwhelms the best of human minds. Given the complexity of medicine and the evolution of it as a science and art, I can certainly appreciate how these unrealistic expectations developed. However, I cannot accept the fact that the system of medical care and medical education is not yet changing.

Patients, on the other hand, have been awed with the rapid advances of medicine over the past 40 years, at least since the discovery of the antibiotics; and not seeing the inner workings of the system, they expect that we can do what we portray on the surface. I firmly believe from my experience that most of the time patients expect that we can take their history, perform a physical examination and perhaps some laboratory tests, and narrow the diagnosis down to a single cause almost every time. This is the mystique that medicine has portrayed over the years, and it has been apparently in doctors' interests to keep the mystique unchallenged. As patients become aware of advanced tools like Problem Knowledge Couplers, however, they will want them used on their problems for several reasons:

- *Patients are concerned* about their problems or they would not be in the office in the first place. They want the physician to be every bit as concerned about their problems as they are. The patients have a vested interest in the outcome of the encounter, much more so than the doctor. They are willing to pay the high price of professional care, but they expect the highest performance in return.

- *Patients want thoroughness.*[*] Nothing upsets a patient more than a physician "brushing the problem off" as unimportant. It has been my experience that they can be quite satisfied with an ambiguous outcome or a non-diagnosis as long as they are satisfied that the approach has been thorough.

- *Patients not only want thoroughness; they expect and demand it.* Because we are professionals, and because of our high fees, they rely on us to be thorough as a matter of course. Although they often accept less, they do not expect less. In fact, patients often expect this to the point that they carry the attitude into the doctor's office that theirs is the only problem that we have to deal with that day.

  The profession has presented itself as the highest form of professionalism and as the noblest scientific endeavor. Hence, the public has come to feel entitled to demand this level of care and legally we are held to that standard. When a patient outcome goes awry, the patient often seeks a legal remedy. They have even been willing to pay our high prices for this entitlement so long as they receive the highest level of concern and thoroughness.

---

[*] A word of definition needs to be said about *thoroughness*. Too often, faced with the pressures of time and liability constraints in practice, doctors and patients believe thoroughness means covering all possible fronts indiscriminately. This is how defensive medicine arises. In contrast, the concept of *thoroughness* represented by couplers involves a thoughtful and discriminating selection of the options. The values underlying this process relate to many issues, some of which are generic and some of which are unique to the individual. Only some of these values relate to cost.

- *Patients are learning to assess the quality of their care.* As they become more educated and more aware of the ambiguities in the practice of medicine, they learn that they need to know enough to protect themselves against poor medicine. Patients today, like never before, have come to question the necessity of surgery, the use of drugs, and the reliability of our opinions. As patients see tools like the Problem Knowledge Coupler, they are starting to become aware that they can to a considerable degree, begin auditing the performance of their doctors, at the very least by asking critical questions, and that it is legitimate for them to do so. Furthermore, a good litmus test on their doctor is for the patient to gauge the doctor's response to such questioning.

This is not only necessary but good for medicine. The patient can see the ambiguities involved and question performance before they are so disgruntled that they hire a lawyer to audit the performance for them. Lawyers only know one way to audit performance, and that is with a lawsuit. Physicians who get upset or, as is so often the case, outright angry when questioned either have something to hide or are terribly insecure in their knowledge. Examples of this are so common that they hardly bear repeating for physicians or nurses, but lest a patient not be aware of this, I would like to cite an actual example.

Case 1

Patient K.M. had presented with a temperature of 105° F and prolonged seizures. The patient's mother had called from the farmhouse. Being appraised of the severity of the situation, I accompanied the ambulance to the farm, started an I.V. in the living room, and immediately gave a dose of the anticonvulsant, valium. On arrival at the hospital, I finished a complete workup and instituted antibiotic therapy after the appropriate blood cultures and spinal tap had been performed. I then took the patient's parents aside and explained everything that I could explain to them in layman's terms, this being my usual custom of practice. I informed them that although I was quite sure that I had done everything appropriate for this case, because of the severity of the illness, I wished to consult by telephone with a pediatric specialist. (I do not as yet have Problem Knowledge Couplers for the workup and management of febrile seizures.) The parents were quite pleased with this. The pediatrician informed me that he had nothing further to offer and thought that the case had been handled very well. I reassured the parents further about the conversation and the remainder of the patient's care went uneventfully. Some months later I was out of town and my practice was being covered by a different physician. Patient K.M. again presented with a high fever and, although he was not having recurrent seizures, his parents were extremely concerned. The covering physician did not explain much of anything to the parents, and as their level of uneasiness grew, they asked about a second opinion. The covering physician then literally ordered them into the waiting room and even went so far as to say that their other children could not come in with them because he had something to say to them. He closed the door and proceeded to tell them that he was a "highly trained professional" who knew what he was doing and, "I do not need second opinions like Dr. Bartholomew." The parents promptly and probably wisely took their son to a distant facility to see a pediatric specialist at that point.

When this story was later related to me, it was painfully obvious that the parents knew that anyone who does not think he or she needs any help or advice and claims to know it all probably has some serious problems. If on the other hand, this physician had simply communicated with them, told them what he was doing, and reassured them from hour to hour during the crisis situation, they probably would have developed a rapport and enough confidence in him to at least let the care go on somewhat longer. Because of his attitude, they strongly suspected that there was something wrong with his care.

The point of this story is that, whereas physicians have over the centuries thought that medical matters were too complicated for lay people to understand, patients in general can understand fairly well what is going on with a given situation even if they do not know the complex medical terminology or the intricate diagnostic and treatment regimens that we employ. Not only can patients fairly quickly grasp the essentials of a case, but with their increasing sophistication they are demanding this type of involvement and demanding explanations of their care. They will no longer simply sit back and say, "Doctor knows best," because often they have seen that doctor does not know best. As Problem Knowledge Couplers are developed for both diagnosis and management of particular problems, patients will become more and more involved in their own diagnosis and management.

My experience using couplers in the clinical setting has given me the gratification that patients' wants and needs as outlined above are continuously met by the couplers. Not only do the patients see the thoroughness involved in the use of couplers, but they sense that we care enough to give them the kind of thoroughness that they feel entitled to. With the coupler's systematic review of details in the patient's life that could be relevant to the current problem, the patient feels that his or her individual situation has been thoroughly examined and all possible conclusions have been taken into account. In management couplers, they further see the many different combinations of therapy and understand that the care of a complex, long term problem requires a detailed understanding of the patient's unique situation, followed by a careful monitoring of the options finally chosen. Even when a diagnosis is still in question, they have, in my experience, been completely satisfied with the outcome of the encounter. In addition, by receiving a printout of the findings and possible causes, they feel empowered to review the situation at home and to watch for signs and symptoms that may aid the diagnostic process in the days or weeks to come. The use of couplers teaches them that there is a time course to disease and not all signs and symptoms necessarily occur "by the book" or simultaneously. By thus empowering our patients with information, as opposed to leaving them in a void, we reinforce their collaborative role as part of a team working toward an understood goal. As we shall see in the next section, it is only when this occurs that the optimum physician/patient relationship is built.

Although the heading of this section is *Couplers from a Patient's Perspective*, let me add one last thought lest anyone get the idea that patients' views are totally separate from physicians'. What happens when a physician or member of his or her family gets sick? He or she demands the best, seeks five or ten local opinions, self refers beyond the local community to a Mayo Clinic type setting, and expects as a matter of course to be given a copy of the medical record! He or she, if there is a specialist somewhere in the country who subsubspecializes in the particular problem, will telephone or visit that specialist in person. This is not a condemnation of this kind of behavior; it is simply human nature. So why should we expect that our patients would want any less? We should be willing to give our patients exactly what we would want if we were the patient. Furthermore, the patients know that there are different tiers of knowledge within the medical hierarchy so we only look foolish by trying to portray it otherwise. More and more, patients are breaking our secret code. We have all been lied to by adults since we were children. We gave up our belief in Santa Claus. Likewise, patients do not believe that "Doctor knows best." As students, we were misled about many things, not the least of which was that we could remember all the facts, pass a test, and practice excellent medicine if we continued to read journals and memorize facts. Perhaps this was true once. Perhaps the explosion of knowledge outstripped the schools' abilities to deal with this change sociologically and educationally. As science expands, we need tools to extend our minds as well. Teachers can no longer answer all of our questions and we know it. We can no longer answer all of our patients' questions and they know it.

Couplers from a Doctor's Perspective

My experience has now made it apparent to me why, from the patient's perspective, couplers are needed. This is not so easily apparent to other physicians. At first glance, couplers appear more time consuming, which they are, and too exhaustive for the routine everyday practice of medicine. It would seem that we need not look for rare things every time. However, this becomes a self fulfilling prophecy because, by not looking for rare things, we do not find them; therefore, they are rare. We become convinced in our own minds they are so rare that they do not warrant looking for, and the cycle has been completed. If things were that simple, we could conveniently make a home "cookbook" for patients to follow, and medical school could be shortened to two years. In truth, the textbook case is so rare that everyone runs to look at it in the medical center when it is found. Patient presentations are not one textbook scenario but thousands of similar, yet unique combinations of presentations that our experience enables us to categorize. The rare patient, however, does not want to be categorized and shuffled off, because it is those rare cases that have to live with the missed diagnosis.

Physician may ask themselves, "Why should I use Problem Knowledge Couplers?" There are, indeed, several reasons why we should use couplers on a routine basis. First, let me dispel the notion that they are extremely time consuming if used properly. Certainly the first few times using a coupler will be time consuming, but no more so than reading a textbook chapter on a given problem. In my clinic we have experimented with nurses (and an occasional medical student doing an elective month in the practice) doing the "pre-workup." This is the bulk of the time consuming process. When I enter the examining room, I have a coupler that is largely done. With a good nurse, a large portion of the common physical findings can be entered in the computer and a note left if something is in question. The physician then rechecks any physical findings that are positive or questionable. This is, in fact, extremely time saving and allows you to, in Dr. Weed's words, "Become a consultant in your own practice." The physician in this setting enters the equation at a higher level of expertise and, instead of spending the whole day gathering mundane data, spends much more time reviewing the complexities of the cases that need that extra caution to the patients' benefit. Furthermore, I must admit that the practice of medicine in this setting is simply more fun. It is more fun because it is more intellectually rewarding, and this in itself is an excellent reason to be using couplers. By having this extra time to spend on more complex cases, the physician can then begin to use the couplers to function at a higher intellectual level than a busy practice usually affords. I charged headlong into the couplers and began learning simply by using them. Because of the timeliness of data that is built into the couplers, and since they are so pertinent by being problem oriented, I do not need to spend 20 or 30 minutes going through indexes of textbooks to find what may or may not be appropriate information.

Using Problem Knowledge Couplers has, for me, become an enjoyable experience, now that I am comfortable with them. The couplers are full of information; I have never failed to learn something new each time I have used one. If this is true for an experienced clinician, think of the value that they would hold for medical and nursing students! Using couplers begins to become a reinforcing loop—because they are fun to use, you use them more. The more you realize that valuable information, beyond your own personal store of knowledge, is being brought to bear on each of the patient's problems, the more secure you feel, the more patient gratification you generate, and the more gratification you have from your practice.

For those who would ask, "Why not go on as we have, making a good living doing adequate medicine for the majority of cases?," I would answer, "Because that is intellectual poverty! Good physicians do not want to be technicians. We enjoy challenges and we love to be right! Gratification from our work is an essential human need and appears to be a very key ingredient to avoiding professional burnout." When I have used couplers and explored all of the possibilities with the patient (the patient or appropriate family members having been at the computer terminal developing the coupler with me and seeing all of the ambiguities involved), I have never failed to be gratified after discharging the patient. I leave the encounter knowing that I have looked at the possibilities; furthermore, I know that the patient and/or family members have seen the great complexity involved and are immensely satisfied that the possibilities have at least been thought about. They leave with a printout to review at home at their leisure. They are told that they are free to take that printout to a specialist and to seek a second opinion with my blessing if they feel a need. I have nothing to hide. In today's malpractice climate, that gives me a feeling of confidence that they are satisfied with the fact that I have done my best. I certainly go home at night with a sense that the day's work has been completed. I am not left with a lot of nagging questions and loose ends that, for me at least, cause sleepless, dream filled nights.

Another use for couplers is medical record keeping. Unless you have owned and operated your own clinic, you may not see all of the hidden overhead expenses that are involved, including medical record keeping. Normally we see a patient, take a verbal history, perform a physical and perhaps order lab tests, and then dictate that history and physical and a summary of the laboratory data. This requires doubling up on our time, once to generate the information and once to regurgitate it into the dictaphone. The information must then be transcribed and filed into the medical record. With the use of couplers in the examining room and a printer at each terminal, all three steps are accomplished concurrently. A final dictation or direct entry can then be made into the medical record portion of the computer program simply indicating that the coupler was run and giving the final impression or impressions and plans. It becomes redundant to regurgitate all of the information at that point since it has already been generated, dated, and printed on the coupler printout. This frees the medical record technician by at least 50% to accomplish other tasks in the office. Therefore, the initial cost of setup will not only be regained in your own time but in your overhead time. Still another reason to use couplers is that they can be tools for avoiding malpractice risks. Essentially all of the reasons stated above are cumulative in acting as malpractice avoidance maneuvers. The best malpractice avoidance tools are excellent doctor/patient communication, comprehensive patient care, and meticulous record keeping. How the patient's or their family perceive the thoroughness of that care is extremely important. There are physicians who have very superficial medical practice skills, and yet their interpersonal skills are so excellent that their patients would never think of suing them. They perceive that the doctor is doing a good job, and most importantly they perceive that the physician cares about them as a person. A computer program cannot change your interpersonal skills, but it can certainly show patients that you are thorough and you care enough to be thorough. In actuality, most physicians do care about their patients but they do not come across that way because they are so busy or because their mind is on serious medical problems and not on social etiquette. They are constantly rushing, which often comes across as a non-caring attitude. They are usually preoccupied with a heavy load of problems they are concentrating on which comes across as being unfriendly. The patients often do not see the amount of time we spend in our inner office thinking about their case, dictating notes, and reading about their problems. In fact, this has been systematically hidden from the patients to carry on the aura that we have all of this information in our head. With the amount of time spent with the patient in the use of couplers as well as the computerized medical record, the patient comes away much more satisfied that they are being cared for in the best possible manner. Furthermore, the use of couplers engenders communication between patient and doctor. Lastly, as I will explain in detail in the section on the computerized medical record that follows, patients who possess a copy of their own medical record have the complete feeling that their physician trusts them and has nothing to hide from them. Informal polling of my patients who have been through any part of the process of generation of their computerized medical record or coupler usage have expressed complete satisfaction and, in fact, admiration of our project.

Couplers and Medical Education

It is well documented that the medical literature is gravely underused by practicing physicians because of both time constraints and accessibility. The efforts to keep current are difficult and poorly accomplished at best. The couplers have the currency of data built into them and, as outlined above, are specific to the problem at hand. Furthermore, the electronic nature of the information can be updated quickly while a textbook is becoming outdated. In fact, information in a textbook is often becoming outdated by the time the ink is dry. If you enjoy teaching medical students and nurses, as I do, then you will benefit from the use of the Problem Knowledge Couplers and the computerized version of the problem oriented medical record system in that teaching. One of the things that dismayed me most about medical school was that it took so long to get a real feel for exactly what the world of medicine encompassed. There are so many synonyms and so many redundant terms or terms that are so similar with only a slight difference in meaning and yet are used synonymously by different physicians in different parts of the country. For all of medical school and most of my internship, I felt that I was only operating in a small portion of the medical world. As I began to see the disorder in our medical terminology and its usage and how this had confused me, I realized that I must not have been alone in that feeling. Until we define our world more succinctly and more thoroughly, the practice of medicine will remain very much an art while at the same time we try to claim that it is a highly refined science. Science can only be done well when the terms of that science are well defined. By using Dr. Weed's system, we have begun to define terminology; we limit the use of synonyms so that all levels of staff, not only doctors and nurses, can interact in a more effective way. This not only facilitates teaching but it makes it more enjoyable for student and teacher alike. The use of couplers in the teaching process begins to define exactly what parameters to look at for a given problem. We teach medical students to do a two hour physical and yet, while fine for learning physical diagnosis, it does not aid them in defining a toe problem. We would spend hours on the eye exam in medical school, and yet I never saw one planter wart the whole four years of medical school. Now I treat at least two per week and had to teach myself to do this! My practice is replete with examples of that nature. The use of couplers begins to hone our skills to the problem at hand and that is the essence of learning. It then becomes much easier for a teacher to see where the student needs more work: time and task become the variables, and excellent performance becomes the constant. In teaching we are taught, and this feedback helps our knowledge base grow. For instance, although I usually learn from a coupler, I have found areas where I have felt that a coupler was deficient. What happens then? At this stage of development, I make a printout of the portion that I feel is deficient and then write my reasons on the printout or make a typewritten critique and mail this to Dr. Weed. Acting as editors, Dr. Weed and his wife, also a physician, evaluate and document the added information and, by editing, update the coupler. Can you imagine the teaching possibilities around the country if all medical schools used couplers and there were one central "Library of Couplers" for editing and building couplers that could support semiannual or annual updates and produce new couplers? The cumulativeness of our combined knowledge and experience would serve to bring the practice of medicine to a level of excellence seen only in isolated elite areas around the country today. The cumulative benefit to the public at large is hard to comprehend.

Living with the unknown is harder than any hard work. I am a stickler for detail. I want to know and perhaps more importantly, I want to know when I do not know. We can only recognize what we do not know by seeing the total picture of what is known about a given subject. It is not good enough to be close. I was awed many, many times in medical school at the quickness with which a diagnosis was made. In actuality I was impressed that professors and residents could make certain diagnoses so quickly and wondered when I would be smart enough to do the same. However, as I began to learn more, I found out that not only did I not know all of the ambiguities, but often my teachers did not know them either. They seemed at least outwardly content to intuit most of the time. The following is a case in point. We had a patient with a vaginal discharge. The professor and an ob/gyn resident in the clinic

244

Kenneth A. Bartholomew

that day heard a one minute history, observed a two minute physical exam, and took a quick look at the saline prep under the microscope. "That is classic Hemophilus vaginalis," they said. (Now known as Gardnerella vaginalis.) Knowing at least something about microbiology at that stage, I asked how they could know for sure if it was that particular bacterium since most of them look alike on a wet mount slide. The answer I got was, "It's classic." They could give me no more criteria than that. "But," I asked, "if it is so classic, why can't you give me more criteria?" What they were really saying to me was that there was a 95% likelihood based on presentation and probability that it was Gardnerella. They probably believed that they were 99.9% correct and were very comfortable with that. What they probably did not realize was that they had made a 100% diagnosis for that patient based on a 95% probability. (In fact, physicians often defend to the death a bad decision, once they have taken a stand.) I was not comfortable with that type of decision making then, and I am not comfortable with it now. The use of couplers will force our teachers and us alike to develop in a very systematic way exactly what criteria we know about a given problem and begin to look in very critical ways at how much we do not know about a problem. Furthermore, we will let the patients see this ambiguity, and they will not expect 100% accuracy in diagnosis and management. This is only logical, since we cannot guarantee them 100% correctness in diagnosis or 100% satisfaction in outcome even with the best management we know how to give.

Another striking example of why couplers should be used in the teaching process is one of the first cases I had while on cardiology rotation as a senior medical student. The patient presented with a heart murmur. I was wracking my brain trying to remember all of the different types of murmurs, how each one should sound through the stethoscope, and where on the chest each one should predominate. Two senior staff physicians and one cardiology fellow listened to the patient and, lo and behold, there were three different interpretations of the same murmur! This was a major turning point in my medical education. I had assumed up until that point that I was not making diagnoses with enough conviction because I did not know enough. While I surely did not know enough and still do not, suddenly I found out that three physicians specializing in cardiology could not tell what kind of murmur this patient had for certain. Yet, during the anatomy and physical diagnosis portions of medical school, we were told to memorize and regurgitate information that we assumed was 100% reliable. Suddenly I found out that only after the cardiac catheterization was completed would we know the answer for sure. I am not saying those physicians should have known what kind of murmur it was by examining the patient; I am simply saying that they should have been honest throughout medical school with their level of knowledge and the reliability of the knowledge that we have to date. Instead, many of them held themselves out as nearly infallible, giving the medical students, the nurses, and the patients the appearance of applied science as being infallible. What then should we expect from patients who have a missed diagnosis or mishap in treatment except a lawsuit? The patients can only assume that someone made a mistake when, in fact, they are not privy to the ambiguity that is involved in the practice of medicine at this stage. The use of couplers in that case would have given us a very good look at exactly what we know and what we do not know about heart murmurs, and everyone would have been operating under the same assumptions. Most importantly, everyone would have been operating with the knowledge that sometimes assumptions have to be made because our knowledge, even under the best of circumstances, is lacking.

The two cases presented above tell of ambiguities in diagnosis, but the ambiguity in medicine does not end there. It is generally assumed that if the right diagnosis can be made, then the right treatment can be applied. A third case, which was related to me by another physician is in order. While in medical school, on an internal medicine rotation, a patient presented with diabetic ketoacidosis. A general practitioner had admitted the patient to the hospital and had instituted a plan of care for the unambiguous diagnosis of diabetic ketoacidosis. While making rounds with an internal medicine resident and an attending physician, the medical students were "allowed access" to the "fact" that the local doctor's care of ketoacidosis, while probably "adequate," did not seem to meet the standard that they would have used. Shortly thereafter they were presenting the patient to a professor of internal medicine who gave a different plan of treatment, which was "superior" to the other three physicians' plans. This intrigued my friend and his medical student colleagues and prompted them to do some research on their own. They read the current journal articles and textbooks and polled several physicians, and then compared all the treatment plans. The only treatment modality that seemed to make any critical difference was the institution of high volume I.V. fluids. All of the gospel on different modes of administration of insulin, special diets, etc., were not agreed upon. Needless to say, this opened those students' eyes to the ambiguity in medical treatment just as the first two cases had opened my eyes to the ambiguities in medical diagnosis. If the medical establishment cannot hide this even from junior medical students, we certainly should wonder why we persist in this type of behavior.

Town and Gown and Continuing Medical Education

I know that I am not alone when I say that the demands of the workload of everyday practice in a small town is such that I am often denied the enjoyment of simply sitting and reading journal articles. I love to read. In fact, I would categorize myself as a compulsive reader. Yet I feel like I am neglecting my medical reading because of the demands on my time to practice medicine. I would like nothing more than to make morning rounds and then spend the fresh morning hours between 10:00 am and noon reading and upgrading my education. However, there are many days when I have arisen at 6:00 a.m. and have had 20 to 30 patient encounters by noon. Where then do you one find time to read to keep your knowledge current? The working answer to this is in Problem Knowledge Couplers. This puts the currency of data right up front with the relevance of that data. We then have at our fingertips what we need to know when we need to know it. Coupler builders and editors must then continuously sift the literature for the best information and put it at the fingertips of the busy practitioners. By doing so, we meet our needs at the same time that we are meeting the needs of our patients, and both parties are gratified. Medical schools are often criticized for not meeting the needs of practicing physicians. For years I have heard about the supposed conflict between "Town and Gown." This conflict exists only because they have different goals. Just as conflict occurs in patient encounters when the goals of doctor and patient are different, so do the conflicts between "Town and Gown" occur when their goals are different. Unfortunately, this need not be the case. Most medical school professors are interested in research and teaching, and most town physicians are interested in doing a good job of practicing medicine, both intellectually and financially. Personally, I see no conflict in the two endeavors since the town physicians can do their job only if taught correctly and kept up to date by the medical school professors. The goals are not different. The final goal is to take care of patients and to do it exceptionally well. Only short range personal goals vary within the context of this overall goal. Therefore, the medical schools need to deliver to the hands of practicing physicians the tools by which to accomplish this task. Is a lecture on the cytochrome P-50 system in albino rats delivered in Paris, France, the type of tool the practicing physician needs? Yes, that type of research needs to be done, in fact must be done, to analyze systems and figure out how they apply to humans. I admire those who can do this. What need not be done is to terrorize students and non-university based physicians with these lectures and then expect them to apply that knowledge in a busy emergency room at 3:00 am with a patient dying before their eyes. Practicing physicians need the information perfected, sorted, and synthesized into a usable format: the Problem Knowledge Coupler is that format. If the professors of medicine at the medical schools deliver that type of tool to the practicing physicians, they will be lauded as visionary. If they cannot sort, perfect, and synthesize, what does that tell us about our level of knowledge? On committees I have been associated with in medical schools, one of the problems that the medical school people see is how to foster communication, and therefore, better understanding between "Town and Gown". I ask you, what better way can there be to foster communication than a working relationship such as the building and perfecting of couplers and the use of these couplers on patient care? There will be an automatic communication system set up and when a problem is encountered with a coupler, a phone call can be generated to the medical school and the problem immediately addressed. In my opinion, the conflict is a conflict that should not exist and exists only because the two groups have not identified their common goal. A lack of communication exists only because of the conflicting goals. Solve one and you solve the other.

Couplers From a Business Perspective

Lastly, a physician must look at couplers from a business perspective. If what I have said above is true, and couplers can be used efficiently from a cost and time standpoint, then couplers become a very wise business tool. The malpractice avoidance portion of that business decision has already been addressed. From a strictly business point of view, what are we trying to accomplish? A successful businessman will continually try to give the consumer the best possible service for a competitive price. Doing so insures consumer satisfaction and therefore insures repeat business. Nowhere is repeat business more important than in a professional setting. If patients are getting the thoroughness and type of personal care that they want and expect, then not only will they become repeat customers, but they will refer friends and relatives as well. This is already happening in my practice. I have had patients bring in relatives from many miles away, who have been followed by very good board certified physicians, because they felt that I had something to offer that they were not getting elsewhere. My review of the physician's care revealed absolutely nothing that could be challenged or criticized, but the patients did not know this. They did not see the ambiguities involved with their care. They were not educated in their care to the extent that they wanted to be educated. Therefore, they did not know if their care was thoughtful and thorough. They have stayed in my practice and I can only assume that it is because they are satisfied that the above needs are being met. The use of Problem Knowledge Couplers, therefore, from this perspective is simply good business. In summary, if all of the foregoing criteria have been met, then we have a system in which the patient's needs and goals and the doctor's needs and goals have fused as one. There is no longer any antagonistic conflict between the patient and the doctor and true teamwork has evolved with one goal in mind, that being total, thorough, and thoughtful patient care with satisfaction generated for both parties. In so doing, I believe that we have reestablished the traditional and time honored doctor/patient relationship but have taken it one step further. It is no longer a parent/child type of relationship but becomes more like a relationship between true partners in diagnosis and management. Instead of the double edged sword it is today, the doctor/patient relationship becomes a tool in itself. Being an instrument rated pilot and a lover of aerobatic flying, I continually see parallels in aviation safety and medicine. I am compelled to close these thoughts by quoting Gerard Bruggink, a retired National Transportation Safety Board Safety In Human Factors expert:

Aviation character is the triumph of humility and common sense over arrogance and overconfidence....Whatever individual traits we associate with aviation character, they all support the notion that character governs the quality with which we apply our skills and knowledge to the task at hand. Character generates the mysterious force that often holds things together when aviation's grand design comes apart at the seams. However, when a spectacular "save" would justify conferring the ultimate in accolades the display of aviation character we limit our praise to stereotyped references to just a few character elements such as professionalism and dedication.

Although the most spectacular test of character lies in the handling of a rare emergency, its unremitting test is the monotony of routine operations. It takes more than certifiable skills and knowledge to tip the scales in favor of safety when invitations to complacency abound. Under these circumstances it is the staying power of character that insures the quality of human performance. If this sounds like a misty notion at a time when we put all our money in engineering, regulatory, and procedural solutions for human error problems, consider some of the occurrences that have embarrassed the industry, worldwide, over the last few years.

Bruggink went on to cover such events such as deadstick landings of two air carrier jets that were out of fuel, crew induced engine flame outs in three others, a crew of two who locked themselves out of the cockpit during cruise flight, loss of control at high altitudes, etc.

I would add removing the wrong kidney, operating on the wrong knee, operating on patients whose cardiorespiratory status was totally malfunctioning, giving a medication that the patient is known to be allergic to, and myriad other examples of high technology losing out to prudent care. Everywhere in the above quotation that the term "aviation" is used, you could simply insert "medical" and the quote would stand unchallenged. Let us then use the tools of our age to meet the unremitting test of monotony of routine interaction so that a routine case does not become an emergency. Let us begin to use tools like computers and Problem Knowledge Couplers to give the type of care that we imply by our words and actions we are capable of giving.

The Computerized Problem Oriented Medical Record

I have always believed in good medical records not only to document what I had done at any given time, but because I saw from the beginning that the medical record was the tool with which to follow the patient's progress and whether or not a given modality improved or hampered the patient's recovery. Dr. Weed published his book, *Medical Records, Medical Education and Patient*

Care, just three years prior to my starting medical school. I can recall reading articles in medical newspapers about him and his problem oriented system. However, in medical school we were not taught (or at least did not appreciate) all the implications of a complete problem oriented medical record. We tried to identify each problem and make a plan for each problem, but, although this was stated as an admirable goal, we were not really held to the task and never really learned the true value of the complete system. When I began practicing medicine, I thought that I had excellent medical records. In fact, compared to many, my records were quite good. One Medicare reviewer even made the comment that "I wish we could use Dr. Bartholomew to teach other doctors how to keep records." However, I could see that something was lacking in our paper system early on. It was difficult to track problems and track laboratory data because of the need to source orient the charts so that lab data was always easy to find in one area of the chart. Furthermore, I began seeing a few years ago that keeping the medical record in the office and giving the patient verbal instructions did not get the job done. Data were constantly being lost at the level where they most needed to be retained, i.e., at the patient's level. It did the patients no good to have me do an excellent workup, keep excellent records, and then give them verbal instructions that they promptly forgot or confused. Patients, especially elderly patients, continually came back with the medications mixed up—taking the wrong dose or the wrong medicine, etc. This is not an isolated problem. This is an extremely common problem throughout the country and the world. I quote from an actual chart:

J.H. brought all but one of his bottles to the clinic today. He had not been cutting his Moduretic in half but had been taking a half tab of Glucotrol. It became obvious after about 15 minutes of reviewing medications with him and then with his wife that he does not pay any attention to his meds. He states that his eyes are not good enough to see the small print and the color of the pills so he lets her do it all.

Therefore, I began giving my patients instructions in writing several years ago. This became very tedious and time consuming. In a busy practice, it became difficult to force myself to do this thoroughly each time. I realized that there had to be a better system of accomplishing this and it was then that I began looking at computerization. I was quite disappointed, however, at the articles about computers and medicine. Each time I would see a journal that had an article labeled "Computers and Medicine," I would rush to pick it up and begin reading. It soon became evident that there was a pattern of articles that were talking about "Computers and Accounting" as applied to medicine. Article after article appeared on various bookkeeping and financial record keeping systems, billing systems, etc. I was disappointed that there was nothing about the practice of medicine and computers. I began that search in 1983, and in 1986 I met Dr. Larry Weed. He was speaking at a conference in

Minneapolis, and I immediately recognized his name and picture from the articles I had seen in medical school. I, therefore, made it a point to go to his talk and was absolutely enthralled by the simplicity of his concepts and the design of his software. It was, in fact, the type of system that I had assumed they would teach us when I entered medical school. I was eager to institute such a system in my practice.

I have a very busy practice; I am the only physician in the county. I had thought for several years that patients should have their instructions in writing, but Dr. Weed carried this one step further. He felt that they should have their entire medical record in their possession. This way they could see how the different variables affected their care and how their actions might affect the different variables. We, therefore, came to the conclusion that one of the goals of our project would be to have my patients possess a copy of their own medical records. I am extremely gratified to report there have been no negative feedbacks from my patients who possess a copy of their medical records and only one equivocal reply. That was from a gentleman in his eighties who stated that he would take the medical record home but he probably would not read it because he would not understand it. However, when asked if he would keep his list of medications tacked to his refrigerator with a magnet, he said, "Absolutely," because he would then be sure to take them correctly. Although he was not excited about having his whole medical record, from his perspective, he was very happy to have the one thing he saw as important for his particular needs. Therefore, I would have to say that the acceptance has been 100%.

Let us now look at how the computerized medical record varies from a paper medical record and how it is used in an operational sense. I will use real patient encounters as examples; these points are real and the problems do need addressing. The classical medical record is what is known as a *source oriented* chart. In this type of medical record, the progress notes are kept in one area in chronological order with all of the patient's problems mixed together as they present over time, and all of the laboratory and x-ray data are kept in a separate area of the chart. Charts have evolved this way because it is administratively convenient and easy to retrieve from the chart. A *problem oriented* medical record, however, has each problem's progress notes and relevant lab data collated under a title for each problem. While it is clinically logical to format paper records in this fashion, it becomes cumbersome operationally to make certain retrievals. For example, if laboratory tests are done for one problem but also have a bearing on another problem, you will have to page all the way through the chart to find all of the laboratory work since it is spread out within the chart under other problems to which it is also relevant. Therefore, it becomes a matter of expedience to place all of the laboratory data in one section, i.e., the "lab work" section, of the chart for ease of retrieval in the future, but without regard to the clinical logic of that arrangement. By applying the technology of the computer age to the problems of medical record keeping, Dr. Larry Weed and Richard Hertzberg have solved both problems. Now each problem has a heading (problem title), but the computer keeps all of the problem titles at the top indentation level and all other types of data pertaining to that problem subsumed to that heading at lower indentation levels, as in an outline. Therefore, you only need to look under those headings if you want to review the progress notes that pertain to that particular problem. The problem list will have all of the problems at the very first level of entry, and you need not look underneath a given problem unless you want to. Counter this with a paper record where you usually have to page through all of the data, and data of varied categories, to find that for which you are looking. An actual problem list appears below.

Top of Record

PROBLEM LIST:

1:	Health Care Maintenance	
2:	Allergies (Xylocaine, Flu Shot, Valium, Ampicillin, Oil Base Injections, Verapamil)	
3:	Atrial Fibrillation	(1-22-87; 2-11-87)
4:	Hypothyroidism	(1956)
5:	Pap Class III - suspicious for malignancy	
		(3-27-85)
6:	Coronary Atherosclerosis	
7:	"Fluid Retention"	
8:	Visual Acuity, decreased	
9:	Urinary Tract Infection, acute	
10:	Neck Injury	(2-25-80)
11:	Appendectomy	
12:	Ovarian Cystectomy (X 2)	
13:	Migraine Headache	(1956-present)
14:	Diverticulosis	
15:	Herniorrhaphy (Bilateral Inguinal)	(1973)
16:	Tonsillectomy	
17:	Actinic Keratosis	
18:	Neck Pain	
19:	Chest Pain	
20:	Weakness	
21:	Shoulder Pain	

Now, let's take an actual problem such as Pap Class III and follow its development over time. We would simply press key #5, and then Pap Class III would come up to the top of the screen. The problem list would disappear (as if it "moved" off the screen to the left). Beneath this we would add the *problem set*, which consists of the following concepts:

Goal
Basis of Diagnosis
Status
Disability
Follow Course—Parameters and Treatment
Investigate Cause
Complications to Watch for

These seven headings are the problem set and are entered under each problem so that each problem is followed consistently using the same format throughout the patient's chart. This not only makes it easier for the physician but also easier for all other users, including the patients themselves, to follow each problem and its related information. The next two levels of entry would then appear as follows.

Pap Class III - suspicious for malignancy (3-23-85)

Goal
   Rule out cervical cancer
Basis
   Pap smear
Status
   Stable
Disability
   None
Follow Course - Parameters and Treatment
   The patient was found to have a Class III Pap smear in 1985.
Plan
   Follow with pap smears q 3 months until negative.
      Pap Class I - Normal - 1986
      Pap Class I - Normal - 1987
      Pap Class I - Normal - 1988
Investigate Cause
   Colposcopy with biopsy - only if Pap smears remain positive
Complications to Watch for
   None at present

In this particular case, the problem was a self limited problem and therefore was quite easy to follow. (We also notice at a glance that the patient did not follow up every three months. That was before we started this project and before she had a copy of her own record.) Another one of this patient's problems, however, is atrial fibrillation, and the list of notes under *Follow Course* is 34 entries long and 7 levels deep. This includes laboratory tests of multiple types. You should then be able to see that each problem can now be followed almost at a glance instead of having to page through all of this patient's laboratory and progress note data. Admittedly there is a little more initial capital investment in the work required at the outset to set up the charts initially to accommodate this structure, but time is saved in the long run over and over again. Imagine a carpenter who does not organize his shop and tools and may waste one to two hours looking for a certain tool till he ends up borrowing it from a neighbor because his own tool is, in effect, lost in the chaos. Countless times, I can recall looking for laboratory tests that I was sure had been done on a patient but I could not find in the record. With the computerized medical record, I can find any laboratory test in a matter of seconds. By using the flowsheet function of the medical record, I simply enter the laboratory test in the parameter section and then do a retrieval request from the whole chart. The computer promptly displays the test results in flowsheet format in chronological order, regardless of the original problem for which they were ordered.

There are other medical record programs that will search for laboratory data in this way, but the Problem Knowledge Coupler (PKC) system has taken this one step further. Residing in the flowsheet program is a function which assigns a number to each of the lab tests. Selecting on that number takes me back into the patient's chart at the point where the test was entered, thereby permitting me to review not only what the lab value or result was, but also when it was performed, why it was performed and what problem it refers back to.

The format is completely variable. There are multiple levels of entry but each level can be bypassed if desired and there is no bottom limit to the chart. A chart can be as long or as short as you wants it to be without wasting computer disk space. Most of the computerized medical records systems that I have evaluated enter a block of space on the hard disk for that patient's chart. That space is taken up whether or not anything is entered into it and, once it is full, you cannot expand it. With the PKC system, this patient's chart is enlarged gradually as data are entered into it just as a paper record would be, but with electronic speed. With the multiple levels of entry, each given encounter or each thought is entered in the form of an outline for a manuscript. The beauty of this is that the flow of thoughts and flow of logic actually have a physical outline to them rather than a continuous unstructured typed page format. A problem can also be upgraded as follows. Suppose this patient is later found to have cervical carcinoma. The problem Pap Smear Class III would then be called up on the screen under "current element". Now the problem statement can be modified by typing M and then respecifying the medical entity to Cervical Carcinoma. We would then modify the description so that we do not lose the original information. It would now look like this on the screen.

Cervical Carcinoma   6/9/89
   (Presented as Class III Pap Smear 1984)

Without this structure, we would have had a list of typed unstructured narrative statements that spoke about Pap smears being normal and Pap smears having Class III findings, spread out throughout the chart. Now, as the problem and diagnosis take shape over time, we can make the record cumulative. This saves an enormous amount of time by not having to redictate another note about the prior Pap smear history; all the relevant information is pulled together in the chart under the problem title and automatically dated by the computer, so that both the chronology and the clinical logic of the problem formulation are clear. A note should be made here about ease of use. Any new task seems complicated when you first begin to learn it. The design of this software is simple and clear. We have been able to implement it without any computer literate staff. If you can read English, you can figure out where to go next on the chart. There is no computer jargon to be learned with this system. It is based on normal language. Furthermore, because it is so simple, like any other tool you use a lot, it becomes automatic. I can find a patient's problem list or I can flowsheet three lab tests simultaneously without ever looking at the screen. Just as touch typing becomes automatic to the point where we do not think about the command going from the brain to the index finger, so it no longer is necessary to think about using the program or to think about the fact that we are using a computer. Our fingers flow around the keyboard just as they do when touch typing because everything is single key entry. In no time at all, the computer is no longer a formidable learning task but a very easily used tool to make patient care more manageable and less time consuming. When that level is reached, and it is reached quite quickly, the computer phobia that some people exhibit abates very rapidly. As I stated above, we started with a staff that was 100% computer illiterate, yet we have never had a problem training someone to use the system, nor have we ever had a problem losing large blocks of data.

The Medical Entity List

Diagnoses, laboratory tests, medications, x-ray tests, and virtually anything else the operator wishes can be stored in a separate file called the medical entity list. Medical entities are kept in a separate file and keyed to the patient's chart so they are available for future searches. For instance, the problem Diabetes Mellitus, Type I, has been entered in the entity list. When you want to enter that problem in someone's chart, simply press #1 for Problem List, keystroke *A* for Add, *M* for Medical Entity, type *Diab* and press the Enter key and all of the entities starting with "Diab" appear at the top of the list. We then press key #1 which corresponds to Diabetes Mellitus, Type I, and the whole entity is entered in the patient's chart automatically in the same format every time and with the correct spelling, etc. It is stored in the patient's chart as the entity number, using only one to five characters and saving disk space, rather than stored by text, using 5 to 40 characters. When entered as a medical entity, we can then at any time search all of the patients with Diabetes Mellitus, Type I. This powerful feature makes this a useful research tool as well as a practice analysis tool. For example, imagine the value of this when a drug that was formerly thought to be safe is now found out to be unsafe and is being recalled from the market. Every patient in the practice who is on that drug can be found in a matter of seconds and each patient contacted individually. This would take weeks or months in a paper record system. Also the record system can be analyzed by record number or birth date. At the time of this writing, we are in the process of doing a mailing for all children who need Hemophilus Influenzae, Type B immunization. We have searched all of the records according to birth date and have searched out only those children between the ages of 18 months and five years and within a couple of minutes have generated a list of all those to whom the letter is to be mailed.

Recently, changes have been suggested in the use of female hormones. Therefore, I needed to search my own practice population for anyone on estrogens, and anyone on progesterones, and anyone who has had a hysterectomy. The computer program can search these separately or in combinations, so I have used the AND/OR/AND NOT function, chosen the AND mode, and all three parameters have been combined into one search and printed out in alphabetical order. This is enormously helpful utility in getting an otherwise time consuming, labor intensive job done. These are just a few examples of how the rapid and accurate retrieval capability can be used to "manage" the clinical aspects of a practice.

The Property List

In addition to the medical entity list, each entity has what is termed the property list. The property lists reside in a file indexed to the entity list. Such items as dose or cost or indications/contraindications/warnings or ICDA codes, etc., are properties. The property file allows rapid access to the important information on a given entity. This file is open ended and anything can be entered into it that you might later wish to retrieve quickly. Currently, we are trying to make a brief synopsis of the *Physicians Desk Reference* (PDR) in the property lists so that when a patient is placed on a medication, the important aspects of a medication can be seen at a glance with two key strokes. Compared to having to look this information up in a book, this retrieval from the property file saves an enormous amount of time. With a terminal in each room, drugs can be reviewed at the time of being prescribed, and generic names, actions, synonyms, warnings, contraindications, tablet or solution strength, and dosage range by weight and age can be reviewed in less than a minute. It often takes five to ten minutes using the book. An actual example follows for Ciprofloxacin HCl.

Cipro (Ciprofloxacin HCl)   (2092)
Synonyms: Ciprofloxacin HCl (Cipro)

Property List:
  Class = = = = = > Fluroquinolone Antibiotic Action = = = = > DNA-Gyrase
  interference

  CONTRAIND. = >   Quinolone Allergy
  CONTRAIND. = >   PREGNANCY AND CHILDREN
  WARNING = = = >   CARTILAGE DAMAGE-immature
      "   = = = = = > CNS disorders
  Precaution = > WELL HYDRATED, crystals
      "   = = = = > avoid alkaline urine
      "   = = = = > renal insuff., decrease
  INTERACT'S = >   prolongs theoph. 1/2-life
      " = = = = = >   Antacids w/ mag. or alum.
      " = = = = = >   probenecid- >1/2-life
  Meals = = = = = >   preferably not with
  Pt. Ed. = = = = >   dizziness, lightheaded
  Adverse = = = >   nausea 5.2% diarrhea 2.3%
      " = = = = = >   vomiting 2% abd pain 1.7%
      " = = = = = >   headache 1.2% restless 1%
      " = = = = = >   rash
  Lab change = > Hepatic, renal, hematol.
  Adults = = = = >   250-750 mg q 12 hours
  Duration = = >   1 week to 6 weeks-severe
  Tabs = = = = = = >   250, 500, 750 mg.
  Reviewed = = >   2/15/88, KAB

Another use for the property list is the use of ICD-9-CM coding for
diagnoses. For instance, Diabetes Mellitus, Type I, has the property
ICD-9-CM = = = = = >250.01. With this in the property list, my secretaries can
simply find the entity Diabetes Mellitus, Type I, and look at the property list
and find the correct code number in less than ten seconds. Additionally, a
Fasting Blood Sugar would have a property listed as *CPT = = = = =>82947.*
When my nurse enters the blood sugar result, he or she can simply write the
code number on the billing slip saving the front office personnel an additional
step. Eventually, if the program is expanded even further, these billing tasks
could be done electronically when the test is entered in the chart. We are also
currently building the property lists for any given lab or x-ray test. An example
of this would be an oral cholecystogram (OCG), an x-ray test of the
gallbladder. When a physician orders an OCG, it then becomes not only the
nurses' prerogative but the nurses' duty to check the property list of that test.
The physician should also have reviewed it, but given that it may have been
a telephone order and the physician may not have been in the hospital at the

time or may not have yet gotten a terminal installed at home, it then becomes feasible to have the nurse check the property list of an oral cholecystogram. The nurse would call up *oral cholecystogram* from the entity list to place it on the patient's chart which could be called up by typing oral or OCG, since oral cholecystogram and OCG are listed as synonyms within the entity list. The nurse would then pick the number off the list that corresponds to the proper entry and Oral Cholecystogram would appear in the chart regardless of which synonym was chosen. With oral cholecystogram now being the current element in the program, simply hitting the letter *C* twice would give the property list of OCG.

Property list of Oral Cholecystogram:

Low Fat = = = = = = = = > Diet for 2 days
Telepaque = = = = = = = > 6 tabs day 1, 20:00 hrs. Telepaque = = = = = = = > 6 tabs day 2, 20:00 hrs.

NPO after = = = = = = > Midnight before test
Diarrhea = = = = = = = = > prevents absorption
Diarrhea = = = = = = = = > excessive, D/C Telepaque
NON-VIS = = = = = = = = = > if bilirubin >3.0[1]
CONTRAIND. = = = = = > Allergy to Telepaque
CAUTION = = = = = = = = = > Iodine Allergy
Reviewed = = = = = = = = > 1/27/88, CW/JM/KAB

Now the nurse can quickly check the patient's bilirubin results after seeing the message

   NON-VIS = = = = = = = > if bilirubin >3.0

If the bilirubin was greater than 3.0, he or she could quickly bring this to the physician's attention and have a test canceled that otherwise would have been a waste of time, money, and x-ray exposure for the patient. The time savings and money savings for the patient is obvious, but in the day of DRGs, it is now in an institution's financial interest not to run useless or redundant tests. With a terminal in the radiology department as well, the x-ray technician would also check the property list for OCG. The technician would then see what the preparation entails and what contraindications might be associated with this test. The technician could then quickly browse the patient's problem list to see if that patient has any contraindications to the test. This type of shared responsibility and shared treatment of the patients is not currently being done in medicine. Lab technicians, x-ray technicians, medical record personnel, and registered nurses are left out of any of the deeper level decision making processes in medicine. Since everything is based on a memory system, it is assumed that the physician is the only one who can make these decisions. However, with a system that empowers the nurses and technicians, we effect not only more efficient patient care, but much better patient care at a higher level of expertise. There are many physicians who do not want to give up this authority or have anyone else able to question their competence. Yet, when a mishap occurs, everyone is looking for someone else to blame. Too often people have their own hidden agendas within their working relationships with one another, MDs and RNs not excepted. If our overall goal is good patient care, then we simply must find the best means by which to effect that goal. From the patient's point of view, there is no conflict between physician, nurse, and laboratory technician. The patient's only goal is to get well.

It is only when we look at goals in the big picture that this suddenly seems so simple. One last word on simplicity of use—something can be simple to use but if it is not convenient it will not be used. There are programs out now that give us a look at drugs, drug interactions, lab tests, and disease information; but when all these programs are placed on one hard disk, people are intimidated against using them because of the need to know how to exit one program and enter another, something that is not always done easily. It often entails exiting to DOS, changing directories, and knowing secret passwords to get into the new program. This can be intimidating to one who knows nothing of directories, subdirectories, and passwords! Richard Hertzberg has solved this problem for users by building all these functions into one program. No exiting to find things, just a few keystrokes from an English menu, and you are where you want to be. Even a separate file on diseases is being started so that you can look up the information about a disease and its diagnosis and management in a few seconds. Knowing a little bit about human nature and its tendency to take the path of least resistance, I believe that this is the only way you will get people to routinely access the information that is available for patient care.

Computerized Medical Records: Philosophy into Action

Now that I have given an operational description of how the computerized problem oriented medical record works on the personal computers, we can look at how we have implemented it in my clinic and community hospital, how it has affected the way we practice medicine and affected our approach to patient care. In order to do this, we have to examine just what the medical record is supposed to be. If you believe that all that record needs to be is simply a hastily jotted note by the doctor to remind himself what he did at a certain moment in time, then you certainly have no use for the tool I am referring to here. In reality, the medical record is many things to many people. It is:

- A flowsheet of data changing over time and affected by interventions such as diet and medication

- A legal document that will make or break a malpractice case in a court of law

- A diagnostic tool for arriving at a diagnosis

- A teaching tool for medical personnel from physician through nurse's aide

- A teaching tool for patients

- An audit trail of the performance of individuals within the health care system, and of the system itself.

Only when we look at the medical record as indeed encompassing all of the above points will we begin to see why it is so necessary to have this tool help us rather than hinder us.

The medical record as the chronicle of changing data over time cannot be argued and the completeness with which it is kept will show what changes occurred with interventions, such as diet, drugs, exercise, etc.

The medical record as a legal document is also without question, and it is the consensus among malpractice attorneys, both prosecuting and defense, that cases literally hinge on the medical record. I will go on to demonstrate later in this discussion that the medical record as developed here is another type of legal tool as well—it is one to avoid the malpractice suit in the first place.

The medical record is a diagnostic tool in and of itself may be questioned by some. Let me illustrate this point from an actual case. Patient R.B., an ex-smoker with chronic obstructive pulmonary disease, was seen by another physician for cough. As best we could ascertain from the medical record for that visit, the medical encounter consisted of the following:

Bronchitis - Tetracycline 250

The diagnosis of *bronchitis* in this case was based on no specific evidence recorded in the record, i.e., no symptoms, physical findings, or tests recorded as the basis for the diagnosis. What was the presenting complaint? Cough? Fever? Sputum production? Chest pain? Shortness of breath? Bloody sputum? We don't know, and the physician probably will not remember after about two weeks. We only know what one doctor's conclusion was based on an unspecified or unrecorded constellation of findings. Was there a history? Was it complete? Was a physical examination done? Was it complete? And furthermore how do we know that the practitioner knew what he was hearing when he auscultated the chest? Finally, did he make a logical conclusion based on the data available at that point in time? When that patient came to see me, I defined the problem as Cough. The past history was listed as

Bronchitis alleged several months ago—Treated with Tetracycline

but the presenting problem was

Cough.

As the story unfolded, it became clear that the patient was developing congestive heart failure, at first manifested only by the ticklish cough as the fluid irritated his lungs. Whether or not there ever was an acute infective bronchitis, we will never know with certainty. With careful following, the medical record then began to reveal the story for anyone to see, not the least of whom was the patient himself. Had good documentation not been a requirement, he may have been treated over and over for *bronchitis* and the diagnosis of *congestive heart failure* never arrived at until he showed up in the emergency room at 2:00 a.m. in the morning drowning in his own fluid.

A good medical record becomes a teaching tool for physicians in seeing how certain modalities affect patient care and what variation there is in the flow of any given problem. A good medical record becomes a teaching tool for the other medical professionals as well. One of the most gratifying outcomes of the project in Faulkton has been watching the growth and development of my medical records technician, Zelda Gebhard. In the last two years she has gone from being a typist sitting in a cubicle typing whatever I spewed into a dictaphone to a real partner in patient care sitting in my inner office as we continue to develop and apply Dr. Weed's computerized medical record system. Zelda herself has admitted that in her first years of being a medical records technician she never gave much thought to what she was typing. Her job was to correctly type, collate, and file lab tests. Since there was no cohesiveness of design or thought processes in a chronologically ordered paper chart, the flow of the problem was not there for her to see, let alone understand. Without the medical training the bits and pieces over time were not appreciated by her and, of course, she did not have time to go back and review all of the prior data. This tool has made her think critically about what she is doing, what we are doing, and why we are doing it. With the computerized medical record, she needed to know what was going on in order to know where a particular note or particular lab test should be entered. She began to see the flow of ideas and just as importantly began to see how we define problems in medicine. Now, it is very easy for her to think critically about the performance of *locum tenens* physicians as she sees the neatness or sloppiness of their thought processes, whichever may be the case. Someone once said that, "To misstate the problem is the greatest sin." Hopefully that has been shown by the *cough-->bronchitis-->congestive heart failure* problem portrayed above. Now, when other physicians work for me, and they make a diagnosis such as strep pharyngitis without having done a streptazyme test or throat culture, Zelda brings this to my attention by asking if this should be listed as *strep pharyngitis, pharyngitis*, or simply *sore throat*. I can see her growing ability to analyze the problem and to apply the rules of clinical evidence to support diagnostic accuracy. It makes me wonder if medical schools have failed overall in teaching doctors to think critically and scientifically about these questions. In this case, this tool has transformed Zelda from a typist to more of a partner in patient care, a change that has been to everyone's benefit, patients included. If she can do this with a medical record technician's background and training, with no clinical hands on experience, just think what it can do for technicians, nurses, and physicians as they begin to mobilize their capacity for critical thinking rather than making hasty assumptions based on partial data with poorly thought out plans. I am further convinced that patients know this intrinsically.

The medical record is a teaching tool for the patients as well. A key element in our project here has been to get as many medical records into as many patients' hands as we can, given the limitations of our minimal budget and our single user system. By possessing a copy of their medical record, the patients also begin to look critically at not just the medication involved but at the total picture of what is going on with their health. They begin to look at each problem and learn to grasp the concepts of how to examine their own record in the framework of, "What is the goal? Basis? Status? How do we follow this problem? What are the complications to watch for?" They can also view their complete problem list as a whole, can ask questions about it, and can even question my diagnoses. Since many of these charts have been formulated with the patient sitting with me at the terminal, most of these questions have already been answered. Keeping a thorough problem list is more difficult with a paper record system. We may fail to take time to add a problem to the problem list. The problem list on the front of a paper record has a way of getting cluttered; we may be tempted to defer in order to see whether that problem is going to turn out to be a minor, self limited problem, not worth a place on the master problem list, or whether it is going to turn out to be a long term problem. We may need time to deliberate how we wish to define it, i.e., *cough* vs. *chronic bronchitis* vs. *congestive heart failure*. Since the problems are often left off the front of the paper chart on the first encounter, they may never get put there for later analysis. The computerized medical record requires that each encounter be problem oriented in order to enter the data and use the system. We must define a problem in terms of the defining evidence actually present.

Do we have the evidence to name it *strep throat* or do we only know it is *sore throat*? Not only does the computer automatically assist us in constructing the problem list, it also prioritizes the problems for us. When we modify the display weight of a problem, we can determine the order in which the computer automatically displays the list, without losing data: the most important problems at the top of the list and the minor, self limited problems at the bottom. By having a complete problem list, we have, at a glance, an overview of what a particular patient's health is like, or at least how often that patient seeks medical advice. For instance, imagine a problem list of five problems and a problem list of 30 problems in two people who are the same age. The immediate Gestalt of looking at these problem lists is that one patient is generally quite healthy and the second patient is either quite ill or at least seeks medical advice very frequently. I do not like to write off patient's problems easily to psychiatric or psychological problems. In fact, it may be that I do not make the diagnosis of psychosomatic illness or depression often enough. However, when I do make a diagnosis of depression or psychosomatic illness, I document my reasons and review the complete problem list with the patient. If, after starting an antidepressant, six other problems on the problem list improve (headaches, insomnia, marital problems, and almost continuous sore throats, earaches, and sinus congestion), then the patient and I can raise the issue of whether there are interrelationships among these problems. This becomes very important in helping patients understand their own problems and to begin to deal with them whether they are anatomical or psychological. If a diagnosis of psychosomatic illness is arrived at by the physician but not agreed upon by the patient, then either there needs to be further testing or further communication. The record has served its purpose in fostering that communication. Will psychosomatic patients hound you to death? I have found the opposite generally to be true. When they do come in they now know they have to define their problem very exactly. If they come in as often, it is because they are getting what they need from the doctor/patient relationship—understanding, caring, and communication.

The Problem Set

The problem set as described earlier encourages the patients to think more critically about their problems. It is not immediately apparent that these concepts—Goal, Basis, Status, Disability, Follow Course, Investigate Cause, and Complications To Watch For—could have an impact on the approach to patient care. However, the fact is that the more I used this problem set, the more I began to realize how important each of these parameters is in the analysis of a given problem. Previously, I thought most of this was self evident. Clearly, each of these parameters may need to be addressed in a given patient. The parameters may change within the same patient from problem to problem, and in fact, the patient's other problems have a great effect on how we approach the seven parameters for a given problem. Therefore, a complete problem list is essential.

Goal

If we do not think about the goal on each given patient, we may not give optimal care. I had not been used to thinking carefully about the goal. I supposed it was self evident or implicit. However, since cures cannot always be effected for every problem, it is very important to consider each goal for each problem individually. Let us look at the patient with hypertension. On most patients, I would write the goal underneath hypertension as follows:

Hypertension

Goal
Keep blood pressure below 150/85

This seems like a reasonable goal. It may be varied a little depending on the patient's age and general condition, but most people would agree that it is a reasonable goal. However, suppose the patient's problem list contains the entity *lung carcinoma, terminal.* Now, what is the goal for the patient's hypertension? The goal is to totally ignore the hypertension, which would take years to cause any complications, and let the patient die in peace rather than being made ill or wasting money on office visits or antihypertensive medications, since the lung cancer is going to kill him before the hypertension does. The goal in this case should be to ignore the hypertension for the sake of quality of life for his remaining days. I have now come to realize that we must establish goals earlier and with more forethought and precision. We cannot set a goal for our patients' medical problems unless the patients participate in goal setting as part of a team effort. Without involving patients in that step of decision making, their uniqueness is left out of the equation. For instance, can we force an 84 year old man to accept treatment for adult onset acute leukemia or cancer of the lung knowing that the treatments are very poor and often make the patient quite ill while not effecting a cure? Or if we have a patient whose problem is *smoking* and we establish a goal of *smoking cessation*, we will simply be at odds with the patient if she has come right out and told us that she has absolutely no intention of stopping smoking. Doctor originally meant "teacher." We need to educate these patients, but it is my opinion that all we can do in this situation is give them the information and let them deal with it. They are the ones who make the ultimate decision and not us. If you harangue a patient too much, they simply stop coming in. Then what have you accomplished? Instead, give them the hard, cold facts in their medical record, and let them decide their own fate. Without giving these factors due thought and without involving the patient, there is no way we can effect total patient care. And we cannot involve patients without sharing the information with them. Therefore, it becomes mandatory that the patients possess a copy of their own medical record.

Basis

The basis for arriving at a diagnosis for a given problem is not to be taken lightly. If during an encounter a patient states that he has had rheumatic fever, a good physician will immediately want to know how that diagnosis was arrived at and whether or not there are implications for long term cardiac health. If the basis of the diagnosis was "severe sore throat as a child," the diagnosis of rheumatic fever will carry much less weight than a basis that shows culture proven strep, acute arthritis, and a new heart murmur. Outlining very carefully what depth of precision we are operating at when we arrive at the basis for a diagnosis not only allows medical personnel to see the level of our expertise but allows patients to understand why these diagnoses were arrived at. For instance, each of two patients may have *coronary atherosclerosis* on the problem list, but the basis for its being there is "chest pain when exercising" in one case and "angiography shows 90% occlusion of left main coronary artery" in the other.

Disability

There is no way we can assess the level of disability a given problem causes without proper discussion with the patient. This depends more upon who the patient is and what they do than it does upon the problem itself. For instance, a ruptured Achilles tendon may have absolutely no effect whatsoever on a cement finisher who spends most of his time on his knees, and yet would be a total disability for a professional basketball player who can no longer walk effectively, let alone run and jump. The occupational realities of the individual patient have a great deal to do with how the medical problem produces disability in that individual.

Follow Course—Parameters and Treatment

We may make exquisite notes and make exquisite plans; yet, if the patients do not follow these plans at home, what real good have we done? As I stated in my opening section, I became aware quite early that this information, given verbally, gets forgotten all too quickly. In fact, there are studies that show that verbal information given in the inner office or examining room is lost up to the tune of 65% or more by the time a patient checks out at the front desk and leaves the office. This has been established on exit interviews—and even if the figure was only 20%, it would be unacceptable. How then can we accept that somewhere between 30% and 80% and, in some patients with memory loss, 100 percent, of the knowledge we thought we were imparting to our patients is lost before it is ever acted upon? As scientists, we absolutely cannot tolerate this type of "voltage drop." Information must be given to the patient in writing for their further review at home. With the computerized medical record this can be accomplished in an extremely time saving fashion. When I used to write out instructions in long hand I was doing double duty. I had to print it out neatly in large letters so that those with visual difficulty could be sure to read it and then I had to go back to my desk and dictate the note. In essence, I generated the information twice. By putting this information in the plan of the medical record, it becomes merely a touch of three keys to print the information for the patient. Let me give you two good examples of why it is important for the patients to have a copy of their medical record and how the medical record is a teaching tool for these patients. Patient J.N. is a one year old who had either a persistent or recurrent otitis media for five months. The mother failed to bring him back for follow up on four occasions from January through June of 1987. In June when we began using this system full time at the clinic and began little by little giving patients their charts, the mother saw my note and my admonition that follow-up on these problems is important or hearing loss could result. When she was able to review the fact that she had missed follow-up several times and the child had recurrent infections vs. infections that were never completely cleared up in the first place, something apparently struck home because she has never missed a follow-up visit since then and we have eradicated the effusions in this child. Hopefully, he will not have any long term hearing deficit because the second problem here, proper parent education, did not go on for two to three years.

The second patient does not have such a positive outcome. Patient J.S. is an older, overweight, smoking, diabetic who over the course of several years never did get to the point where she was all that interested in stopping smoking, controlling her blood sugar, exercising, or losing weight. She would take her medication for high blood pressure, and she would take her insulin, but that is as far as she wanted to be involved. Despite recurrent admonitions that she do so, no change in behavior was affected. After seeing the progress notes that very succinctly stated that she had not been exercising, that her weight had either been stable or going up rather than down, seeing her blood sugars ranging in the 200 range, and documenting no cessation of smoking, I made the comment in the record, "The patient is obviously not that interested in getting these problems under control," and she agreed. The patient recently had a mild stroke, and in the hospital she said, "I know it is my own fault and I should have done those things before and I am absolutely going to do them now." It would have been much better had she done them several years ago and prevented the problem but at least with this type of care and openness of communication the patient did not blame me for the decline in her general health. She now sees very clearly where the responsibility lies and who has control of the variables, and it is my contention that only when this is done universally in medical practice will the malpractice crisis be ameliorated.

Complications to Watch for

This section of the problem set is specifically intended for the patient's information. Patients often complain that doctors do not tell them what to expect in a given problem. In fact it has been the basis for a large number of successful malpractice cases. Having the complications to watch for in writing allows them peace of mind to at least know some of the major things to look for. Our patients who have a copy of their medical record and are on the anticoagulant Coumadin, for instance, know exactly when they should be calling or coming in. This saves untold unnecessary calls. Each of the above examples were problem specific but there are three more general examples of problems in the medical record that instruct patients—Allergies, Medications, and Health Care Maintenance. Let us look at the first four problems on all our problem lists.

Problem List

- Incomplete database (on every patient's problem list until erased by physician)

- Health care maintenance

- Allergies

- Medications

First, let us look at how we have formulated a patient's health care maintenance problem and what it might entail.

Health Care Maintenance

> I DO NOT WISH TO BE KEPT ALIVE BY ARTIFICIAL MEANS IF
> THERE IS NO REASONABLE HOPE OF MY RECOVERY.

Immunizations Tetanus-Diphtheria: booster every 10 yrs Diphtheria/Tetanus Toxoid, absorbed 8-8-89; Flu Shot Yearly Age 65 / Chronic Disease
    Influenza Immunization 10-2-87; 10-14-88; 10-26-89;
Overseas Travel
  - Cholera: Immunization only approximately 50% effective and suggested
      only for high risk workers or areas. Their tour company demanded
      that they have this.
          Cholera Vaccine: 7/16/88 <0.5 cc subq now and again in 3
             weeks>

Cholera Vaccine: 8/5/88 0.5 cc subq

Malaria: Chloroquine Hydrochloride 300 mg elemental (500 mg of the phosphate) once weekly - start one week before trip.

Traveler's Diarrhea: Doxycycline Hyclate <1 po bid X 10 days if severe diarrhea develops and an MD cannot be located <KAB/zg>

Seat Belt Use Limited

USE THEM! They can save your life!

Diet   Low Sodium Diet Low Cholesterol and Saturated Fat Diet

Physical Exam & Blood Tests Annually
Breast Self Exam Monthly Breast Exam Annually by Physician Mammogram Annually: Mammography 1/26/88 IMPRESSION: MINIMAL DUCTAL HYPERPLASIA. NO RADIOGRAPHIC EVIDENCE OF MALIGNANCY ON TODAYS STUDY.

Mammography: 11/89 FINDINGS: PATIENT HAS VERY BENIGN APPEARING FIBRONODULARITY IN THE MAIN PORTION OF THE BREAST PARENCHYMA. THERE IS POORLY DEFINED DENSITY PROJECTING MEDIALLY AND INFERIORLY IN THE RIGHT BREAST WHICH IS STABLE AND UNCHANGED FROM THE STUDY 1-26-88. RECOMMEND ANNUAL FOLLOW-UPS.

Call In January For Exam and Tests Pap Smear Annually Pap Class I -Normal 1/09/87 Call in January for Exam and Tests Pap Class I - Normal 1/26/88 Call in January for Exam and Tests Pap Class I -Normal 1/11/89 3+ endocervical cells, trace rbc present, atrophic.

Call In January For Exam and Tests— —

Risk Factors:

Family History of Colon Cancer Family History of Breast Cancer

Family History of Diabetes Mellitus— —

Health care maintenance is a good illustration of the cumulative value vs. fragmentation of paper records. With this system, once it is done, it is done. You know exactly where to look for information, and it takes less than five seconds to do so. In a paper record it keeps getting covered up or cluttered up.

Certain standard problems always appear on the problem list. For example:

Allergies/Sensitivities/Adverse side effects:
        Penicillin = = = = = = = = = = = = = = = = = => Hives
        Ceclor = = = = = = = = = = = = = = = = = = => Hives
        Feldene = = = = = = = = = = = = = = = = = => GI Bleed

Each medication is displayed on the problem list under the problem for which it is a treatment. But also, a medication section is actually displayed as a separate item on the problem list, for the administrative convenience of being able to review all medications quickly, and so that all current and discontinued medications can be reviewed at a glance. This takes the appearance of the following:

Medications

    Current Therapies
        Indomethacin (Indocin)   12/23/88
            <25 mg po tid with food>
        Calan (Verapamil HCl)   8/22/89 <SR
        - 240 mg daily>
    Discontinued Therapies— Enalapril Maleate
        7/03/88
            <5 mg q hs>
    Procardia (Nifedipine)   5/20/88
        <10 mg po tid>

Finally, the medical record can be used as an audit trail to track the performance of the health care system as a whole. The health care system can be looked at as a single physician, or clinic or the health care system in the United States as a whole. While it may be true that physicians do not want their performances audited, it is now becoming a fact of life that it is being audited on a routine basis. Medicare peer review is a fact of life, and insurance companies in the last three years have adopted auditing of performance as a standard for reimbursement. The structure of the medical record described here serves as an audit. Unfortunately, the style of *post facto* audit carried out by the federal government on Medicare patients often takes the form of fingerpointing and backbiting three to four months after the patient has been discharged and the intricacies of the case have long been forgotten. This is like testing someone on biochemistry, then moving on to physical chemistry and not giving them their test scores in biochemistry for four months and expecting them to have gained anything by the testing experience. Audits should be done on current patients under active care with current decision making fully documented in timely records. The atmosphere should be educational, not adversarial. It should incorporate suggestions for improvement and should be backed up with objective documentation. The physician being audited should not be made feel intimidated by a punitive atmosphere but should feel stimulated and intellectually challenged by the process. When I undertook this project with Dr. Weed, I welcomed the idea of having someone with knowledge and experience examining my charts, I found I could relish the learning experience; I can not say that I ever relish the experience as practiced by the PRO four months after the fact by anonymous auditors. Performance audit is becoming a standard fact of life in today's practice of medicine; it is time we have the tools to do it properly.

I will illustrate with an actual case from my medical records. Patient L.P. presented for care in our clinic while I was on educational leave and told the *locum tenens* physician that he was feeling weak. The physician did a battery of tests and one of the problems that he placed in the medical record was *high serum iron*. He stated that the etiology of the high serum iron was unknown, but he was stopping the patient's daily ingestion of iron sulfate supplements that he had been on for years. The physician had failed to do a rectal examination and failed to find that the patient was bleeding into the gastrointestinal tract. Therefore, as the patient digested his own blood, his serum iron shot up temporarily while he was, in fact, losing large amounts of iron in his stools. His blood count dropped precipitously and two weeks later the same physician, who had just stopped L.P.'s iron, now gave him a shot of injectable iron because he was, on this occasion, thinking strictly of the anemia that had now surfaced. (But he had apparently not referred back to the problem list and reviewed what he had just done two weeks earlier.) Over the next two weeks, the patient began having black and then grossly bloody stools and presented to the hospital for admission with significant anemia and weakness. Luckily the patient had not bled to death in the meantime. That physician was doing "incident medicine," reacting to each incident separately. Had that physician used the medical record as a diagnostic tool, he may have started to put together the presenting signs and symptoms and come to the correct diagnosis sooner. If a person is basically a sloppy thinker then perhaps no tool can help him, but the tool may give the patient the ability to seek a second opinion elsewhere, and a second physician can then put together the data and make a correct diagnosis. In this situation a physician who was not used to practicing comprehensive medicine but who was forced to use a good medical record system (via dictaphone) had his audit trail laid out before him. Since auditing of performance is becoming a fact of life with Medicare and insurance companies, it is in their best interest as well as the patient's to have the proper tools with which to do this. Throughout all of this discussion, the

concept of patient involvement, and possessing a copy of their medical record
has hinged around patients being involved in their care. I am continually
plagued with patients going to a specialist and getting a $2,000 workup and
then dropping in over my lunch hour to ask me to explain what went on (for
free) since, "The specialist was too busy to explain anything to me," or "They
don't explain things in plain English like you do." As we have a population
of patients who become more and more aware of the problems involved with
medical care and who become more educated about medical care, the patients
will soon be demanding this kind of client participation and information and
their own records in hand to negotiate their care among providers. In the past
year I have been to three conferences at which the problem of quality
assurance has come up. This is the talk about town right now since the
government and medical insurers are trying to figure out exactly how much
bang they are getting for their buck. These third party payers have decided
that they are not going to pay unless a certain quality standard has been met.
The name has evolved over the past few years from quality control to quality
assurance and now to quality assessment because no one could control or
assure outcomes. However, the strategies talked about over the past years on
how to control, assure, and assess quality are all after the fact. They are all
like the PRO reviews that do large studies and point fingers if a patient
encounter falls outside of an accepted range. This does no good for the
patient who has already been through the system because it is an exit
assessment. We do not have any entry level quality assurance. It is high time
that we in medicine develop and use entry level quality assurance guidelines
so that patients are consistently receiving quality, from input through to
outcome. If this was done on the entry level, millions and millions of dollars
now being spent on exit level surveys would be unnecessary. Problem
Knowledge Couplers and computerized Problem Oriented Medical Records
are examples of tools that are ready to be put into place. Unfortunately,
Medicare is currently studying whether or not to make cookbook protocols for
establishing practice guidelines. The reason we have not had cookbook
medicine over the decades is because it does not work but it does not
acknowledge the unique variables that have to be factored into total care.
There is inherent danger when individuals are rigidly categorized into
inflexible protocols. If physicians do not have this fully in mind, they will not
pick up the early warning signs of a treatment plan gone awry. The use of
couplers on the other hand is designed to factor in the very specific individual-
ity of a given patient. The use of a comprehensive medical record will pick up
the flow of multiple interacting variables that must affect decision making.
Modifications of treatment, tailored to the individual patient, are what good
physicians now try to do, but are limited by the unaided capacity of recall and
handling a complex task off the cuff at the time of performance. That is
exactly why those of us who are pilots, especially instrument rated pilots, use
very rigid checklists before ever taxiing out on a runway let alone flying into
fog shrouded mountainous terrain. We use these checklists because we want

to stay alive, and we know the difference between a safe pilot and an unsafe pilot is the difference between a smart pilot and a dumb pilot. Commercial pilots do these things without a second thought because they have to get into the airplane with the passengers. However, physicians often charge headlong into a complicated case without integrating a complete history or physical, or a complete checklist or a comprehensive medical record. One wonders if they would do so if they had to get "in the airplane with the patient." We all know that we sometimes forget the simplest things when we are in the middle of a complex interaction and chide ourselves afterwards for doing so. These things happen as a course of human nature, and the medical fraternity is not immune. We need better tools to protect ourselves and our patients from these hazards. We practicing physicians need to take charge of new and better ways of assuring quality so that government bureaucrats, many of whom have never practiced a day in their life, do not take over completely. Who is in the best, in fact the only, position to do this? We can do quality assurance because the government says we must, or we can do it for the right reasons—because we are the patients' advocates and we want the right answers for the patients' sake.

The Next Step

Use of couplers by multiple personnel, the use of a computerized medical record, medication and lab testing properties, and disease information at our fingertips, and patients possessing a copy of their own medical record—all of these are do-able tasks. I have been both blessed and cursed by having to practice alone in a small town. I have had to treat patients from 32 week preemies with no spontaneous respirations to 102 year old patients with heart failure. I have had to treat colds to cancer. I have been inwardly beset by great uncertainties about my proficiency, and I am realistic enough to know that there is no way I can know everything. But it begs the question to say I should not be doing all these things, because for Faulkton, South Dakota, and many communities like it, there is no choice. Without new tools and new premises for the entire system, those of us on the frontline in practice along with the government bureaucrats and the academic centers are all in a double bind. Conventional continuing medical education (CME) curricula alone will not do it. The literature is replete with data to show this. Therefore, my present reality demands that I involve myself with a new pattern of practice using new tools that protects me from my mistakes and alerts me in a timely fashion when I need help. I hope to continue to do what I am doing and where I am doing it, and even to have more free time in the future. I can only do this with the type of help that is available in the modern computer age. I now know enough to know that I do not want to practice medicine for the next twenty-five years without these tools.

Eventually, we will have a local area network with the clinic and hospital on the same system and a terminal in each exam room, the emergency room, the coronary care unit, the nurses' station, and eventually a portable computer that can be plugged into each room in the hospital. Hopefully I will soon have a terminal at home so that I can access patient data immediately when I get a phone call at night. Eventually all patients in our little community will possess a copy of their own medical record. Over time they will learn how to use their record and they will know that their own record in their hands is their ticket of admission to our clinic. (I have had a few patients come to the clinic without their record and, by the second or third visit, throw up their hands with embarrassment when I walk in the room at having to say to me, "I know, I forgot my record.") The medical record will be generated with the patient beside me at the terminal and any questions that they have at that time can be dealt with then and there. If it is a new patient or a very lengthy encounter I will dictate it, but since I can type fairly fast, I like to enter the information while the patient is still with me. The work is then done and they have a copy to take with them. This saves me time later by not having to dictate the note and it saves me office overhead by not having to generate the information twice. It definitely saves me time in not having nearly as many phone calls. It also saves me time in not having a patient's family stopping in to ask, "What did you tell Dad? His memory is getting so bad." The patient now can share the information with the family and they become additional members of the team; they can help with the information gathering later if necessary. These are not trivial or mundane in the day to day running of an office practice.

It will also save me time by getting instructions to the pharmacy. By having the patient take a copy of their current medications and the problem list to the pharmacy, we are all operating on the same wavelength and medication interactions can be avoided. This particular winter brought home the time saving advantage beyond question. The Midwest was hit by a widespread and severe influenza epidemic, and hospitalizations were running four to five times normal throughout our whole area. In one 48 hour period I had 12 admissions to the hospital. The paperwork went like clockwork because I had past histories, medication lists, family histories, etc., at my fingertips at the keyboard for each patient. I did not get behind on any of my paperwork, and it is hard to describe how good that feels after a 16 hour day. This is what I knew would eventually happen, but I now can say it with the assurance of one who has been there. In the near future when we have the multiuser system in place, when a laboratory test or x-ray is ordered, it will be the duty of the technicians in those departments to review the property lists associated with each test, procedure, or drug in the entity database to make sure that there is no contraindication or problem that would interfere with the test being completed reliably and safely. The completed test data are then promptly entered into the computerized chart, thereby saving time in the front office and in the physician's office. The information will be entered in the correct place because the lab requisition will have the problem for which the test was ordered written on the requisition. The beauty of the system also is its flowsheet capability: if a lab technician entered the data in the wrong area, (i.e., under the wrong problem), thus "losing" them, the flowsheet method could be used to retrieve the "lost" data, which could then be moved to the proper location, all in less than a minute. When we have a fully integrated, multiuser system and a patient comes in with a new problem, the personnel will have already the patient through the coupler by the time I see the patient. I can then enter the care process at a higher level of expertise, with all the data already in front of me.

Few people understand the complexity and volume of data that needs to be addressed each time a patient encounter takes place. The volume of data on a chronic patient becomes so large that it becomes unmanageable, and therefore lost, just as the volume of data in the medical literature is already unmanageable and lost to the average practitioner, as Edward Huth pointed out in an editorial in the *Annals of Internal Medicine*. Excellent workups and treatment plans unique to a given individual on a given hospitalization become lost in the stack of charts. The same information often has to be regenerated again because the physician does not have time to read over a four inch thick chart. With the computerized medical record system, we can bring all of the problems and important data to the top levels of the record where they are accessible for review at a glance. Therefore, with the couplers making scientific data from the literature accessible, relevant and timely, and the computerized problem oriented medical record system making each individual patient's unique problems and treatment plans available at a glance, we now finally have control of the overwhelming volume of data that needs to be accessed each time a patient encounter occurs.

We are currently trying to effect this in Faulkton, South Dakota, and we have not done it with hundreds of thousands of government dollars. We have done it on a few thousand dollars and on daily maintenance of records at an overhead cost that I can live with. In the fall of 1988, when I gave a presentation on the Weed system, one doctor stated that these records, including *Entities*, and *Properties*, took too much maintenance to get going. That is like saying people should not fly because it took so long for the Wright brothers to build their first airplane! When implemented this way, it breaks down the barriers of inpatient and outpatient care which, after all, are artificial barriers since it is the same patient no matter where he or she happens to be sitting (or lying) at the time. We can then do away with the concept of an inpatient chart and an outpatient chart and begin having records that are cumulative which in turn lend themselves to patient care that is cumulative and has continuity. I cannot stress the term cumulative enough; it comes up over and over again in the development and institution of this system, because care is so fragmented in the current medical system, and it so badly needs to be cumulative to effect efficient, cost effective and accurate patient care. The original theories and now the actual computerized version of the POMR and

Problem Knowledge Couplers are the best tools that I have seen to effect this change. As patients become more sophisticated, they are beginning to demand this type of cumulative and continuous care as well as the documentation of it. Physicians can usually get a patient to accept their treatment plans by selecting, slanting, or even censoring the information they choose to give patients. For instance, if a surgeon wants to perform a hysterectomy on a woman who has fibroid tumors (a benign condition of the uterus), all he or she needs to do is say, "We should take this out to make sure that the growth is not cancerous." The mere mention of the word "cancerous" will have that patient so panicked that she most likely will consent to an operation without hesitation under those circumstances. That is not informed consent. That is misinformed consent. Only when patients possess their medical records and can have access to tools such as Problem Knowledge Couplers will they begin to be truly involved in their own care. It has long been the courts' rulings that patients have the right to self determination; but self determination cannot be accomplished without information. It has long been proven that it is unwise to carry out medical care based on one encounter here and there. Much wiser are those who make well thought out decisions based on carefully followed changes in condition and course depending on prior changes in therapy. This can truly be accomplished if patients have their medical records to review and if consulting physicians have the records to follow as well.

The right to self determination and the importance of patient involvement is delineated by patient I.R. This patient had a problem found on physical examination termed *breast mass*. I performed a mammogram that was equivocal and obtained a surgical consultation. The first surgeon wanted to do a biopsy with mastectomy to follow if the biopsy was positive. I spoke with the patient about the current thinking of lumpectomy with radiation vs. simple mastectomy vs modified radical mastectomy. Because of her reluctance to undergo a mastectomy, a simple biopsy was first performed and based on the pathology report the problem of breast mass was now upgraded to *breast cancer*. At this time, the first surgeon definitely wanted to do a mastectomy, but the patient was still unwilling to undergo a mastectomy and now knowing something about lumpectomy with radiation, she wanted a second opinion. Therefore, she was referred on, and the pathology slides were sent with her. The second pathologist felt that this was not carcinoma but only an abnormality in the duct tissue; two other pathologists agreed. This patient was saved a disfiguring surgery. Had she had no knowledge of the different treatment modes she might never have asked for the second (independent) surgical opinion in the first place. This patient also learned something about the medical care system and that is that breast cancer is not always breast cancer. One wonders how many times this happens throughout the United States every day! Another patient had a diagnosis made of malignant melanoma, and when I explained all of the possibilities and suggested a second opinion based on the child's age, it was found that he did not have a malignant melanoma but simply a juvenile mole that had some characteristics that mimic malignant melanoma.

As cases like this become common knowledge, the general population will not stand for being left out of the decision making process. I mentioned earlier that I would comment further about this system being a legal tool. If we practice medicine in the way outlined above and if we involve the patients on a personal and professional level, they begin to see what is known and what is not known in the medical field and how much ambiguity there is in the practice of medicine. As patients begin to understand that physicians cannot control output without controlling input, they develop a more realistic idea of what they can and cannot expect from the system. They see how important their role is in the overall picture. They see that we are trying to do a thoughtful and thorough job, that there are huge gaps in medical knowledge, and that they have a lot of the control in their own hands. If they have been working with you in a teamlike approach rather than being dictated to, how likely is it that they will sue you if they do have a poor outcome? I think that it is rather unlikely unless you have totally missed a diagnosis or totally botched a surgical procedure. Patients know that doctors are not infallible; that is almost a common joke among patients. Yet if they see us as quite fallible, why is it that we continue to portray the myth that we know everything and they cannot possibly know anything about medical care? A few years ago when I was at the annual meeting of the American Cardiology Society, I witnessed approximately 30 to 50 physicians rushing to the smoking area to have a cigarette between talks. When you witness a sloppily dressed, diabetic physician smoking and eating sweet rolls while telling his patients how to live, the patients often become like our children—to quote Dr. Weed, "They can't hear our words because our actions are screaming too loudly." Another thing that is happening much less frequently in my practice (and in the future will hopefully cease to happen altogether!) is that nurses, friends, and relatives will not be stopping my patient's medications. This has happened untold numbers of times in the past. Patients will come to the clinic often worse for the experience, having stopped the medications because a friend or daughter or relative who is a nurse had them stop a medication because someone else had problems with it. This is another form of "cookbook" medicine. A tragic example of this occurred while I was still in training. A young girl had lost her kidneys due to a streptococcal infection from pierced earrings. Her father donated one of his kidneys and she was doing fine but friends encouraged her to live nothing but a "natural life" and told her that steroids were very unhealthy. She stopped her steroids and rejected the kidney that her father had risked his life to give her. She, of course, had to go back on dialysis. This type of free advice occurs all of the time with well intentioned but uneducated friends and relatives. In my patient population, the patients know why they are getting their medications. They have been educated as to the ambiguities involved and having their medical record they can review why they were placed on medication in the first place. Additionally, they are taught to discuss all changes with me; therefore, these encounters are becoming very infrequent and hopefully will soon cease all together.

In this matter of patients possessing a copy of their medical records, I shall present one final example that embodies everything that we are trying to do which can and should be a real example of how our medical system should work in the future. Patient D.H. developed atrial fibrillation and was chemically converted with Digoxin. She was seated at the computer terminal when her medical record was generated, and she was given a copy to review. She understood the need for digitalis blood levels and was taught to check her pulse daily. She was then released with a copy of her medical record in hand. Shortly thereafter, she and her husband left on a trip for Texas. They had gotten only as far as Kansas when one morning she awakened with the sensation of her heart palpitating again. She immediately checked her pulse and found it to be irregular at a rate of 125. She called the local hospital emergency room and was told that she would be met by a cardiologist when she arrived. As she walked into the emergency room, the cardiologist introduced himself and she proceeded to hand him her medical record and state that she was in atrial fibrillation, that she had a Digoxin level one week prior which was within therapeutic limits, and her pulse was now irregular at approximately 125 beats per minute, "and here is a copy of my medical record. Here is my problem list and my list of current medications." She reported that the cardiologist appeared almost literally to take a step backwards and he admitted to her afterward that he had never had a patient present herself in such a succinct and forthright manner and had never had a copy of the medical record handed to him in this manner. Within two minutes he knew exactly what was going on with this patient, exactly where she had been, and the fact that Digoxin was no longer working for her. He then knew exactly what step he needed to perform next instead of wasting one to two days redoing everything that we had already done and then coming to the conclusion that she needed a different medication.

Contrast this to patients who do not know anything about their problem, who have been left ignorant by their physician, and who wait until they are about ready to pass out from the lack of blood flow to the brain before they go to an emergency room in a semishocked condition. They don't know anything about their health care. They don't know the names of their medication, they didn't think to bring them along, and they do not know if they have ever had a blood level performed. That patient takes one to two days to workup and make decisions on vs. the patient who turned two days into two minutes by understanding her medical care and having her medical record in hand. Although I have multiple examples of benefits from patients possessing a copy of their medical record, this example is the most dramatic and shows the totality of the situation. It is the experience that galvanized my belief most firmly that patients should possess a copy of their entire medical record.

The last two medical students who have rotated through my facility have been intrigued and amazed at the capabilities within this system. It did not take them long to see the difference between working up a patient with data already in the computer and a new patient to the system. One of them, in an essay to the dean and medical education supervisor, asked why tools like this were not available for students already and "Why are we dragging our feet?" I am sure that many patients wonder the same thing. It is now becoming possible to implement a system that involves

- Patient cooperation

- Participation by nurses, technicians, and medical records personnel

- "Second opinion" input from relevant journal articles kept current in the couplers.

And, as our experience proves, it can work without huge outlays of money.

14
Comments of Other Medical Practitioners

Implementation of Problem Knowledge Couplers in a Primary Care Practice

Charles S. Burger, M.D.

I met Larry Weed and the concept of the Problem Oriented Medical Record as a medical student at Case Western Reserve University Medical School in 1963. The logic and elegance of that system were apparent to me then, and in the 27 years that I have been using it in clinical practice I have not heard an argument against it that holds up.

After postgraduate training in internal medicine and a tour in the Army, I joined Harold Cross and John Bjorn at the PROMIS Clinic in Hampden, Maine, in 1971. These two men had taken the concept of the Problem Oriented System and implemented it in a primary care setting, thereby quieting those critics who said it was impractical and would not work in the real world.

The next ten years were spent refining this "defined system" on paper. Protocols of care and flow sheets were developed and refined. Patients were given their records, and performance audit was instituted. We began to drown in paper!

In 1981 Larry appeared with a computer and the first Problem Knowledge Couplers. We looked and were intrigued. They had the same simple elegance of the Problem Oriented Medical Record System. However, they seemed impractical, time consuming, and disruptive of the usual patient flow. The results of the coupler session did not integrate into our record, and we were overwhelmed with the number of possible diagnostic and management options that poured out. We felt uncomfortable with this new tool and therefore did nothing with it.

But I felt challenged. Going head to head with the computer on any given problem always produced the realization that my mind could never equal its power and thoroughness. I could try and be an intellectual John Henry but to what benefit? For several years, I dabbled, trying the couplers on occasional patients. I learned to use the editor to build couplers and my appreciation of the power of this system grew.

In 1984, I left the PROMIS Clinic with the long term goal of fully integrating the Problem Knowledge Coupler (PKC) system into my new practice. We have been progressing slowly and patiently towards that goal, living with the inevitable frustration of having to move back and forth between the old and new paradigm.

It soon became clear that injecting a computer and a new paradigm into the old system without careful preparation would not work. The entire organization from the receptionists to the business office had to understand the concept and see how they fit into the implementation of the new system.

I started by developing couplers for use in areas where we performed repetitive functions. I began by developing couplers to process questionnaires for physical examinations. In addition to organizing the positive responses into appropriate categories (current systems, past medical history, potential problems, etc.), the coupler may recommend suggestions for further testing or examination to the medical assistants who complete most of the examination. For instance, a positive response to the question regarding history of early familial coronary disease prompts the instruction to draw a lipid profile. These "lab action" options were developed after review of the literature and documented as much as possible.

Next came routine well adult examinations performed by nurse practitioners and medical assistants. This coupler makes recommendations and provides information for patients based on lifestyle factors, physical examination, and laboratory results. The patient is given a copy of the results before he leaving the office. This has become a major preventive care tool in our practice.

For the last four months we have been perfecting a triage coupler used by our receptionists to assist them in evaluating patient complaints over the phone. Previously the receptionists had used simple written protocols to guide them, but situations were often too complex and many decisions were tossed back to me for my own inconsistent responses. With the triage coupler, more information is gathered. Options are then presented to determine: how soon the patient should be seen, the appropriate provider (nurse practitioner, medical assistant, physician), the length of the visit, and lab work to be obtained prior to the visit. The coupler provides information regarding home treatment for those patients who do not need to be seen.

As we began our first crude attempts of implementing the triage coupler, we were amazed how this tool stimulated discussion about how we make decisions at the front desk. Receptionists have kept notebooks of problem areas and we discuss these on a weekly or even daily basis. We have had to rethink our philosophy on medication refills. Comments have been added to guide decision making when alternative options are presented. Once a problem is clarified, updating of the system can occur immediately so there is immediate feedback of the improvement in the system. Very little is written about this triage process in primary care but, to the degree possible, I have tried to support the coupler's management decisions with information from the literature. What started as a very crude tool four months ago has now become extremely sophisticated.

Medically untrained individuals are now making triage decisions with a high degree of sophistication backed by a coupler that incorporates my 20 years experience in medical practice and, as much as possible, information from the medical literature. As the system is constantly refined, I am less often bothered by questions on how to handle a given complaint. A new receptionist can be trained much more rapidly to reach a high level of competence at triage. There is no question in my mind these individuals with this coupler will do a more consistent and thorough job of complaint evaluation than I would without the coupler. There is enormous satisfaction in knowing that one's efforts are cumulative and everyone is contributing to a system that is becoming better all the time.

The most difficult area in which to fully implement the couplers has been in routine office visits for diagnosis and management. First, couplers do not yet exist for many of the common problems that one sees in primary care practice. This requires the staff and myself to operate via two different modalities. Getting the additional couplers built, therefore, is of primary importance. Second, the computer must be like any other tool that we use frequently in clinical practice. Like the stethoscope, for example, it needs to be readily available in all clinical areas. The financial obstacle to achieving this is dropping all the time as hardware costs diminish. Third, we need a new level of sophisticated medical assistant who is skilled in history taking and physical examination and trained to enter appropriate information into the coupler. Much of the historical information can be gathered by the patient through the use of a questionnaire for each complaint, which is filled out prior to the patient's being seen. Lastly, the difficulty of changing old clinical behavior patterns should not be underestimated. They have been engrained through education and habit.

Why go through this difficult process? The most obvious answer is that our obligation as physicians is to provide the best medical care possible and that goal is impossible without the use of this system. Couplers guarantee a thoroughness of information gathered and consideration of all diagnostic and management possibilities that cannot be achieved with the human mind alone. It becomes a tool for continuous learning. As we demonstrated with the triage coupler, rather than replacing thinking, couplers stimulate it. We continuously focus on the process of care, feedback our experience to improve the system, and learn about items in the coupler which we do not understand. The effort is cumulative, and the system becomes better all the time.

What a relief to know that, with each patient interaction, we bring the best medical knowledge available to bear on that particular diagnostic or management problem! The patient is now drawn into the decision making process, which becomes a shared responsibility as we sit together considering the options.

The patient response has been uniformly positive. A patient, after having been run through the respiratory diagnostic coupler several years ago, summed it up nicely: "Now you fellows won't have to guess anymore." Patients no longer have to wonder whether we have thought of everything. For those patients who wish to be drawn into the process to an even higher degree, the couplers become a wonderful teaching tool particularly in the management of chronic problems. They can have access to the same information as the physician. From the patient's standpoint, this is a very empowering system.

With this system in place, we can also begin to look at tasks and responsibilities. Access to information through the computer has broken down hierarchies in all organizations where computers have been introduced. There is no question that this will occur in medicine as well. We have clearly demonstrated over the past 20 years that individuals with no medical background can be taught reliably to perform the majority of physical examinations. Estimates are that nurse practitioners and physician assistants can reliably provide 70% to 80% of primary care now delivered by physicians. In a well defined system where people have access to information and the decision making power of the computer, nonphysicians will more easily rise in the system. The implications of this are profound for the future of the medical establishment.

It is clear, based on our success thus far towards implementing the full use of the Problem Knowledge Couplers in our practice, that the main obstacles against the implementation of such a system on a wide scale will not involve practical reasons, but rather political considerations.

Computers in a Private Practice in Hampden, Maine

Harold D. Cross, M.D.

I have been in private general/internal medicine practice since 1958. Since startup of this practice, a goal for all patients has been to define all their health problems prior to deciding on management, if required, of each problem. This sequence is used to treat problems within the context of each individual patient's unique personal situation.

The approach to achieving this goal of defining the problems has been modified in major ways over these past 32 years. The main modifications have been increased patient and staff involvement in data collection (the most time and energy consuming aspect of care) and the use of computers in data collection and problem evaluation.

Changes in Practice. Changes, as reflected in the way we have scheduled blocks of time on the appointment books, are illustrated below:

- Physician interview/examination

    - During the first ten years: M.D. time, 1.5 hours; patient time 1.5 hours
      (This approach is still used in crisis cases.)

- Self administered paper/pencil questionnaires, and staff physiological/lab testing/protocol
    - Plus physician component of exam and interview
    - For the next 17 years: MD time, 1 hour; Patient time, 3 hours

- Patient given duplicate record to keep, read, and audit
    - Started in 1978, continued over the past 12 years

- Patient/computer interaction for part of initial database (Wellness Coupler) and use of diagnostic couplers for specific problems, e.g., dizziness, headache, hypertension, back pain, knee pain, etc., plus items in [b] above.

What have been some of the results of some of these changes?

- Effect on problem solving efficiency and patient attitude
    - Compared to patient and staff generated data bases, the physician directed history/exam is less defined, less consistent; consequently, it misses more medical, social, familial, and behavioral problems. Time and fatigue factors have a negative effect. Patients feel pressured to answer questions that they have not thought about and are not well prepared to answer. This results in tension, untruthfulness, and an overall slowing down of the problem solving process. Defensive or guarded reactions occur when sensitive areas are involved. Patients' suspicions are sometimes aroused by the interrogator's intonations, pauses, or facial expressions. This can be counterproductive and often leads to multiple followup visits—in effect, counseling sessions to work through, explain, or deal more fully with a problem.

- Effect on patient attitude

- The patient becomes a problem solver. Patient administered questions require more of the patients' time, but they facilitate thoroughness, accuracy, and honesty. Since there are no personal interview nuances, overtones, and ambiguous body language, patients tend to be less defensive. The patient does not know the person who is responsible for the development and design of the questions. Once they have read and then responded, their mindset is altered and actually opened to possibilities beyond their own initial concern, e.g., "tired blood" or "low thyroid," which they may have locked onto as the cause of their fatigue. Having completed a health questionnaire that deals with the desired historical database, the patient, in this practice, responds in a different fashion than when the information is elicited by a direct interview. The most notable difference is that the patient is now in a problem solving mode, not defensive, but open and interested in the various possibilities. After all, that patient came in to find out what was wrong and what can be done about it.

  With patient questionnaires, the number of follow-up visits needed to resolve and/or clarify problems in the two to three months immediately after the examination was cut in half. Most required none, compared to the two to five visits in the immediate post-physical examinations done by physician alone. Physician time was reduced to 0.5 hours by this approach; database was more extensive, and more was accomplished in this time period with fewer followup visits and less physician time used after the physical examination. About 15 to 20 minutes of the physician's time is spent completing the physical exam, the rest in defining each problem and the goals and plans for each. The physician functions more as a consultant (like an attending or visiting professor on rounds), and less as a data collector.

- Patient possesses/uses his or her medical record
  - Since 1978, patients have received a duplicate record of their history, physical examination, laboratory findings (including EKGs and other physiological testing), problem lists, recommendations (plans), and most importantly progress notes. (X-ray reports results are included as information under the problem oriented progress notes.) Patient oriented terminology is used. An instruction written on the outside of the record folder advises the patient to carry the record with him or her to every medical encounter, not only with our practice but to all other providers they see or other medical care facilities they may need to go to. Compliance with this has only been partial. Nevertheless, there are many who do take pride in having their own records and in being regularly updated on their progress. Having their charts with them facilitates

their care as they move about within the health care system and reduces duplications of tests and procedures—and presumably also costs.

- Use of computers
  - Computers that the patient and physician directly interact with are for us a major change. People respond to or process the written or video screen word differently than the spoken word in the interview setting. It has been my observation that patients read/process the video monitor screen questions several times faster than questions in a person to person interview. (I estimate this to be four to five times faster.) For example, it is common for the patient to answer 100 to 200 questions about the nature of their headache in five or ten minutes, covering 40 causes of headache. Why is there such efficiency? I submit the following reasons:

- The questions have been carefully worded, not just "off the top of my head"; the wording is improved and refined as users gain experience.

- The questions are processed in a non-threatening, non-pressured fashion, at the patient's own rate. There does not appear to be any "intimidation."

- Most patients start to get interested, and this involvement speeds the interrogation process along.

- Only one screen at a time is displayed, avoiding the distraction of how much more lies ahead to do.

Effects on Practice

Patients

- Patients participate more in health care planning. They are more involved in defining their own health problems; viewing their data on the monitor as well as participating in some of the direct entry of data makes their own data clearer, easily viewed, and legible, and shared simultaneously with the provider. Patients appreciate being treated respectfully, as equals.

- Learning is enhanced by involvement, use, and repetition. To quote one patient user of the headache coupler:

"Responding to the coupler questions need not be done by a physician, but can be done by the patient, thus requiring little of the physician's time. That is precisely the way I used the "Headache" Coupler a year ago and even today, when I sense the onset of a headache, I can remind myself of the findings that were on my printout."

- I have not observed any particularly negative experiences, with the use of the computer by patients in this practice, other than negative remarks in anticipation of using the computer. Once they are into it, it is commonplace for the patients to talk freely to the machine, to me, or to one of my assistants.

Physicians

For the physician concerned with delivering quality medical care, the most oppressive and limiting factor in delivering such care is the inability of the human mind to remember all that one needs to at a given moment of action. The knowledge couplers bridge the memory gap. I do not expect anyone to believe this who has not actually tried to use one or who has not built one. It may take six months to build a diagnostic coupler for headache, but with its use, a physician can now accomplish a preliminary evaluation of a patient for all of 40 possible causes on the first pass. This can be accomplished in 30 or 40 minutes. A result of using this diagnostic tool (the Knowledge Coupler) is that it drives the physician user to be a more careful examiner, learning simple, inexpensive examination procedures at the outset.

Physicians are now the consultants using the guidance provided by the knowledge coupler. They can direct their energies, expertise, and time to coach the patient, and be a mentor in providing input to the decisions that need to be made, goals that need to be established, etc. This is refreshing, exciting, and fun! It is my concern that medical knowledge can make a difference for the patients that come under my care—that they are evaluated for all possible causes, not merely the most likely ones, simply because whatever it is that particular patient has is 100% for him or her, even though it may be only 25th on the list of probabilities for the population.

Problem Knowledge Couplers in Psychiatry

Willie Kai Yee, M.D.

The use of computers in psychiatry is probably now on the breaking point of an exponential curve. Software for diagnosis and record keeping is now available to the profession, in addition to the more commonly seen functions such as billing and word processing (*Psychiatric News* 1987). What follows is a discussion of the use of the Problem Knowledge Coupler in psychiatric practice.

The Conceptual Background of the Problem Knowledge Coupler System

The Problem Oriented Approach. Patients do not walk in the door and say "I have an affective disorder." A diagnosis of affective disorder is made in response to some problem that the patient has. A coupler that would cover affective disorders would start with a common complaint such as "fatigue" or "loss of interest." These complaints could lead to a number of diagnoses, of which affective disorders would only be a portion.

Using Problem Knowledge Couplers in Psychiatry

Suitability to Psychiatry. The Problem Knowledge Coupler (PKC) system was developed for use by anyone, regardless of specialty or professional discipline, who wishes to discover and solve medical problems. The Screening History and Review of Systems Coupler is useful in establishing a complete list of problems for psychiatric patients. The Wellness and Health; Assessment and Guidance Coupler assesses various aspects of the patient's lifestyle, including nutrition, exercise, sleep habits, and management of stress. This coupler is useful in therapy when lifestyle factors are present which may be contributing to the patient's symptomatology or poor functioning. The recommendations of the Wellness Coupler may be used in the treatment of a variety of conditions as therapeutic tasks to be done between sessions. Cognitive and behavioral approaches, particularly, benefit from the output of this coupler.

Psychiatric Couplers. Couplers for psychiatric problems are presently under development. Couplers for the Management of Depression, the Diagnosis of Anxiety, and the Diagnosis of Personality and Character Disorders have recently been completed. In keeping with the philosophy of the PKC system, medical causes of these problems are covered as well as psychiatric causes .

The Effects on Psychiatric Practice. The use of the PKC system in a psychiatric practice has a profound influence on the way that psychiatry is practiced. This is in large part due to the conceptual basis of the PKC system, which was developed out of a recognition of the necessity to change the way that medicine is practiced. I believe that the need for a change in practice of psychiatry is now apparent as it was in medicine when the Problem Oriented Medical Record (POMR) and PKC systems were developed. This orientation distinguishes the PKC system from other psychiatric software now available. Most of those are aimed at doing more efficiently or accurately some function that is already being done without computers. Although the PKC does aim at more accurate diagnosis and management, its integration into practice has effects that go far beyond efficiency or accuracy.

The Patient-Psychiatrist Relationship. The most profound alteration becomes apparent the first time the psychiatrist sits down with the patient to review the results of a coupler. This side by side posture can be seen as a metaphor for the alteration in the relationship that is taking place. The psychiatrist and patient are now involved in a *collaborative* relationship, with both parties having access to the information from which a decision could be made. Since couplers are structured to present multiple options, e.g., less frequent diagnoses or less commonly used treatments, there is no longer a "treatment of choice" for a given condition. The ambiguity that physicians, including psychiatrists, face all the time is now confronted by both patient and provider. The hierarchical structure of medicine, in which a single diagnosis or treatment is authoritatively prescribed, is replaced by a relationship which acknowledges uncertainty and the trade-offs which must be made when any decision is made.

Integration of Psychiatry and Medicine. The use of the PKC system brings the practice of psychiatry closer to medicine. Nature does not respect the distinction between psychiatric and medical causes, and neither do the couplers. One recent study indicates that 9% of psychiatric patients have an underlying medical disorder (Hall 1979). Another study, surveying chronically mentally ill patients found 53% of the subjects had undiagnosed medical problems (Farmer 1987). The use of the coupler system in diagnosis places a greater emphasis on medical causes and gives the patient and psychiatrist more power and responsibility in their management. This integration of psychiatry with medicine has been recognized as a desirable trend and openly promoted by the American Psychiatric Association in recent years.

The Literature. If a psychiatrist reaches the point of *building* as well as using couplers, his or her approach to the literature changes. First, the lines between specialties become irrelevant as soon as a problem orientation is adopted. If one begins with anxiety as a problem, the solution may be found in gynecology or immunology as easily as psychiatry. Heaven help the patient who *starts out* with the wrong specialist! As psychiatric couplers are built, one recognizes the need for the inclusion of literature well beyond the boundaries of the "psychiatric literature."

Second, as literature is reviewed for "parsing" of its information into a form that the computer program can manipulate, issues of crispness, the acknowledgment of uncertainty, and the interaction with other phenomena become prominent, along with traditional issues such as the adequacy of research design. One can now read with a clearer and more skeptical mind, and can concentrate on the quality of the information rather than memorizing it so that it will be available when needed. This has serious implications for medical and psychiatric education (Weed 1987).

Malpractice Risk. I believe that the routine use of couplers in psychiatric practice also provides considerable protection to the psychiatrist from litigation. First, the integration with medicine offers greater assurance that underlying medical conditions will not be overlooked. It is our legal as well as ethical responsibility to be certain that medical conditions that can cause psychiatric problems are examined. Failure to do so is a certain invitation to malpractice suits. Second, the process of reviewing a coupler with a patient insures that the information on which a decision is based is accurate, and that both patient and psychiatrist are aware of the risks and benefits of a given course of action.

Present Trends in Psychiatry and Medicine. This altered relationship with the patient is part of another trend in psychiatry and medicine. Consumer participation in medical decision making is now advocated as an essential process in the improved delivery of medical care (Ferguson 1980). The recognition and implementation of this process with the use of accessible expert systems such as Problem Knowledge Couplers can benefit patient, practitioner, and society. In the psychoeducational treatment of schizophrenia, for example, the provision of adequate information to the patient or family members is the key to an altered relationship with the clients, one which employs them as allies, rather than passive recipients of treatment. In the field of schizophrenia, at least, the effect has been a dramatic improvement in relapse rates (Anderson et al. 1986).

15
Problem Knowledge Couplers and Their Use in Dentistry

Louis M. Abbey, D.M.D.

In a recent report assessing dentistry in the year 2000 (Kaldenberg et al 1990), a distinguished panel of experts representing all aspects of the profession listed computerized diagnosis and treatment planning as one of the innovations that was widely cited and discussed during their forum. This is but one reference to what is now becoming a frequently forecasted component of future dental practice. Until recently, however, computerized diagnosis and treatment planning was considered farfetched and "ideal but impractical" by many in dental circles looking at trends that would influence the way practice would evolve in the next century. One fact is evident, however: we are educating dentists today who will spend the vast majority of their practice lifetimes well into the next century, and we are not preparing them for the technological revolution and knowledge explosion that they will experience.

Everything that has been said about expanding knowledge bases, limitations of human memory, and the compensations we make for these limitations applies unaltered to the practice of dentistry. Dentists are independently practicing health professionals who treat their patients with medical and/or surgical means. Dentists regularly prescribe a large armamentarium of medications. They administer local and general anesthesia and perform complex surgical procedures that often compromise (at least temporarily) patient's cardiorespiratory systems. Although most of their patients are ambulatory, dentists treat people who have serious systemic diseases, complicated medical histories, and who are taking medications on which their lives depend. A growing number of dental patients have artificial or transplanted organs and may have highly contagious diseases such as hepatitis or AIDS.

Socioeconomic trends suggest that as the 21st century gets underway, dental patients will be more affluent, living longer and retaining more of their teeth.

Thus, these patients will be demanding more dental care over an extended period of time. If knowledge doubles every five to seven years, then dentists stand no chance of keeping abreast of the knowledge base they must master to serve these patient's diagnostic and treatment needs into the next century.

The Problem Knowledge Coupler System is perfect for dealing with diagnosis and treatment in the practice of dentistry. Dentistry and medicine differ in that the dentist is often more challenged by deriving the treatment plan than by deciphering the diagnosis. It is just the opposite in medicine. Systemic diseases vary widely in their clinical presentation, often complicated by coexisting conditions and multiple, superimposed signs and symptoms. Much of the challenge of diagnosis in systemic medicine is managing and choosing appropriately between a confounding array of diagnostic aids, all of which seem to lay some claim on the correct answer.

Patients present to dentists with clinical problems involving teeth, oral mucosa, periodontium, and/or jaws. The dentist uses a very limited array of diagnostic tools to analyze and determine the cause or causes of patient's problem(s). Descriptive radiography is perhaps the most widely used diagnostic tool in dentistry. Most information obtained in dental radiography is morphologic rather than quantitative. Dentists rely extensively on tactile, visual, and auditory senses and on their ability to communicate with patients to obtain history, signs, and symptoms associated with a problem. Laboratory tests, though used frequently enough, are confined primarily to complete blood count and bleeding and clotting examinations. Additionally, dentists often rely on laboratories to screen for infectious disease. The biopsy and histopathologic examination are perhaps the most widely used second echelon means of obtaining a definitive diagnosis once a lesion has been detected. It is the dentist's responsibility to be aware of and take appropriate means to manage occult systemic disease, drug interactions, contraindications, alterations, and necessary precautions and complications that may involve known systemic diseases or conditions. The database of information concerning these areas is expanding at an exponential rate.

For the dentist, the diagnosis may be quite evident but there may be several confusing avenues toward therapy. In some cases, therapeutic choices may involve irreversible procedures that preclude switching choices after therapy has begun (e.g., once the tooth has been extracted it cannot be placed back into the alveolus). Numerous therapeutic choices open to patients depend on socioeconomic factors, patient education, and determination. Treatment planning for the dentist often involves an array of options based on patient centered factors that must be clearly delineated and communicated to patients at the time of presentation. This perplexing situation often results in patients being offered fewer choices than are actually feasible and doctors making decisions for patients.

The databases on individual dental problems are often relatively small and well contained compared to some of those on medical problems. Smaller, manageable databases facilitate the speedy response of computer systems and simplify coupler construction. Most of the information needed to diagnose common dental problems is quite well established and not extremely controversial. Problem Knowledge Couplers seem to fill a long felt void in dental care both in diagnosis and management, but particularly in management. Given this wide application, however, personal experience attests that dental educators, practitioners, students, and administrators do not necessarily rush to embrace the concept of applying technology to problem oriented health care.

Coupler Philosophy and Dentistry

Christopher C. Weed (1982) wrote about the purpose of the Problem Knowledge Coupler:

> The purpose of the Problem-Knowledge Coupler is to provide in an external form a reliable, responsive mechanism for guiding the [dental] care provider by coupling the uniqueness of the patient's situation to the body of relevant medical[/dental] knowledge during the initial stages of diagnosis and management, where the completeness of one's planning is most crucial and most difficult to achieve without aid.

Within the curricula in dental education, the overwhelming portion of time is devoted to treatments. All of the subject matter is categorized according to specialty. This results in courses in periodontics, restorative dentistry, surgery, pathology, etc. (similar to medicine). Classes in dental school are dominated by the following pattern of information transfer:

> Today we will take up the subject of disease X. Disease X is defined as ABC. Here is a picture of a person with Disease X. The clinical characteristics are 1, 2, 3, and 4. Disease X is treated with treatment Y.

It is not surprising then that dental school graduates are well versed in the names of diseases and conditions and their treatments, clearly delineated along specialty lines. Patients, however, do not present with names of diseases pinned to their shirts. Brian D. Monteith, Chairman of Prosthodontics at the Medical University of South Africa recently commented that dental education currently represents an overriding preoccupation with solutions, with really very little attention being given at all to identifying the relevant problems (Monteith 1990).

This has been borne out by Morris and Bohannon (1987), in their study on the quality of dental practice. They meticulously surveyed 300 dental practices in the United States, representing all specialties, geographic and demographic areas, and levels of income. They found out, for instance, that 83% of the records made provision for recording periodontal status, yet only 18% of these practices actually recorded the information. Sixty-one percent of the records provided the opportunity to record occlusal analysis; only 7% did so. Fifty-three percent of the records provided space for recording a treatment plan, but only 24% of the sample recorded such a plan. In contrast, however, they found that nearly all of the records sampled from graduates since 1974 accurately recorded treatments and fees. Morris and Bohannon conclude that "a wide gap exists between the way faculty believe dentistry should be practiced and the way it is practiced." Perhaps the underlying reason for this can be found in a dental curriculum that is preoccupied with providing answers and too little concerned with problem analysis.

It is not surprising, therefore, that the philosophy and purpose of Problem Knowledge Couplers stand in contradistinction to a large part of the current foundations of dental education in this country. The sad result is that when a tool like the Problem Knowledge Coupler is presented and demonstrated to dentists in practice or to faculty in schools, it represents such a radical departure from their basic orientation that the applicability of the system is shrouded in noncomprehension. Some will offer that couplers are for an ideal world but they could not possibly work in the real world of practice. It is a mistake to assume that the logic and aptness of Problem Knowledge Couplers will be immediately apparent to the dental community.

The Problem Knowledge Coupler System for diagnosis of patient problems allows the user to focus on the problem, thus reducing distraction. It organizes questions and answers and permanently records the information so that time is used more efficiently, eliminating repetition and making question sequencing more logical. When using this decision support system, the clinician has the entire database concerning a given problem at his or her disposal rather than just the part that can be remembered at the time. The database on any given problem can be updated instantly making it possible to have the most current knowledge available. Since the whole database is utilized to analyze any group of findings obtained at a session, the clinician is relieved of the problem of tunneling and focusing which often leads to premature hypothesis formation, elimination of causes on insufficient grounds, and ultimately to a mistaken diagnosis or inappropriate treatment. Using the combinatorial reasoning process rather than functioning on Bayesian logic and probabilistic reasoning, the Problem Knowledge Coupler System always presents the clinician with all of the choices suggested by a given combination of findings leaving the full power of decision making in the hands of the doctor. Most of the rule based systems that use probabilies establish the likelihood of a given cause as being the basis for a patient's problem. This reasoning assumes a problem has a single cause. More and more evidence is mounting that many patients' dental problems are the result of more than one cause interacting to produce a series of symptoms usually unique to that one patient.

Computer assisted decision support using the Problem Knowledge Coupler System could significantly influence the way dentists practice. Diagnostic routines could be completed faster and with more confidence, permitting more immediate patient treatment, education, and counseling. The continuous cuing that takes place when using the couplers can reinforce and enhance the practitioner's knowledge base and increase diagnostic acumen. Records produced using the Problem Knowledge Coupler System have a similar organizational structure allowing for orderly review of the patient's diagnostic and treatment experience. This type of record can facilitate rapid review and forwarding of consultant information, eliminate unnecessary duplication of diagnostic investigations (e.g., radiographs), and promote significant cost effective measures while increasing quality of care.

Integrating Problem Knowledge Couplers into Dental Education

There is no question that educating dentists and practicing dentistry in the next century will involve a shift from a disease/treatment model to a problem oriented approach to patient care. This paradigm shift will necessitate using the tools of modern computer technology. It is equally clear, however, that a fragmentary, piecemeal approach to this transition will be counterproductive if not destructive to the effort. Since this conversion would represent nearly a 180° shift for most present day curricula in dental education, it is impossible to imagine that it could be accomplished effectively in any manner but a uniform commitment and action on the part of faculty and administration.

Personal experience can attest to the difficulties encountered advocating problem oriented, patient centered dental care using Problem Knowledge Couplers in a didactic or clinical environment where the vast majority of the faculty subscribe to a disease/treatment centered paradigm for patient care. Commitment to this paradigm is neither well constructed nor scholarly. Rather, it is often pursued because "that's the way we've always done it and we've done all right so far." Students quickly learn where the majority of faculty place their emphasis. This realization is translated into studying the facts and memorizing the lists for the majority and neglecting the problem oriented emphasis advocated by the minority. In some cases, it can even lead to complaints that the teaching by certain faculty is out of step. Administrative pressure may begin to build for the problem oriented faculty to conform to the system.

The problem oriented approach to teaching dental students demands more interdependence between faculty and students. Consultation is encouraged, and cooperative approaches to solving patient problems are the rule. This behavior depends on consistency and faculty reinforcement across the curriculum and tends to stifle competition and individual star performance. The disease/treatment centered model emphasizes memorization and independent problem solutions often carried out in isolation, a behavior reinforced by the "rugged individualism" so valued by the society in general.

Building Problem Knowledge Couplers within the research/productivity centered university environment is not without inherent risks. The average time necessary to build a coupler, including the knowledge net, is usually two to three months, given the varied schedules of university faculty. A faculty member must take on such a project as his or her research effort to justify the time commitment. The discouragement comes when the faculty member applies for internal or external funding to purchase a computer and the Coupler Development System for the project. Most internal and external research committees are not prepared to handle such requests and end up rejecting the applications as "not real research." Even if the faculty member has a computer, perhaps even purchases the software out of personal or discretionary funds, often the department administrator is critical of the lack of funding simply because of the time commitment involved. Once couplers are built, few publications able to stand the scrutiny of the tenure and promotion committee are interested in a paper that may arise from the coupler project. Faculty quickly learn the narrow scope of what is considered "productive scholarly activity."

With one or two couplers working, there is a need for collegial review. This is the time to approach other faculty to review the couplers for content. Usually they are willing, but few are familiar with the philosophy and use of couplers. Teaching colleagues the background required so they can use couplers with enough facility to render an honest review often takes nearly as much time as it would take to teach them the development system. If a colleague reviews one coupler successfully, the faculty member who developed the coupler might suggest tentatively that they cooperate on a conjoint project for the next coupler. Any enthusiasm generated usually disintegrates when colleagues discover the time/effort commitment and how radically they must alter their approach to diagnosis and treatment planning.

I continue to be convinced that the future of Problem Knowledge Couplers in dentistry lies with students. If students were to spend a large portion of their preclinical years constructing couplers for diagnosis and management of the problems encountered in clinic, they would have a coupler library with which to begin their clinical practice. Such an effort demands full restructuring of the curriculum, faculty commitment, and consistent reinforcement at all levels, particularly among top administrators. Here again, personal experience has proven that one or two junior faculty beating the problem oriented drum to students or faculty are virtually ineffective.

Another dental education avenue that has met with some small success is recruiting interested students. During their second or third year, students often express an interest and willingness to learn knowledge net building and Problem Knowledge Coupler construction. This mentoring system is very gratifying to the faculty member and individual student. It is not, however, an effective way of integrating couplers into the curriculum. Dental education is too "lock step" with only scattered free hours. Students tend to overestimate their ability to make commitments. This will continue until the dental curriculum includes more time built in for independent study and elective courses. Many students still have only limited familiarity with computers. Enthusiasm runs high, but few come with any concept of the theory behind problem oriented diagnosis and treatment because it is so radically different from the rest of the curriculum. It takes time to break through the traditional faculty/student protocols so that students begin to consider themselves colleagues. Coupler building requires confidence and self directedness, which can emerge only after relationships evolve from traditional student/teacher to peers with different levels of experience.

Most students feel they cannot afford the time, but the few who can usually find only an hour or two per week (including the research time), which is generous considering the current dental curriculum. This kind of sporadic time for coupler building is not particularly effective or productive whether the builder is a faculty member or a student. In one year's work, including some vacation time, a student working with me has managed to build one coupler in rough draft stage.

I have also had the opportunity to train two faculty colleagues in coupler building. Considering that both had to begin by mastering basic computer skills, and neither could spend more than two hours at a time in training, it took most of four months before they were able to plan, design, research, and build a coupler on their own. The mechanics of coupler building are not difficult to master. I have designed a three hour workshop in which I have participants build a very simplified diagnostic coupler. This is only an introduction, however, and certainly does not prepare faculty members to strike out on their own in an efficient way, particularly when they find they are working without much collegial support. Further, most faculty who express interest are in junior positions seeking credentials to obtain tenure. They soon realize that they must spread their precious time thinly if they expect to do "research" as well. In addition, they learn all too quickly that it is nearly impossible to carry the coupler building skills back to a skeptical department. This experience augments what has been said previously about the need for a schoolwide commitment to use Problem Knowledge Couplers in dental education. In my own personal experience, using only the sporadic hours that were available to me and starting from page one of the manual distributed with the Coupler Editing System, it was a year before I felt very confident that I knew how to build couplers efficiently in both the diagnostic and management modes.

At Virginia Commonwealth University School of Dentistry, we now have one computer and six coupler databases available for use in our patient screening and emergency clinic. These have been available for students to use with patients for nearly one year. This system is used sporadically for medical and dental history taking, physical examination recording, and dealing with patient problems, such as toothache and periapical radiolucency. Students are warily curious and reluctant to use the system without a faculty member present, but are quite enthusiastic with supervision and guidance. All students rotating through the service do see at least one coupler session with a patient and participate in a seminar that deals with Problem Knowledge Couplers and their application in diagnosis and treatment planning. After a coupler session, student response has been enthusiastic, curious, and laudatory in regard to the information content. Some have been skeptical and argumentative, taking issue with the content particular couplers and offering suggestions for improvement. The most frequently expressed summary comment is that they hope such a system is readily available for them when they are in practice.

Experience has yielded nothing short of universal patient acceptance of computer use and Problem Knowledge Couplers in diagnosis and treatment planning. The one word most characteristic of patient response is "thorough." Patients seem to be under the impression that when their dentist uses a computer they are unquestionably receiving the highest quality health care.

One factor that stands out after a year of using couplers in the clinical setting. Problem Knowledge Couplers and the patient and doctor traffic and work patterns they demand do not fit easily into the clinic routines. The traffic and work patterns in a clinic using a paper record system are very different from patterns evolving from a problem oriented, patient centered clinical setting using couplers and computers. This is compounded, for example, by the need for space to accommodate new and sometimes bulky equipment (i.e., the computers) or with concerns for infection control. This is a challenging area for study and needs much work. Introducing couplers and computers into the traditional dental office environment is clearly disruptive and awkward and cannot be done without thorough study of the changes that will be necessary to accommodate the new approach to care. If overlooked, this aspect of the paradigm shift could be fatal to the entire effort

Increasing familiarity and ease with building couplers inevitably yield insights into how they can be used in novel ways within the educational environment. It takes little modification in the building routine, for instance, to construct couplers that can be interfaced with case presentations in the classroom or seminar. Two screens and a means of overhead projection for the computer are all the additional equipment needed to augment the standard audiovisual equipment commonly found in classrooms. The information can be built into the database in such a way as to present the case information on a text screen while projecting transparencies of the case on the other screen. The imaginative use of findings, causes, comments, and options results in a case presentation, review of the findings, pathophysiologic interpretation of the findings, and differential diagnosis. A similar structure can be designed to present cases for treatment planning. This style of presentation has enabled us to place increasingly more emphasis on problem solving skills and less on memorizing endless lists of facts and descriptions. It has also provided an effective means to detail how the basic sciences figure into the understanding of patient problems, differential diagnosis, and therapy planning.

Problem Knowledge Couplers and Private Dental Practice

The reaction of the dental community to Problem Knowledge Couplers has been far from hostile. In fact, most audiences are sincerely interested and express how much help such a tool would be for them. They admit the knowledge deficit and are amazed at the thoroughness and accuracy of the system. But when the idea of placing a system in their office is broached, many of the traditional barriers arise. Most often the argument goes something like this:

The system is wonderful and would surely be a boon to my practice and peace of mind, BUT...

- It could never fit into the flow of my office routine.

- How could I take the time to train all my staff?

- I would only use it with my more difficult cases.

- Why should I get a system like that if I am going to refer the cases anyway?

- I really think it would take too much time to use this system with my patients.

And the list could go on and on. The impression is that the established dental practitioner is not ready or willing to undertake such a paradigm shift, despite the findings of Morris and Bohannon.

Another argument often heard from private practitioners concerns liability and whether having a computerized diagnostic system will leave them more open to lawsuits. Another variation on that theme is that if they installed such a system in their practice, what would be the effect on the usual and customary standard of care in their community? There seems to be no clear answer to these questions. Legal experts say the issue has not been tested before the courts. It would seem logical that using a knowledge tool such as the Problem Knowledge Coupler System would confer no more liability than using a current textbook. Some informal opinions from attorneys concur.

From the standpoint of risk management, however, it would seem that using a tool with access to the most current knowledge about a problem and using an instrument that greatly enhances record keeping and documentation would only strengthen the practitioner's position and minimize risk. It may even be that some day insurance companies will offer malpractice insurance premium discounts to dentists who use a knowledge management/decision support tool.

Use of Problem Knowledge Couplers in Other Areas

Problem Knowledge Couplers have potential for use in almost any area where
problem solving is necessary and the solutions are complex involving many
variables attributable to multiple causes. When combined with laser videodisc
technology, CD-ROM and read-write optical disks, Problem Knowledge
Couplers offer many possibilities. They are potentially useful in training
situations especially where problem solving and critical thinking are being
taught using case simulations. This same principle applies to continuing
professional education.

Problem Knowledge Couplers have strong potential for use in areas where
auxiliary personnel are the first line contact persons in emergency and triage
situations. For example, in situations where a medical or dental paraprofes-
sional is in charge of a health facility when dentists are not readily available
for consultation, Problem Knowledge Couplers can aid in decision making
when it is necessary to distinguish between true emergencies and problems
that can be postponed. Management couplers can be used in treatment
planning and are especially useful when planning therapy for complex cases
involving vague pain situations (e.g., TMJ or myofacial pain) or several
different specialty areas, such as endodontics, periodontics and prosthodontics.

Centrally stored and maintained knowledge bases could be electronically
linked to distant facilities to provide consultation services avoiding costly long
distance transportation. It seems possible that patients could carry their dental
records with them on floppy disks or have them stored in a large central
facility being immediately accessible from terminals anywhere in the world.

The Computerized Problem Oriented Dental Record

We have had some preliminary experience with development of a preliminary
model for the computerized problem oriented dental record. This record
keeping system addresses the three major reasons for record keeping in health
care:

- To maintain a concise, chronological account of the patient's presenting
  condition, subsequent problems, and treatment rendered

- To provide the basis for quality of care review

- To be a cumulative source of clinical data for research and evaluation
  of therapeutic modalities.

The design is focused on the patient's problems and the record draws
attention to the primary areas of concern for each patient. Each problem is
dealt with in a structured format of *basis, status, plan,* and *procedures.* This

structure immediately guides the reviewer, consultant, or researcher to the elements critical to an evaluation of any problem management. A brief review of the problem will answer the questions

- Why was it considered a problem in the first place?

- What is the current status of the problem?

- What was the therapeutic or management plan?

- What were the procedures carried out in response to the plan?

A clear, concise, consistent, and organized record is provided by using a custom built vocabulary that can be augmented by personally added comments. If paper records are required, printouts are consistently organized and clearly printed, eliminating the need for deciphering handwriting. This record system will facilitate speedier, more comprehensive, and more accurate quality of care assessment.

A significant advantage would be achieved if the computerized problem oriented dental record could be linked electronically with Problem Knowledge Couplers. Currently, though coordinated through common terminology and similar functions, the two systems are electronically functionally separate. Another advantage would be to alter the source code and build in more flexibility as to the systems on which the programs will run and the configurations in which they will run. This would pave the way for porting the system to mini and main frame computers and allow for multiuser configuration whether on a central system or on linked PCs. One of the chief advantages of both of these systems, which will be even more evident if they are linked, is that the systems are oriented and designed with the patient's problems as the main focus. With this focus, and an open program architecture that is amenable to upgrading, modification, and adaptation to different operating environments, the chances of the system becoming obsolete are kept to a minimum.

Ideally there are three distinct components to health care practice:

- Problem diagnosis and treatment

- Patient record keeping

- Fiscal management.

The Problem Knowledge Coupler System and the computerized problem oriented dental record are the first two components. If both were fully electronically integrated and then further integrated with a superbly designed fiscal management system, total practice management merging diagnosis and treatment, record keeping, and fiscal management would be possible.

16
Problem Knowledge Couplers in Veterinary Medicine

Phillip D. Nelson, D.V.M.

Clinical education in veterinary medicine has been a difficult proposition for veterinary medical schools. When medical education first began, there was no division of preclinical and clinical years. The student and the degreed clinician were clearly both students of medicine exploring and investigating the wonders of life and the possibilities of therapeutic intervention. The degreed clinician used each patient to formulate and test some hypothesis and was allowed to watch the results of this living experiment. Many secrets were still to be unlocked, many bacteria were yet to be found, viruses were too small to be thought of, and alcohol was the most effective safe disinfectant available. The clinician of the day was akin to our investigator in the laboratory. And the wonder was that the student was a firsthand witness to the factual ignorance of the doctor. Clinicians did not teach what caused a particular disease (for in truth they did not know), but rather how to determine that a particular disease was present (diagnostic skills) and what was then the most effective treatment. The student learned clinical diagnostics and applied anatomy at the bedside. The student learned what the important questions of the day were and more importantly learned how to answer them.

Simultaneous developments in related fields set the stage for the drama that medical education is playing out today. Each newly discovered fact in medicine allowed researchers to ask new questions and discover the answers at an ever quickening pace. Although the transference of knowledge has never equaled the pace of its discovery, the rate at which new breakthroughs were being published quickly outstripped the average clinician's ability to assimilate them. It did not take long before consumers realized that some doctors possessed more specialized knowledge than others, and began to demand performance based on the collective knowledge of the profession, rather than the individual.

And, thus, we have arrived at the major dilemma facing medical educators and medical students today.

Is there any wonder why specialties developed? The wonder is that the generalist survived—particularly in veterinary medicine. In the not too distant history of veterinary education, it was often touted that the graduate of the day could perform as a clinician, or a researcher, an academician, or in industry all as a result of the training received in veterinary medical school. Well, if that were ever true, it is now a baldfaced lie! Even within clinical practice, the mixed practitioner is becoming a rare breed. With society's ever increasing demands of the practitioner, how can we possibly expect the new practitioner to be knowledgeable to a degree of litigative competence for all species?

When graduate DVMs are hired by the poultry industry, they are retrained in an intensive program that results in a veterinarian who suits their purposes. Is this an indication of failure of academia, or an astute understanding of what is possible in the present standard veterinary curriculum? Should a graduate veterinarian choose to work in meat inspection, a six week intensive training course is required, regardless of performance in school. Why? In clinical practice the litmus test has long been whether or not the graduating veterinarian was been given the opportunity to perform a spay, and can it be done in half an hour. Clearly it is evident that academia cannot inoculate every graduating veterinarian with extensive details or technical expertise that allows the individual to perform in every possible arena! Industry and government agencies have long recognized the problem of the inverse relationship of knowledge depth and breadth, and have demonstrated their understanding by practice if not by verbalization. It is time that academia recognize the problem, change its approaches (and thus its product), and stop the false advertising.

Our present system of rounds and lectures is designed to expose the student to medical knowledge deemed critical to the practice of medicine. The irony is that a goodly portion of this critical knowledge cannot be agreed upon by a majority of clinical educators in the field today. The amount of knowledge required of a given student depends on the given clinician, his or her area of interest/specialty, the uniqueness of the information, the amount of time available on a given day, and a myriad of other factors. The veterinary medical student feels an emphasis on being able to *memorize answers* rather than being required to *demonstrate an ability* to determine the proper set of questions that should be investigated; and once determined, demonstrate an ability to investigate.

The clinical educator faces a similar dilemma. It is not the intent of the clinical educator to require rote memory, but rather to stimulate independent thought and, through familiarization with important concepts, impart knowledge. Good intentions, however, are frequently lost in action predicated by patient, client, and career demands. The demands placed by the clinical educator on the subordinate members of the system can quickly sabotage the most honorable intentions!

The Great Experiment

In 1984, Tuskegee University attempted to develop a number of Problem Knowledge Couplers (PKCs) via student assistance for the eventual incorporation into its clinical instruction program as an initial effort to mitigate the deficiencies mentioned earlier. The original and laudable attempt to make PKCs an integral part of clinical instruction must be credited to Dr. Tsagye Habretamariam, who is Director of the Biomedical Information Management Systems at Tuskegee University's School of Veterinary Medicine. It was largely his vision and guidance that led us to the lessons learned and the successes eventually attained.

We took a class of approximately 60 students and divided them up in groups of three or four, assigned each group a development topic, (e.g., bovine diarrhea, equine infertility, canine alopecia, etc.), and placed each group under the supervision of a faculty member who served as content expert.

The students were given several classes in which the approach to interpreting scientific literature was discussed. The particular format required by the knowledge network was explained, and the students were instructed to search the pertinent literature on their assigned topic, parse the information, and repackage it in the format needed for data entry into the knowledge network.

This information was then to be reviewed by the faculty supervisor (content expert) and, if found to be accurate, passed along to data entry personnel for entry into the knowledge network. The information would then be repackaged into the appropriate PKC by the students and a few faculty/staff with PKC expertise. We undertook what turned out to be a horrendous project! Four of the 21 PKCs initiated were completed. It was an experience that taught us many things. The problems were not with the PKC software but rather with our scheme of PKC development. Lessons were learned by faculty and students. It was extremely rewarding to observe fourth year students gain enlightenment of the issues of controversy in scientific literature. It was simultaneously disconcerting that the majority of the students reacted as if they were detecting inconsistencies and theories presented as facts in scientific literature for the first time in their career—after three years of medical education! This was clearly a reflection of how the rigors of the curriculum had forced the student to swallow any information offered without questioning it, as a survival tactic.

Our problems in developing PKCs were numerous. The faculty involved had difficulty ignoring precepts and tendencies that they had spent years internalizing. When contradictory information was found by the student, it was not uncommon for faculty members to express their biases and pressure the student to include only information consistent with their beliefs and practices. The desire to control information that might be entered into the knowledge network appeared to originate from the erroneous concept that the Problem Knowledge Coupler would provide the diagnosis at the end of the coupling session. With this concept in hand, a faculty advisor might have felt compelled to ensure that the information upon which the "ultimate diagnosis" was made was consistent with information normally used to make a particular diagnosis. Aside from the obvious effect that personal bias undoubtedly had on information initially presented for data entry, the major effect was a limitation of general factual information being gleaned from the literature. It was thought, going into the project, that this would be a rapid way of generating a large knowledge net for each of the major veterinary species. Instead, information that involved pathogenesis, therapy, and pathophysiology was virtually ignored. The information collected was largely limited to clinical signs, diagnostic tests, and to some extent the etiology and treatment of a particular disease syndrome.

We quickly realized our folly. Although this information was adequate (barely) for diagnostic PKCs, we discovered that additional information was desirable to "flesh out" the couplers or to build management couplers. This meant a duplication of effort in reviewing certain articles twice in order to find information pertinent to the task at hand. Our experience underscored the importance of collecting all the data of relevant articles without regard to potential use in a diagnostic or management knowledge coupler. Instead, additional information should be viewed as added depth to the knowledge network that may become helpful in future coupler development.

The students posed different problems: misinterpretation of information, incomplete searches of the literature, impatience at having to classify entities and facts, and impatience with the detailed nature of the information required by the network software. It became obvious very soon, that the process of gathering, reordering, and entering the pertinent information was much too arduous a process for veterinary medical students who were simultaneously undergoing the rigors of completing the fourth year of veterinary medical education. It was also much too long a process that resulted only in the development of the knowledge network—not the PKC, which required considerable data manipulation itself.

Lessons Learned

It was relatively easy to convince the students that an alternative premise of medical education might result in a more fulfilling learning experience. Discussions with the students were filled with admissions of common mistakes made by faculty. By the end of these discussions, the students were ready to participate in our great experiment and eager to contribute to the positive changes in medical education.

The most important lesson learned, was that we as medical educators cannot (and should not) use student labor, time, and effort to establish the groundwork for needed changes in the system, particularly when that system continues to operate by the very principles being challenged. Convincing the faculty to change its basic premise of medical education was an entirely different matter. The underlying emotions incited by this issue collectively formed a major obstacle in producing and implementing PKCs in our system. Faculty concerns about proposed changes in instructional delivery and the development and utilization of the PKC in particular were many. It should not be surprising that a call for changes might be taken as a personal affront by faculty who have invested in the present system. Some faculty voiced deep concerns about time and effort being committed to projects such as the PKC development project, and the miniscule contributions that this project would make to their curriculum vitae. This concern was ultimately the most important concern that established the platform from which all other concerns and disagreements would be mounted. Unfortunately, the system of medical education does not equally reward and recognize those individuals who deliver innovative, quality education as those individuals who have demonstrated an aptitude and talent for research, and/or administration. It was a very difficult argument to counter.

It is clear that the administration must provide career incentives for faculty personnel who dare to tread along such a treacherous path. It is also clear that successful implementation of any new methodology requires the elimination of the old system and a full commitment to making the new system work. This requires unwavering administrative support. There were many concerns expressed about placing too much responsibility on the computer, and distracting the student from learning what is really important, (clinical skills, animal handling skills, skills in formulating plans, etc.). This is not a concern unique to our faculty. It is a common skepticism among many medical professionals when confronted with the possibility of computer intervention in the diagnostic arena. The Problem Knowledge Coupler requires proficiency and accuracy in technical skills and clinical assessment. The clinical investigator must be able to ascertain the presence or absence of the clinical findings included in the questionnaire of the coupler. The clinical instructor is able to use this program as a quality control measure in order to determine the degree of proficiency of a student's clinical skill.

There was general disbelief that the process of making a diagnosis could be broken down into elemental steps, fed into a computer, and then combined again into a discrete diagnosis. This was again based on the idea that this diagnostic software package would provide "the" diagnosis for a particular patient after a coupling session.

Another Try = The Little Experiment

In 1986 a more moderate plan of PKC implementation was instituted with the following goals:

- Production of PKCs that address clinical signs commonly seen in our clinic

- Utilization of PKCs in clinical instruction

- Comparison of student performance between PKC use and PKC nonuse in the clinical setting using standard evaluative instruments and procedures.

It was decided that PKC production would be scaled down to a few faculty who expressed interest in participating in the program and to offer student assistance to provide compensation for student efforts. Armed with a grant from the Department of Health and Human Services, we began our "little experiment." The bulk of the development work occurred during the summer months. In 1988, after six full months of development, six PKCs had been developed. These PKCs were added to four PKCs developed by Mississippi State University's School of Veterinary Medicine and placed in the clinic September 1, 1988.

What transpired at this point was a matter of compromise between theoretical ideals and practicality. It was recommended that appropriate PKCs should be incorporated into the normal procedure of clinical case investigation.

Data Collection

When a patient entered the clinic with a clinical sign for which a PKC was available, the duty clinician was asked to instruct the student to use the appropriate PKC after a history, physical examination, and collection of the laboratory minimum database had been completed. The student would complete a coupling session based on his or her findings and print out disease rule outs. These disease rule outs were used as the basis of discussion in rounds. The discussion addressed the appropriateness of the diseases included in the list, the exclusion of diseases that one may have expected, the order of probability or, at least, the order of disease investigation, and diseases that, upon first glance, seemed inappropriate for the patient.

Rule Out Evaluation (DDx)

Usually, the discussion would progress to focus on two or three of the more probable diseases, the relative clinical signs that placed these diseases on the list, and the clinical signs that were not given by the coupler that may have been present in the patient. The student was evaluated for his or her ability to accurately elicit/detect and classify pertinent historical, clinical, and laboratory data/abnormalities. (Were the abnormalities/findings prompted by the coupler correctly selected or omitted?)

The Diagnostic Plan

At this point the discussion would focus on the diagnostic plan proposed by the PKC. The discussion would address appropriateness and relevance of test procedures suggested, completeness of test procedures, test procedures omitted, and relative cost vs. effectiveness.

Results

The use of paid student assistants solved the problem of initiative (another victory for capitalism). Even here, small lessons were learned. It was much more productive to use time periods during which students were heavily involved in their curricular pursuits (fall and spring semesters), for knowledge network development. The manipulation of entities to build a PKC proved too rigorous and cumbersome for a distracted student working up to 20 hours a week. After assigning the students several articles, an acceptable pace of literature perusal and conversion to knowledge network format was determined. Compensation was based on meeting the mutually agreed upon goal (usually seven to ten pages per hour) depending on the complexity of the subject matter. Until typing skills were given a chance to improve, the student was paid at an hourly rate. Gradually, the student was paid by the fact entered into the network. This included all associated new entries of entities, synonyms, relationships, classifications, etc. This proved a much more equitable system of compensation.

The students involved seemed to enjoy thoroughly the process of discovery and appeared to enjoy equally the learning process of parsing information in order to obtain the true meaning of the literature as opposed to implications, or ill conceived assumptions and/or comparisons. Whereas building of the knowledge network seemed to be an enjoyable experience, the development of the PKCs proved troubling. The bulk of PKC development occurred during the summer months when data entry assistants were available on an eight hour a day basis. The students were constantly admonished to set aside any preset notions, ideas, or learned behaviors about making a diagnosis until all information was entered.

PKC Review

Many times, particularly for diseases that are ill defined in the literature, or cannot be suspected/confirmed without exotic tests), the resultant set of clinical signs may include signs that would not cause the experienced clinician or even the "expert" of the disease to think of that particular disease. This proved to be a perennial problem with faculty who were asked to review a first draft PKC. Most disapprovals would begin with inconsistencies of disease clinical entities of the computer vs. the experience of the clinician. When asked to provide corroboration via documentation, these views were rarely substantiated. This, however, did not stop continued criticism based on the same unsubstantiated (but strongly held) views. In general, faculty were reluctant to support any software that might aid in diagnostics, and particularly when it suggested diagnoses based on unconventional clinical criteria.

In using the PKCs developed, a number of behavior modifications had to be made. The most common reason for nonuse of a given PKC was that the duty clinician or student forgot it was available. Although there was a list of PKCs at the PKC station, even the PKC station was often forgotten. It soon became obvious that incorporation of PKCs into the normal diagnostic procedure would only be accomplished by the same rigorous and continuous demands made by the clinician and medical records personnel used to ensure that a history and phyical examination are completed. In other words, we had to make the PKC a common and integral part of the diagnostic process; so much so, that it would automatically be thought of at some point in the diagnostic process.

The breadth and number of available PKCs again thwarted our efforts. The narrow topics that PKCs address (i.e., feline anemia, feline alopecia, canine alopecia, canine cough, bovine diarrhea) predicates a nearly complete library of clinical signs in order to ensure interaction between clinician/student and coupler. (Every time the PKC station was checked, and an appropriate PKC was not found for the case in question, the experience served as negative reinforcement for future PKC use.)

Subsequently, we became aware that since PKC evaluation is predicated on PKC use, and PKC use is predicated on the development of an adequate range of coupled problems, PKC development became our top priority. In order for a fair and effectual evaluation to take place, the initial effort of development must be made. Our use of the limited numbers of PKCs available in veterinary medicine suggests that our efforts may be worthwhile. Although objective data are not yet available, the impact of the PKC on the student's dicovery process and the clinician's instructional modality appears to be positive. We are currently in our initial evaluation phase. It is expected as research continues, as the network grows, and as the number of couplers increases, the positive effects on clinical instruction will become clearly evident and easily documented.

Summary

The PKC can relieve concern over loss of pertinent details and simultaneously provide accountability for the process undertaken by the individual responsible for the case. The diseases offered as possible causes provide exactly what is required by the student who is suddenly faced with the entire book of medical knowledge without a table of contents (the patient): the appropriate portion of the table of contents. The clinical instructor need not worry about an inordinate amount of time wasted, because the PKC directs the student to the very literature that the clinical educator would eventually provide. More importantly, the student quickly realizes the clinical similarity between diseases, efficiently becomes familiar with current literature, and can actively participate in the investigative process at an earlier point in his or her career. The emphasis of learning shifts from memorization of seemingly isolated details to the demonstration of the ability to investigate. The computer serves as a perfect memory extender and allows the clinical instructor to further emphasize accountability on history taking, physical examination, and sample collecting skills. The PKC aids in this arena also. The student must be able to detect aqueous flare, or a grade II/IV cardiac murmur, or suprascapular lymphadenopathy in order to be able to invoke the assistance of the coupler.

Tuskegee University is utilizing the Problem Knowledge Coupler (PKC) to provide an emphasis on information gathering, accountability for technical and physical expertise, and information that is clearly relevant to an individual case that a veterinary student might be involved with. Clinical rounds are still being held, but with less student confusion or apathy. They are used with the lecture and rounds format because they encourage analytical and interpretive skills, problem solving, and decision making.

We believe that the PKC is a first generation computer aided diagnostic software that has immense potential for practice and clinical education.

Appendices

A

Preface to the 1969 edition of Medical Records, Medical Education, and Patient Care

Lawrence L. Weed

If communities were the size of cells and if hospitals, pharmacies, laboratories, patients, and physicians were the size of subcellular particles, no doubt they would be the subjects of a great deal of research, and much more would be known about their interrelationships and pathophysiology. But the apparent ease with which the organization of medicine itself can be observed has discouraged examination of it and has even made the idea of that examination seem somehow naive and unscientific. Research and planning at the community level may be troublesome. Others besides you observe and are affected by what you are doing, and they are eager to point out imperfections when they see them. To deal with indirect evidence and the abstract at the molecular and microscopic level is not only sophisticated and intellectually satisfying but is a good deal safer, for imperfections are discernible to but a few, and the investigator himself sees flaws only in proportion to his capacity to develop and use analytical methods to reveal them. It is not surprising that so much of our nation's intellectual power has been directed out to space or in to the double helix, where rewards are well defined and the frustrations of dealing with a society that often seems essentially irrational and uncontrollable are largely absent. It is true that failures occur at the sophisticated levels, too, but they are made in tolerable obscurity and rarely under conditions of frustration and social unrest.

All of us would like to correct this imbalance, to see the organization of medicine well studied and well ordered, without, at the same time, shifting the weight of research and planning so far that the undeniable benefits of a concentration on specialized subject areas are lost. Indeed, not only would the standard of medical care aspired to in this volume be impossible without medicine's long history of the closely focused and theoretical study of the science of health and disease, but it is precisely in the effort to apply the fruits of that research effectively and broadly and to order and integrate the elements of it that this volume has been prepared. We cannot help solve society's everyday problems by putting people under electron microscopes or out into the Van Allen belt; we can help not only by the intelligent use of the tools of systems analysis and sociology but also by a basic realization that to improve the quality of the practice of everyday medicine is worthy of our best efforts.

Two fundamental steps in working effectively at the community level are establishing a practical system of communication for use in caring for all people and fixing the standards for such a system so that problems and progress can be defined. Central in the present system of communication is the medical record, upon which patient care, much clinical investigation, and medical education depend, and even unrefined standards lead to the conclusion that it is in need of immediate attention. In its current state it is an instrument full of serious faults, being sometimes irregular, diffuse, subjective and incomplete. Developed standards for the preparation of the medical record do not exist. Where would biochemistry or physics be if reports of their progress depended on journals without qualified boards of editors administering developed standards? One may conjecture that progress in such fields would seriously have been retarded. There is in existence at the present time no body of literature on how to structure the medical record, particularly progress notes on long-term problems, and so there is no framework within which discipline can develop.

My thesis is that this situation can be remedied. The medical record need not be simply a static, *pro forma* repository of medical observations and activities grouped in the meaningless order of source—whether doctor or nurse, laboratory or X-ray department—rather than with respect to the problems to which they pertain; it can be problem-oriented, and thereby it can become a dynamic, structured, creative instrument for facilitating comprehensive and highly specialized medical care. But in addition to being problem-oriented, the medical record must be concise, cogent, and complete, not diffuse, superficial, or fragmentary, for the latter characteristics lead to care out of context. The medical record must serve the experienced physician and yet be intelligible to the medical student; it must serve the student and yet not frustrate the practicing physician; it must be adaptable to computerization but not require it; it must give freedom of expression to the most perceptive and experienced physician, yet must establish form and order to prevent personalization of the record to the point at which subjectivity impairs communication. The medical record must serve the patient as well as the physician, so it must be equally intelligible to all physicians, since patients are likely to require the services of many physicians and as much as possible the progress of the patient among them must be easy and without confusion. The medical record must completely and honestly convey the many variables and complexities that surround every decision, thereby discouraging unreasonable demands upon the physician for supernatural understanding and superhuman competence; but at the same time it must faithfully represent events and decisions so that errors can be detected and proper corrective measures taken when lapses in thoroughness, disciplined thought, and reasonable follow-up occur. The medical record must be the natural extension of the basic science training of the physician; in short, it must be a scientific manuscript.

The pages that follow present specific steps in record-keeping that attempt to satisfy these sometimes paradoxical requirements. They can be satisfied. The contradictions in aims are apparent, not real, as intelligent use of a well-structured, problem-oriented medical record will reveal.

I note that, as will readily be apparent to the reader, the records presented as examples in the text have not been revised retrospectively for the purpose of quotation here. They contain jargon and unnecessary abbreviations, and the quality of the medicine practiced and the logic displayed in the pursuit of solutions to problems are not always exemplary. Many of the problem lists are not in the exact form prescribed; and many of the progress notes, though problem-oriented, do not contain concise analytical descriptions and conclusions. However, all are real and consequently are actual, not imagined, referents to day-by-day medical practice, and all are instructive stages in the direction of the system recommended.

Most of the examples used here represent care for acute, hospital-type problems, even though the text emphasizes the need for more attention to ambulatory care and preventive medicine and demographic approaches in defining and dealing with problems. Appendix E and a forthcoming volume by two general practitioners using problem-oriented records will better illustrate this emphasis.

L. L. W.

B
Introduction to the 1969 edition of Medical Records, Medical Education, and Patient Care

Lawrence L. Weed

The beginning clinical clerk, the new intern, and the practicing physician are confronted with an apparent contradiction. Each is asked, as a "whole" physician, to accept the obligations of meeting many problems simultaneously and yet to give to all the single-minded attention that is fundamental to developing and mobilizing his enthusiasm and skill—for these two virtues do not arise except where an organized concentration upon a particular subject is possible. It is this multiplicity of problems with which the physician must deal in his daily work that constitutes the principal distinguishing feature between his activities and those of many other scientists. The multiplicity is inevitable, but a random approach to the difficulties it creates is not. The instruction of physicians should be based on a system that helps them to define and follow clinical problems one by one and then systematically to relate and resolve them. Doctors vary tremendously in their capacity to deal competently with widely varying numbers and types of challenges in medical practice. We must therefore sort out physicians in terms of what they actually do competently for patients and not in terms of how they trained, what specialty group they joined, or how well they fared in qualifying examinations. In other words, the basic criterion of the physician is how well he can identify the patient's problems and organize them for solution.

What is done in medical education to prepare the physician for a lifelong scrutiny of the records on his patients? The answer is, very little, for in many medical schools, as in many specialty training programs, elaborate provisions are made for transmitting the facts of basic science and clinical medicine, but little is done to transmit to the student the scientific methodology that will eventually permit him to deal with complex biological systems successfully.

What is this methodology? The scientist defines a problem clearly, separates multifarious problems into their individual components, and clarifies their relationships to each other. He records data in a communicative and standard form and ultimately accepts an audit from objective peers by seeking publication in a journal. Basis scientists are neither better people nor better scholars than physicians; they do not pursue more scientific or intrinsically "better" problems. They are simply subject to better monitoring by a system that mobilizes the criticism of their peers throughout their lives. Clinical medicine, on the other hand, substitutes qualifying examinations at a single point in a career for a lifelong process of recurring audit and it must frankly be admitted that the customary methodology of medicine fails to provide the kind of structures context that promotes objectivity, sharpens skills, and permits progressive self-evaluation.

To focus the comparison more sharply, let us look at the clinical specialty board candidate and the basic science graduate degree aspirant. The latter, after spending the first year or two mainly in course work, devotes an increasing proportion of his time to his thesis, to which all his other activities ultimately become secondary. Conferences, seminars, normal free time—all are set aside, if need be, because it is by his thesis that the candidate scientist will be judged. The thesis reveals both what he knows and what he is capable of doing with what he knows. Each day, as he works, his preceptor and his colleagues can study and criticize his data as he records them in his note-books. Finally, everyone who sits on his examination board reviews a copy of his thesis, which is written in a very standard form so as to simplify critical analysis, as a precondition of acceptance. If he receives his degree, he proceeds to a new problem, completes his research on it, prepares his report, and submits it for publication to a journal whose editors exercise the right to establish standards of form and content and may require him to write his paper several times. As a consequence of this process, he develops a respect for order, logic, and consistency and cooperates with his critics without feeling that his creativity and originality are jeopardized by their guidance. It would not occur to the scientist to protest to the editors that there is much "art" in his laboratory work that never can be recorded and that the editors have to see him at work in order fully to appreciate him.

The clinical specialty board candidate, on the other hand, submits to examinations in which he is asked to recall memorized facts. No thesis composed of analyses and defenses of his cases recorded on a specific form is required of him. Instead, he is given an informal oral examination on the basis of a preselected case; preselected data are presented to him in a setting in which patients are normally "worked up" in the clinic and in the ward. The strategy and completeness of his own search for the data, the depth of his theoretical understanding and the delicacy of the analytical capacity that will permit him to make sound therapeutic decisions, and his ability to sustain quality and energy in his daily attach on all types of problems, esoteric and mundane, are poorly evaluated by such examining procedures.

In clinical situations there is in effect not a single thesis, but there are a thousand of them. Little time can be devoted to each, and the physician is confronted with biological variables that are exceptionally difficult to enumerate and control and that are complicated by concurrent human and social problems. The need for organization grows with increasing complexity and pressure of time. Yet the intellectual discipline addressed to clinical problems is often superficial; documentation may be haphazard; systems are ill-defined; and no audit ever takes place.

Figure 1 is a partial sequence of notes extracted from a complicated, unstructured record of a patient with a long list of problems. Facts are presented in language that suggests difficulties in many systems, but the record is so confused, is such a tangle of illogically assembled bits of information, that one cannot reliably discern from it how (or whether) the physician defined and logically pursued each problem.

A double standard exists. We invoke discipline when we prepare the manuscript concerning laboratory research, and we abandon discipline when we write final progress notes, such as these, on the care of patients. The care itself may suffer. The confidence of those students who observe our failure to discipline ourselves also suffers.

We can help student systematize their clinical experience by means of their clinical records; we can demand that they present the data they accumulate on each problem in a consistent, well-organized form, clearly delineated. That this can be done is shown by an extension of the record in Figure 1; this extension, presented as Figure 2, was prepared by a second physician, who assumed responsibility for the same case. Under the new physician, the situation abruptly changed, and the titles of each of the progress notes at once began to make clear the total nature of the case. For example, if we focus on a single problem (#2b. RLL pneumonia), we are immediately able to assess the quality of patient care. We know what attention is or is not being paid to the patient's symptoms, physical findings, and sputum characteristics. We can observe what steps have or have not been taken for the physical management of the patient and in particular what has been done, if anything, to assure the proper drainage of his chest.

If we fail to provide a system for—and to demand order from—students and physicians, then we should not be surprised if they reveal anxiety and confusion in the management of complicated cases. The recourse for many of them is to seek shelter in specialization, where single-mindedness is acceptable and multifarious problems may be ignored.

The education of a physician for specialized and for total care should be based on his own clinical experience and should be reflected in the records he maintains on his patients. An educational institution should set the pattern for the physicians's professional development, and the pattern should be based not on grand rounds, conferences, and journal clubs but on a detailed scrutiny of the clinical experience of students, house officers, and staff, as the clinical records reveal it. The education of a student, a resident physician, or a senior

9/10

Patient received 40 units of regular insulin yest. because of B & 4+
urine sugars. Got 2000 cc Amigen yest. & 500 cc D5W. Was
febrile all night up to 40 at 8PM; this gradually came down to 39.
8PM yest. suctioned & coughed up č return of ½ cup of thick
white sputum-cultured. also blood cultures. Was in must. tent č
mucomist overnight. At 4PM yest. had B-R base. Sputum smear
unremarkable-WBC's but no bacteria.

9/10-12:30

10 o'clock urine 2-3+/0. Given 10 U. reg. ins. at 12:30 PM. Temp.
down to 38? Suctioned N.T. c little return. However during
suctioning pt. vomited 100-150 cc green fluid. Proximal jejunostomy tube draining well now.

9/11-9 AM

Urine 3+ given 10 U reg. insulin. Pt. was hiccuping all night &
this AM. Levine tube passed č 900-1000 cc bileous fluid removed.
Jejunostomy tubes have been draining minimally. Will have Levine
tube down.

                    [Three pages of similar notes follow until 9/26]

9/26

Last night 10PM had seizure like behavior and acting strange.
Apparently hallucinating. Blood sugar didn't register on destrostix.
Had been given 10 units reg. insulin at 8 PM after IV glucose
returned to nl. This AM vomited up brown black fluid 300 cc +
for occult blood. NG tube had been out since 5PM yest. NG tube
replaced & some material small amt. withdrawn. Pt. now NPO č
NG tube to Gomco.

9/27

Still febrile-Ampicillin ig qid-continued; Blood cult. drawn to check
if septicemia still present. Chest X ray today shows infiltrate in (R)
lower lobe. No effusion. Sputum grew out pseudomonas but Dr. -
--- elected not to treat this.

Figure 1. Unstructured patient record.

10/2-6PM

#1 Chronic Relapsing Panc.:

b. Diabetes: will continue moment to moment Rx of spot

urines for now. Today c̄ only 10 regular insulin pt.

spilling mainly 2-3+.

Plan: BLD sugar tomorrow

c.   Panc. insuff.: will begin Cotazyn-B

#2 Complications following Laparotomy:

c. Post op ileus: KUB tomorrow. Pt. now tolerating ice cream

and occ. candy. bs. poor; s̄ gross distention; stool

passes regularly → fistula

Imp: prob. resolving now

Plan: KUB and continue small feedings

d. Sepsis: afebrile now on Ampicillin. see flowsheet.

Reculture tomorrow.

b.   RLL Pneumonia: Film of 9/28 shows some ↑ in this process.

Will repeat P.A. chest tomorrow & cultures.

e. Colonic-Cutaneous Fistula: Continues to drain semi-formed stool

several times per day; the problem is that stool drains

into granulating abd. wound.

Plan: culture stool; Remove some non-func stay sutures;

Freq dressings & consider colostomy bag for fistula.

10/3

#1 Chronic Relapsing Panc.:

c. Panc. insufficiency: Cotazyn-B will be begun

(special purchase) and will evaluate effect

on absorption and/or stool content by measuring amt. of fat

Figure 2. Problem-oriented patient record

f. <u>Pain</u>: pt. still requires freq narcotics. Neurosurg will
   eventually perform epidural block and depending
   upon results will consider cordotomy.

<u>#2 Complications Following Laparotomy:</u>

b. <u>RLL Pneumonia</u>: Chest X-ray today shows marked resolution
   of previously described infiltrates; pt. has been
   afebrile-sputum recultured (see #2).

c. <u>Post op ileus</u>: KUB today shows little improvement from
   film of 9/29. Ba in same position in colon which is
   distal to fistula. Despite this X-ray findings will
   continue to feed (see #2f). Bowel sounds poor and
   abd. seems slightly more distended. Will give oil retention
   enema to try to clear distal colon.

d. <u>Sepsis</u>: Pt. has been afebrile, cultures repeated today;
   o (M) heard today; has been on Ampicillin x 9 days.
   Although potential still present this problem is under
   relatively good control.

e. <u>Colonic-Cutaneous Fistula</u>: all stay sutures removed today and
   wound is well granulated but constantly bathed c̄ stool.
   Colostomy bag applied to try to control this drainage.
   Etiology of fistula? but my be serving decompressive function.

f. <u>Malnutrition</u>: Total protein = 6.1 c 2.1/4.0 = A/G in 1965.
   Wt. has ↓ from 141# →113# since adm.

   <u>Imp</u>: little resolution of ileus, in fact, most of food stays in stomach
   probably; this remains the main problem; other as above fairly well
   controlled except malnutrition.

   <u>Plan</u>: as above plus give gastro-graffin per NG tube and watch progress;
   <u>avoid surgery</u>.

Figure 2. (Continued).

physician becomes defective not when he is given too much or too little training in basic science nor when his clinical load falls below an ideal standard but rather when he is allowed to ignore or slight the elementary definition and the progressive adjustment of the problems that comprise his clinical experience. The teacher* who ultimately benefits students most is the one who is willing to establish parameters of discipline in the not unsophisticated but often unappreciated task of preventing this imprecision and disorganization. Avoiding irrelevant displays of fact, he must continually emphasize the enumeration, evaluation, integration, and continuing audit of all the patient's problems.

Problem-oriented medical records can become a vehicle for converting a broad philosophy of education into specific, attainable goals. Through the creation of a proper record and the proper management of that record, the physician's actial performance in given areas can be exposed to critical evaluation in the same way that the scientist's work is evaluated by journal editors; the physician can be assisted to demonstrate thoroughness and reliability in the formulation of all the patient's problems; and he can be guided in the exercise of sound analytical thought, coupled with good clinical judgment, in establishing patient-care plans and in following up patient progress in each problem area.

Special cases encountered within the daily routine will always provide an unsurpassed opportunity to instruct and evaluate the physician. The same combination of variables rarely repeats itself in textbook fashion in any one case, and the manner in which the student or physician finds his way among each new combination of variables within the constant framework of sound physiological principles and avoids premature diagnostic and therapeutic decisions is the best measure of his performance and growth. Progress notes and operative notes are replete with teaching opportunities, because they are relevant to the current intellectual and emotional concerns of the student or house officer who wrote them. No matter how elegant the teacher's presentation, its effect may be severely reduced if it has no connection with the student's problems at the time. The teacher will be more likely to achieve solid educational goals if he approaches the student through the specific realities that confront him at that point, using terms consistent with the student's level of understanding.

The techniques for putting this approach into effect are not difficult, so long as the teacher agrees to present facts and principles as adjuncts of concrete experience, entering the student's mind that is confirmed by tradition, that passes for education, but that, when the student is confronted with a particular set of variables and needs to take meaningful action, may crumble and leave him anxious and confused. Furthermore, teaching that is not based upon real

---

*Teacher, as used in this book, includes everyone from the intern who helps the student to the full professot who teaches at many levels.

physical and biological problems requiring specific solutions denies not only the student but also the teacher the progressive opportunity to correct the unsound theories, the false generalizations, and the outright errors that abound in every field of knowledge. The solution of real problems is, I believe, the foundation of student morale, and by no means impedes development at the theoretical level but perhaps even enhances it.

Until our basic commitment is to the teaching of discipline and a rigorous approach to medical problems, instead of non-problem-oriented feats of memory, not only will we be unable to take advantage of the enlarged capabilities of the new generation of premedical students and reduce what is now an intolerably long training period but also we may sink deeper into the quagmire of raw information upon which our footing is already insecure, for the number of facts the memory-oriented faculty can impose upon the minds of students is limitless. The problem-oriented record, combined with almost any patient with complex problems, is uniquely suited as a vehicle for teaching approaches and essential skills, leaving libraries and computers to supply raw information and rapid retrieval. In this approach, the training period can simply be defined as that time necessary for a student to demonstrate, through a series of patient records, competence in dealing with new medical situations, using the literature and laboratories as needed.

If the role the medical record will play in his education is carefully stated to the student, the goals become clear to him as well as his teacher, and precise goals are fundamental in effective education. There must be one standard of quality for all kinds of patients: for the patient in the emergency room, the ward, or the recovery room; for the general surgical and medical clinic patient, as well as for the patient in the specialty clinic; and for all of the problems of any given patient, the mundane disorder, the esoteric diagnostic problem, the minor illness, or the major illness. The total job that needs to be done, and not merely the areas of the individual physician's or student's special interest, should be confronted head-on.

I recognize that no mere system of recording data will dispel the tragedy and confusion that surround the desperately ill. As Dr. Dickinson Richards has said, "So often the patient and doctor are waging an unequal struggle against a bitter and irrevocable fate."** Uncontrollable forces are omnipresent in the lives of all of us, excessively so in the lives of some. No system can in itself alter this human condition, but if we do our best to define all the patient's problems and to follow them up one by one, we can, with a clear conscience, set aside medical chores for a moment and be physicians in the broadest sense—and that presumably is what brought many of us into our profession in the first place. There is nothing more tragic than the "brilliant" specialist, overconfident of his knowledge and techniques, who, failing to

---

** D. W. Richards, "Homeostasis: Its Dislocations and Perturbations," *Perspectives in Biology and Medicine,* 3:238, 1960.

comprehend the nature of his responsibility, fails also to treat the trusting patient in the light of his total needs.

In the practice of medicine, both intellectually and "artistically," the greatest constraint on the realization of our potential as physicians is not system, which makes data meaningful and immediately comprehensible, but disorder, which obscures forever original patterns of thought and insight. Demand for explicit expression does not impair the quality of our perceptions; it sharpens and preserves that quality for others to build on.

The Patient's Record

If we are to organize the patient's record logically and efficiently, four basic elements of that record must be recognized:

1. *The Database.* Ordinarily present in the admission note, this may include any or all of the following: chief complaint, patient profile and related social data, present illness, past history and systems review, physical examination, and reports of laboratory.

2. *The Problem List.* On the patient's admission to the hospital, a numbered list of problems is drawn up, containing every problem in the patient's history, past and present. New problems should be added as identified.

3. *The Initial Plan.* The next step is the preparation of a list of plans—diagnostic and therapeutic orders—for each problem, keyed by number to the original problem list.

4. *Progress Notes.*

    a.   *Narrative Notes.* Each progress note is related directly to the list of problems and should be numbered and titled accordingly. Operative notes and notes by nurses and paramedical personnel are to be included.

    b.   *Flowsheets.* "Flowsheets" containing all the moving parameters should be kept on all problems where data and time relationships are complex. The flowsheets and the progress notes constitute the follow-up phase of the record-keeping process and, as such, are the dynamic center of the medical record.

    c.   *Discharge Summary.* No patient should be discharged until the house officer of the hospital has written an adequate retrospective note on each numbered problem on the patient's list.

These elements may schematically be represented as follows:

I. *Establishment of a Database*   II. *Formulation of All Problems*
    History   Problem List
    Physical Examination
    Admission Laboratory
    Work

III. *Plans for Each Problem*   IV. *Follow-up on Each Problem*
    Collection of Further   Progress Notes: Title
    Data   and Numbered
    Treatment
    Education of Patient

C
Samples of Introductions
to Individual Couplers

Lawrence L. Weed

Problem Knowledge Couplers

The following appendix presents a representative selection of introductions to existing Problem Knowledge Couplers. One will note that the basic structure of the coupler system allows the results of coupling to be organized in groups, and the form these groupings takes varies with the nature of the original problem.

If one were to examine the references for each of the linkages in each of the couplers, one would recognize that the 30 couplers now available have come out of a western, biomedical, allopathic environment. To the extent this may seem provincial to some, it does not represent any limitation in coupler building software, but rather the orientation of the builder. Our goal must be, given a problem, to have a set of couplers that accommodate not only people from different schools of training and thought (allopaths, osteopaths, chiropractors, homeopaths, acupuncturists, etc). The patient should be able to see himself or herself in these different contexts and have available the references for the linkages in each. Such a broadened and demystified view of solving problems will open up the possibility that the benefits from various cultures of providers and patients can complement one another as opposed to competing and casting doubt upon one another. At the very least, use of these tools by all groups will encourage corrective feedback loops in the actions of everyone.

Key to Coupler Introductions

HISTORY:
   Screening to Discover Patient's Problems   Coupler 5

Coupler 1

Acute Abdomen
Revised 9/25/90

Introduction. In the Acute Abdomen Coupler, as in many other couplers, the results of *coupling* are displayed in groups in the Index of Causes. In this particular coupler, the basis for the grouping is as follows:

Group 1—Physiological/Anatomical diagnoses (e.g., diaphragmatic irritation as indicated by the finding *shoulder pain*)

Group 2—Risk factors for a given disorder (e.g., risk factors for acute pancreatitis as indicated by the finding *alcoholism*). It is important to clearly separate in one's mind the risk factors for a disease from the actual evidence for the presence of the disease. Otherwise, a patient can be thoughtlessly thrown into the wrong diagnostic category and evidence for the true diagnosis is ignored until it is too late.

Group 3—Specific clinical diagnostic entities

Having examined the patterns and *matches* in each group, one should then see how consistent the physiological statement is with a specific clinical diagnosis, usually giving special attention to those specific diagnoses that explain the physiological state of affairs.

The *risk factor* classification may be helpful when two or more clinical diagnoses seem equally likely on the basis of actual clinical findings. One should first pursue the one for which the patient is at risk, all other things being equal.

The groups on the Index of Causes are separated by a blank line. In any given patient, one to several groups may appear. At least one finding that points to at least one member of a group must occur in a patient if a group is to appear at all. Then within that group, the diagnoses are ordered in terms of the absolute number of findings present.

Coupler 7

Guidance for the Medical Management of Hypertension
Revised 4/09/90

Introduction. The coupler, Guidance in the Medical Management of Hypertension, is concerned with reducing risk factors as well as choosing drugs. Unfortunately, studies have shown that many physicians give far too little attention to the former before plunging into the use of drugs.

Many patients who have a diastolic above 95 and no evidence of target organ damage may, after 3 years of observation, have a diastolic below 95 just by paying attention to matters such as salt, weight, exercise, smoking, and stress in daily living. Furthermore, patients should be aware that merely lowering a pressure with drugs may not change their risk of coronary disease, although there is evidence it will reduce the risk of stroke, heart failure, and renal disease.

Before the patient gets involved with any specific drug therapy, it should be remembered that lowering the pressure by itself may produce undesirable effects such as dizziness; any drug with the same therapeutic effect could do the same thing, so one should not be too quick to call it a bad side effect of a particular drug and switch drugs too quickly. Also, it is now known that physicians, patients, families, friends, and employers of patients have different views about the effects of drug treatment, with friends, families, and employers noticing more irritability, depression, etc., than the physicians and patients observe.

Having discussed the above issues, we can now focus on drugs. A great deal is known about many of the mechanisms involved in regulating blood pressure. Many drugs have been discovered or developed which affect those mechanisms. Unfortunately, in a given unique individual, we do not know, most of the time, which mechanism is at fault, so there is much trial and error in working out a good program of drug management. Which drug is used at the outset should be related to what is known about a particular patient and what is known about the side effects of a given drug. For example, there is little point to giving an antihypertensive agent that makes ulcers worse to a patient who already has ulcers, even if the drug has a good record for lowering the blood pressure in the hypertension population. Also, there is little point in giving too much of one drug to the point of adverse side effects, if we could have given much less of each of two or three drugs that operate at different points in the physiology of blood pressure regulation and which individually produce fewer side effects. But it would be equally unwise to saddle a patient with two or three drugs if one could do the trick. We may not always be lucky enough to have selected the right drug on the first try in this difficult matching process.

This coupler is a useful first pass in the matching process described above. After eliciting information about the unique patient before us, it will use that information to provide the *pros* and *cons* of various drugs for a particular individual. Then, after comparing the drugs in the above terms, the patient can factor in how he or she feels about the cost and the number of doses a day that are necessary for each drug. The patient should pay careful attention to the directions from the manufacturer regarding dose and cautions. Unfortunately, information about how effective the drugs are on lowering mortality and complications on large series of patients will not be available in most instances. The newer and more expensive drugs have not been studied long enough yet, and even the older drugs like the thiazide diuretics with their long term effects on blood lipids may have disadvantages yet to be revealed, although right now they seem to be the best bargain for initial therapy in purely monetary terms. And in medical terms they have proven to be a particularly good choice in many elderly and black patients.

Working out a regimen for a unique individual is a research project, and it is one in which the patient must be intimately involved. In the long run, no one can compete with the patient in having the understanding and control of the relevant variables. So our job is to get the patient in command and intelligently responsive to the data as they emerge. The printout of coupler results facilitates such an approach.

No option will fit a unique individual perfectly; trade offs will be necessary. The printout of coupler results will give the patient a very concrete beginning with very explicit choices. The medical provider's job will be to help the patients get through that initial exposure to professional jargon and to help them negotiate the explicit choices and the inevitable ambiguities and trade offs. After the very first visit the patient should take the complete printout of results home with the choices that were made well marked on the initial printout. At home they should study it until an understanding slowly develops.

Of course, they will also take their own pressures or have a family member do it, keep the flowsheet up to date so that eventually the specific data will speak to them, and they will start making specific recommendations on their own, always backed up by the provider. For a problem that will exist for years, a few months is not too much time to invest to truly understand. Once patients do understand, they will know the jargon on this subject as well or better than any professional. It is like learning any new job: it takes time to learn the ropes and the lingo before you feel at home with it all. It is true that many patients will not want such involvement, but at least this coupler should convince them that no one can do this for them if the best possible management within the framework of their unique set of characteristics is to be achieved. It is far more difficult for a physician to get on top of the details of hundreds of patient's lives (details that are so crucial to making sound "professional" choices) than it is for a patient to get on top of the details of one printout of his or her coupler results, no matter how formidable that first printout may seem.

A few pointers about reading the printout of coupler results:

- The first management options suggested, based on the patient's unique choices, relate to habits and lifestyle, such as smoking and exercise.

- *Pros* and *cons* for each drug option are then presented. Ideally, one would like to have one or more drugs appear that have no cons elicited by the unique patient's responses to the coupler choices. Unfortunately this may not happen too often, so the patient and the physician must take the time to systematically look at each option and decide which cons are the most tolerable among the drugs that have desirable pros for them.

Once both patient and provider see the options and the trade offs presented in this way (something that the unaided mind could never do for the average busy practitioner), they will realize how arbitrary, and at times biased or incomplete, the opinions of experts may be. The full energies of everyone now can be directed toward getting all the facts at the outset and at negotiating the ambiguities that inevitably result when unique individuals are matched against the various options that medical science has created.

Coupler 8

Knee Problem
Revised 6/21/89

Introduction in file. In the Knee Coupler, as in many other couplers, the results of *coupling* are presented in groups on the Index of Causes. The groups are separated by a blank line. At least one finding that points to at least one member of a group must occur in a patient if the group is to appear at all.

In the Knee Coupler, one group is made up of management options as opposed to diagnoses, e.g., "arthroscopy is indicated." If certain findings are present, particularly in an acutely injured knee, it is important to take certain steps regardless of what other findings may be present on history or physical examination. If any members of this group appear at all, they appear right at the beginning of the Index of Causes.

In the Knee Coupler, all the specific diagnoses are in a single group and are ordered in terms of the absolute number of findings present in a given patient for a given diagnosis. As in all the couplers, it is important for the users to take the time to consider the various possibilities and read the comments. In a very short time one has a very broad view of the situation with no burden on the user to recall and process many variables on the spot.

Coupler 15

Chest Pain
Revised 9/04/90

Introduction. Helpful hints about the Chest Pain Coupler:

1. It is important in the patient with chest pain to establish at the outset the physiological state of affairs and the likelihood of a life threatening problem. The first three sequences on the initial display were designed to do that. After using each of the first three sequences of the coupler, one should *couple the findings*, study the results, and then erase the results before starting the next sequence. (One erases by picking the choice "F: Other functions," which is at the bottom of the initial display. That brings up a display with the choice "E: Erase findings" on it.)

2. Sequences 4 and 5 should be used together. After the coupling process, one will note that the suggested *causes* come up in groups, and within each group the causes are ordered in terms of the absolute number of observed findings.

   Group 1—The first group includes those diseases that may require immediate and ongoing attention.

   Group 2—The second group relates to risk factors for coronary disease if any happen to be present.

   Group 3—The third group contains all other causes included in the coupler.

   Risk factors for coronary disease were separated from the findings that indicate the presence of the disease, so that patient and provider alike can be alerted to a possibility without falling in the trap of actually diagnosing the disorder on flimsy evidence.

3. In a very short time one can examine which findings are present for a given cause and which ones are not present, as well as read the comments that help both provider and patient assess the likelihood of the disorder fitting the patient's unique situation.

   It is unwise to become too preoccupied with the presence or absence of a single finding at one moment in time. Rather, one should look at patterns formed by many findings and the evolution of those patterns. Problem Knowledge Couplers facilitate this without placing an undue burden on the mind for recalling, organizing, and recording large numbers of relevant variables at the time one is seeing and evaluating a patient.

The groups on the Index of Causes are separated by a blank line. In any given patient, one to several groups may appear. At least one finding that points to at least one member of a group must occur in a patient if the group is to appear at all. Then within that group, the diagnoses are ordered in terms of the absolute number of findings present.

Coupler 17

Memory Loss and/or Confusion/Cognitive Impairment
Revised 10/12/90

Introduction. In the Memory Loss and Confusion Coupler, as in many other couplers, the results of *coupling* are presented in groups on the Index of Causes. The groups are separated by a blank line. In any given patient, one to several groups may appear. At least one finding that points to at least one member of a group must occur in a patient if a group is to appear at all. Then within that group, the diagnoses are ordered in terms of the absolute number of findings present for each cause.

It will be noted that on the first display of the Memory Loss Coupler, there are five *sequences of questions*. The first sequence does not lead to a specific diagnosis, but rather helps the user determine whether there is dementia or not. After running through this sequence, the user should *couple the findings*; instead causes "Evidence for Dementia" and/or "Evidence Against Dementia" will appear. After reviewing this information and printing what is desired for the permanent record, these results should be erased. Erasure is accomplished by typing "F" as shown at the bottom of the first display, "F: Other Functions." This leads to a choice "E: Erase results".

The second sequence should be handled in exactly the same manner as the first. This sequence helps the user determine the evidence for and against depression. Memory loss and confusion associated with depression may be corrected by treating the depression and its causes.

The third and fourth sequences help the user determine the specific cause for the problem at hand. Coupling should be done after both sequences have been used. The results of coupling may occur in one of the following possible groups.

Group 1—The first group contains those causes that may indicate an emergency situation requiring monitoring and immediate action.

Group 2—The second group contains those diagnoses for which only one finding is present in the coupler. When such a cause appears, it may not be the sole cause for the problem, but it has to be considered at least as a contributing cause and treated accordingly.

Group 3—The third group is the remaining causes in the coupler.

The fifth sequence should be used after the results of the earlier sequences have been digested and erased. This final sequence helps the user understand some of the subtle differences among the dementias that result from various degenerative diseases of obscure etiology. All this, of course, is done in terms of the findings of the unique patient under consideration.

Coupler 22

Abnormal EKG: Interpretation
Revised 11/5/88

Introduction. In the Abnormal EKG Coupler, as in many other couplers, the results of *coupling* are displayed on the screen in groups in the Index of Causes. The groups of causes are separated by blank lines. In a given patient, one or more groups may appear. At least one finding, pointing to at least one member of a group of causes, must occur in a patient if a group is to appear at all. Then, within that group, the diagnoses (causes) are arranged in a particular order - an order which is determined by the total number of findings present for each cause.

The groups in the Abnormal EKG Coupler are characterized as follows:

Group 1—The members of this group are not causes of disease in any clinical sense. However these are reminders of common electrocardiographic technical errors that may be confounding factors in the interpretation of a particular abnormal electrocardiographic finding, e.g., reversal of the leads.

Group 2—The members of this group include drugs, metabolic disturbances, chest wall deformities, and physiologic states, e.g. athletic conditioning, that are all factors that may modify the interpretation of certain EKG findings. Examine each member of this group to see whether such confounding factors might be present in a particular patient, e.g., hyperkalemia, to account for particular abnormal electrocardiographic findings. If such a factor is not present, then one must look for other explanations for the EKG abnormality.

Group 3—This group includes abnormalities of rhythm and mechanism.

Group 4—Specific EKG PATTERN diagnoses appear in this group. EKG pattern characteristics alone are used as evidence for inclusion in this group. One should compare one's tentative conclusions from this group with the results shown in Group 7 which includes diagnoses based on clinical evidence as well as EKG evidence.

Group 5—Qualitative statements about QRS electrical axis are included in this group. As one studies the findings under a member of this group, one should examine the comments for relevant facts about the modifying influences of age, body habitus, obesity etc.

Group 6—Risk factors for various disorders are included in this group. It is important to distinguish risks for a given disorder from the evidence that the disorder is actually present in a particular individual. If one is *at risk* (i.e., manifests findings which are risk factors) for a given disease, but lacks positive evidence (findings present) which point to the presence of the disease at that moment in time, then one should consider that the patient may be in an early stage of disease and further points on a curve by monitoring for defined parameters over time is indicated.

Group 7—This group includes diagnoses based on a combination of clinical and electrocardiographic evidence manifested by this particular unique individual.

The pattern concepts of electrocardiography accessible by the use of the standard 12 lead scalar electrocardiogram, used in the average primary care internal medical office practice form the basis of the information in this coupler with its clinical correlations.

The diagnostic considerations for the arrhythmias are predicated on the use of the standard scalar EKG, in the average office primary care office setting, in which HIS Bundle tracings are not normally available.

Coupler 25

Assessment and Management of an Acute Asthmatic Attack
Revised 10/22/90

Introduction. The Coupler for the Management of the Acute Asthmatic Attack has both diagnostic and management aspects. Instead of creating two separate couplers, there is a single coupler using the basic *diagnostic coupler* framework. After *coupling*, the Index of Causes that appears contains both the classification groups for the severity of the asthmatic attack as well as *cautions and indicators* for various drugs and actions. As one chooses any one of the *severity* groupings that a particular patient's findings evokes, one will see, as in the other couplers, the *findings present* and the *findings not present*. The *options* choice at the bottom of the screen leads one to appropriate management options for that particular level of severity of asthmatic attack.

One may wonder why one needs to classify the patient into a severity group, when one could have the coupler just take each abnormality and couple it directly to a specific treatment, e.g., oxygen for the cyanosis, bicarbonate for the low pH, etc. One could do that, but by using the approach here, the user immediately gets an overall sense of where the patient stands and where he might be headed without being dependent on the value of any single parameter. Also it is helpful to see on one display the whole group of management options that should be considered. One can then go from there and focus on the treatment for each specific finding present. Of course unique patients may have some findings that place them in one group and others that place them in another. If the spread is great and the pattern unusual one should suspect that something other than a pure asthmatic attack is going on.

If one is going to be in the business of managing asthmatic patients, one should always have readily available the means to do FEV1s and PEFRs. It is important to have such objective measurements as a baseline before too many treatments are set into motion.

Have some familiarity with the coupler before actually using it with an acutely ill patient, so there is no delay in acquiring and entering the appropriate data when time is of the essence.

When actually using the coupler with a patient, one should be careful to examine all the items on the Index of Causes that appears after coupling.

Group 1—The first group will give guidance as to whether hospitalization is indicated.

Group 2—The second will indicate severity, as discussed above.

Group 3—The third will alert one to evidence for infection.

Group 4—The fourth will give cautions about steroids and theophylline if they are appropriate to the unique patient in question.

Group 5—The fifth and final group alerts one to a particular individual's risks for a fatal attack, indicators that a severe attack may develop, and indications that one should suspect more than simple asthma.

Coupler 28

Hyperlipidemia Management
Revised 9/24/90

Introduction. The management of hyperlipidemia requires attention to many details applied in a systematic way over a significant period of time. Since the coupler guides the user in eliciting and processing those details, the main task left to the patient and the medical provider is taking the time to examine thoroughly *the results of coupling.* Many management options may appear for a single individual, and there is no substitute for examining each one and deciding whether and how to act upon it. To facilitate this, they have been organized so that specific issues have been raised in the following order:

1. Cautions about interpreting values from different laboratories.

2. Urgent measures for the individual whose lipid values are sufficiently deranged to require immediate therapeutic action.

3. Specific recommendations about the use of alcohol.

4. Pointers to and comments about secondary causes of hyperlipidemia that are raised by the presence of certain findings in a given individual.

5. Guidance as to when certain findings should lead one to consider further analysis for unusual lipid disorders.

6. Guidance about the details of diet and when failures at this level should lead to consideration of drugs.

7. The *pros* and *cons* of an exercise program for a given person.

8. Characteristics of a unique individual that emphasize the importance of dealing with the lipid problem in a serious and organized manner.

9. Guidance as to when one should use the couplers for Hypertension, Obesity, and Wellness.

10. A series of pros and cons for each of the possible drugs for a particular lipid disorder in a unique individual.

11. Background or basic science information about lipid physiology that may help the user have a better understanding of the mechanisms of the particular abnormality that is present in a given patient.

Coupler 49

Urticaria/Angioedema
Revised 11/22/88

Introduction. The Urticaria/Angioedema Coupler covers both acute and chronic cases. The decision to have one, instead of two, couplers was based on the following:

1. The dividing line between the two types of urticaria is arbitrary and not always clear in a given case.

2. A case of chronic urticaria can be exacerbated by one of the agents that causes acute urticaria. The user must be alert to the possibility of a multifactorial situation.

3. The time required to go through the coupler is small compared to the time a physician may spend pursuing the problem in a less thorough and organized manner.

In the Urticaria/Angioedema Coupler, as in many other couplers, the results of coupling are presented in groups on the Index of Causes. The groups are separated by blank lines. In any given patient, one to several groups may appear, depending on the choices made by the particular patient. At least one finding that points to at least to one member of a group must occur in a patient if a group is to appear at all. Within a given group, the diagnoses are ordered in terms of the absolute number of findings present for each cause.

Group 1—Contains those diagnoses which are more urgent and require careful and continuing attention if there is any possibility that one or more of them is present.

Group 2—Contains the four broad categories (Drugs, Foods, Environmental Factors, and Infections) which are the common offenders in many patients. Comments about each of the specific findings, e.g., "cold," are directly under the findings as they appear after coupling. Just a quick glance at this group and the findings under each category shows in some patients how multifactorial the situation can be.

Group 3—Contains all those specific habits and diseases for which only one finding is necessary to consider it a serious candidate for the cause if the presence of the finding is associated with the urticaria.

Group 4—Contains those disorders which may not have been diagnosed yet, but which are good candidates for the source of the urticaria because of the other findings in the patient that are occurring concurrently. In other words, the urticaria may just be an early finding that should be alerting one to a significant underlying disorder.

Group 5—Contains many details relevant to the patient at hand concerning the use and cautions for antihistaminics.

Group 6—Contains details about the paradoxical effects of antihistaminics when the patient is an infant or a child.

Group 7—Alerts the user to which patients are *at risk* for certain disorders.

Group 8—The members of this group are not diagnoses, but rather suggestions as to how to proceed further in that patient that has none of the findings one would ordinarily use to implicate a given cause of urticaria.

Group 9—A physiological grouping that may be of interest to the user.

Coupler 50

Anxiety, Panic, and Phobias
Revised 3/1/90

Willie Kai Yee, M.D.

Introduction. This coupler assembles what is known about the multileveled phenomenon of anxiety into a form that permits rational assessment and treatment. Such an assessment includes an evaluation for the presence of medical conditions that can present as anxiety.

Before using this coupler, the patient should have a thorough medical evaluation, including the Medical History, Physical Examination, and Wellness Couplers, and laboratory screening including complete blood count, urinalysis, chemistry profile, and thyroid function tests. This coupler does not attempt to diagnose illnesses or anxiety secondary to medications (there are well over 100) that can easily be detected by a proper workup. Certain medical conditions that may not be uncovered by such an assessment (e.g., pheochromocytoma), or conditions that may warrant discussion in the context of the evaluation of anxiety (e.g., hypoglycemia) are included.

In addition to being a symptom of a medical condition, anxiety may be regarded as a reaction to specific situations, or a psychiatric disorder in and of itself. The use of the term *anxiety* to cover everything from an everyday experience (worry) to incapacitating psychiatric illnesses makes anxiety subject to extremes of over- and underestimation and treatment.

It could be argued that all patients are anxious, since they are worried or at least concerned about some aspect of their health. Treatment of everyday anxiety with medications is not recommended. Following the above recommendations will identify those in who may benefit from nonpharmacological interventions. This coupler will then evaluate those in whom anxiety is excessive, and who can benefit from treatment. These patients have the highest prevalence rate of the psychiatric disorders and one of the lowest overall utilizations of services.

In the Anxiety Coupler, as in many other couplers, the results of coupling are presented in groups on the Index of Causes. In this particular coupler, the basis for the grouping is as follows:

Group 1—Since anxiety is being evaluated here in the broadest possible context, this group will direct the user to measures which should be taken in the evaluation of the anxious patient, following the principles of the PKC system including the assessment of specific lifestyle and risk factors.

Group 2—Medical conditions which may present with anxiety or may be significant factors in aggravating anxiety or in which anxiety may require specific management. These conditions should be assessed and, if necessary, managed before treatment of anxiety is started. This section includes some conditions which may need to be discussed with patients, even though absent or insignificant, because of patient concern or misinformation.

Groups 3—The Anxiety Disorders and important related mental disorders as described in the *Diagnostic and Statistical Manual, Third Edition (Revised)* of the American Psychiatric Association (*DSM-III-R*).

It is recommended that the user have at least a casual understanding of the principles and structure of the *DSM-III-R* before making definitive diagnoses and treatment decisions based on this coupler.

[Sources to follow ...]

Coupler 51

Depression: Assessment and Management
Revised 4/14/90

Willie Kai Yee, M.D.

Introduction . This coupler is designed as an aid to the management Major Depression and Dysthymic Disorder (in older, pre-DSM-III, and non-psychiatric literature, these may be referred to as "endogenous" and "neurotic" or "minor" depressions, respectively). Depressions caused by medical or other psychiatric conditions may require treatments which go beyond the scope of this coupler. Bipolar ("manic-depressive") Disorder, for example, may be uncovered in the course of treating a depression, and requires a different emphasis. Depressions caused by medical conditions or drugs usually require that the underlying condition be addressed directly. This is not always possible (e.g., the patient may require a medication with depressive side effects), and the management of such depressions is therefore covered in this coupler.

Other disorders manifesting depression that may not be appropriate to the use of this coupler include:

Reactive attachment disorder of infancy or early childhood
Organic mood disorder
Residual schizophrenia
Avoidant, Dependent, and Self-Defeating Personality Disorders
Uncomplicated bereavement

Wherever possible, this coupler uses the terminology of the *Diagnostic and Statistical Manual of Mental Disorders, Third Edition - Revised (DSM-III-R)* of the American Psychiatric Association. Some terms still in use by nonpsychiatrists are not used in *DSM-III-R*. For example, Major Depression replaces the term "endogenous" depression, since research has shown that the occurrence of what appears to be a precipitating psychological event has little bearing on the course of a depression, once the depression has met the specific criteria for Major Depression. It should also be noted that the *DSM-III-R* also attempts to be atheoretical, and although the cause of depression is now generally held to be biological in origin, etiology is included in *DSM-III-R* diagnoses only when specific organic factors are known or suspected.

When non-*DSM-III-R* terms are used in this coupler, they are enclosed in single quotation marks, e.g. 'atypical depression.'

Professionals who treat depression may approach it from widely varying viewpoints, sometimes represented in the press as heated ideological disputes and professional rivalries. The author of this coupler believes that these differences may have their roots in the professional training of the provider rather than demonstrations of effectiveness. In this coupler, psychological and pharmacological treatments are viewed not only as compatible, but as complementary, and even synergistic. This view is supported by a growing number of psychiatrists, and clearly analyzed in the recent work of Karasu.

The PKC system is particularly suited to solving problems involving variables taken from multiple perspectives and avoids both paternalistic narrowness and ideological fragmentation.

Since the term depression can cover everything from a common feeling state (sadness) to a clearly defined psychiatric disorder (Major Depression), the range of applicable treatments is appropriately broad. This coupler is constructed on the assumption that an evaluation including the History and Physical and Wellness Couplers has identified those factors that may be causing the patient physical and emotional distress, and has provided measures that may alleviate that distress and contribute to the patient's well being. Additional measures are recommended by this coupler commensurate with any additional degree of depression and evidence for psychiatric disorder.

The management options in the coupler represent the best summary of the literature that can be made at this time. There are many areas of the field in which adequate research has not been done, and there are situations in which common clinical practice may go beyond or lag behind what is in the published literature. In these areas, options representing sound clinical judgment are made. Where unresearched or controversial treatments are recommended, this is indicated in the coupler. On the other hand, where present research indicates that some widely held practices and opinions are unsupported, the findings of the research are the basis of the recommendations made.

This coupler provides options from which a reasonable treatment plan can be made, and most cases will not use all the options presented.

The management options in this coupler are divided into numerous categories and, based on the unique choices for the individual patient, are ranked in the following order:

Procedures which should be implemented immediately or kept in mind as assessment proceeds

General interventions which may increase the patient's sense of well being, and which may be sufficient to alleviate some depressions

Psychotherapeutic interventions which have been shown to be effective in the treatment of depression

Guidelines for the pharmacological management of depression

Indications for the use of general categories of antidepressant medications

The pros and cons for specific antidepressant medications. Those with the fewest or least noxious side effects are listed first. This ranking is of necessity somewhat arbitrary, but is done to provide the basis for an orderly review of available medications. Since most of the drugs recorded in this coupler may be used to treat most depressions, the *pros* listed here are intended to help identify medications with specific advantages for the particular patient. The *cons* listed for a given drug are not meant as a comprehensive review of all possible adverse reactions, but contain precautions that should be noted in particular cases.

Adjunctive medications used in the treatment of depression

If a decision to use an antidepressant is made, a discussion of the results of the coupler session should be supplemented with a discussion of the specific drug or drugs being employed. The USP Drug Information for the Patient or the APA Patient Medication Instruction Sheets are recommended as an aid to this discussion.

[Sources to follow ...]

References

Foreword

Sacks, O. 1983. *Awakenings*. New York, E. P. Dutton.

From the Editors

Weed, L. L. 1969. *Medical records, medical education, and patient care.* Chicago: Year Book Medical Publishers, Inc.

Introduction

Berry, W. 1977. *The unsettling of America: Culture and agriculture.* San Francisco: Sierra Club.

Boorstin, D.J. 1983. *The discoverers.* New York: Random House.

Bjorn, C. J., and H. D. Cross. 1970. *The problem-oriented private practice of medicine: A system for comprehensive health care.* Chicago: Modern Healthcare Press, (Mcgraw-Hill Publications Company).

Dawes, R. M., D. Fust, and P. E. Meehl. 1989. Clinical versus actuarial judgement. *Science* 243:1668.

Gaumer, G. L. 1984. Regulating health professionals: A review of the empirical literature. *Milbank Memorial Fund Quarterly Health and Society* 3,62.

Heilbroner, R. L. 1972. *The worldly philosophers: The lives and times and ideas of the great economic thinkers.* New York: Simon and Schuster.

Hurst, W., and K. Walker eds. 1972. *The problem-oriented system.* New York: MEDCOM Press.

Hurst, W., and K. Walker eds. 1973. *Applying the problem-oriented system.* New York: MEDCOM Press.

Inlander, C. B., L. Levin, and E. Weiner. 1988. *Medicine on Trial*. New York: Prentice Hall.

Kern, L., and M. E. Doherty. 1982. Pseudodiagnosticity in an idealized medical problem-solving environment. *Journal of Medical Education* 57:100-104.

Lawson, I. 1974. Comments on the POMR. In *Problem-directed and medical information systems*, ed. M. F. Driggs. New York: Inter-continental Medical Book Corporation.

Sloan, D. 1979. The teaching of ethics in the American undergraduate curriculum, 1876-1976. *Hastings Center Report* 9(6):21.

Sneath, P. H. A., and R. Sokal. 1973. *Numerical taxonomy: The principles and practice of numerical classification*. San Francisco: W. H. Freeman and Company.

Tolstoy, L. 1942. *War and Peace*. New York: Simon and Schuster.

Tversky, A., and P. Kahneman. 1974. Judgment under uncertainty: Heuristics and biases in medical decision-making. *Science* 185:1124-1131.

Wason, P. C., and P. Johnson-Laird. 1972. *Psychology of Reasoning*. Cambridge, Mass.: Harvard University Press.

Weed, C. C. 1982. Problem-knowledge couplers: Philosophy, use, and interpretation. Vermont: PKC Corporation.

Weed, L. L. 1964. Medical records, patient care, and medical education. *Irish Journal of Medicine* 271.

Weed, L. L. 1969. *Medical records, medical education, and patient care*. Chicago: Year Book Medical Publishers, Inc.

Weed, L. L. 1975. *Your health care and how to manage it*. Vermont: Essex Publishing Company.

Weed, L. L., and R. Y. Hertzberg. 1983. The use and construction of problem-knowledge couplers, the knowledge-coupler editor, knowledge networks, and the problem-oriented medical record for the microcomputer. In *IEEE Proceedings of the Seventh Annual Symposium on Computer Applications in Medical Care*, 831-836. New York: IEEE Computer Society.

Weed, L. L. 1985. Problem-knowledge coupling. *Mt. Sinai Journal of Medicine* 52(2):94-98.

Weed, L. L. 1986. Knowledge coupling, medical education and patient care. *Critical Review of Medical Informatics* 1:55-79.

Weed, L. L. 1987. Flawed premises and educational malpractice: A view toward a more rational approach to medical practice. *The Journal of Medical Practice Management* 2(4):239-254.

Chapter 1

Covell, D. G., et al. 1985. Information needs in office practice: Are they being met? *Annals of Internal Medicine* 103:596.

Dawes, R. M., and B. Corrigan. 1974. Linear models in decision making. *Psychological Bulletin* 81(2):95-106.

Dawes, R. M. 1979. The robust beauty of improper linear models in decision making. *American Psychologist* 34(7):571-582.

Huth, E. J. 1989. The underused medical literature. *Annals of Internal Medicine* 110:99.

Inlander, C. B., L. Levin, and E. Weiner. 1988. *Medicine on trial.* New York: Prentice Hall.

Markham, B. 1983. *West with the night.* San Francisco: North Point Press.

Poirier, S., and D. J. Brauner. 1988. Ethics and the daily language of medical discourse. *Hastings Center Report* 18(4):5-9.

Putsch, R. W. III, and M. Joyce. 1990. Dealing with patients from other cultures. In *Clinical Methods*, ed. H. K. Walker, W. D. Hall, and J. W. Hurst, 3rd edition. Boston: Butterworths, 1050-65.

Wasserstein, A. G. 1988. Toward a romantic science: The work of Oliver Sacks. *Annals of Internal Medicine* 109(5):440-444.

Weed, L. L. 1969. *Medical records, medical education, and patient care.* Chicago: Year Book Medical Publishers, Inc.

Welty, E. 1983. *One writer's beginnings.* Cambridge, Mass: Harvard University Press.

Williamson, J. W., et al. 1989. Health sciences information management and continuing education of physicians. *Annals of Internal Medicine* 110:151.

Chapter 2

Farmer, S. 1987. Medical problems of chronic patients in a community support program. *Hospital and Community Psychiatry* 38:745-749.

Hall, R. C. W., et al. 1979. Differential diagnosis of somatopsychic disorders. *Psychosomatics* 381-389.

Stravinsky, I. 1947. *Poetics of music in the form of six lessons.* Cambridge, Mass: Harvard University Press.

Chapter 8

Bok, D. 1984. Needed: A new way to train doctors. (President's report to the Harvard Board of Overseers for 1982-1983). *Harvard Magazine* 86(5):32.

Codman, E. A. 1918. A study in hospital efficiency: As demonstrated by the case report of the first five years of a private hospital. Boston:Todd Publishers.

Nelson, G. E., S. M. Graves, R. R. Holland, J. M. Nelson, J. Ratner, and L. L. Weed. 1976. A performance-based method of student evaluation. *British Journal of Medical Education* 10:34-42.

Weed, L. L. 1982. Problem solving: Can we teach it?, eds. D. P. Connelly et al. *Clinical Decisions & Laboratory Use* 1(18):159-181.

Weed, L. L. 1986. Knowledge coupling, medical education and patient care. *Critical Review of Medical Informatics* 1:55-79.

Weed, L. L. 1987. Flawed premises and educational malpractice: A view toward a more rational approach to medical practice. *The Journal of Medical Practice Management* 2(4):239-254.

Chapter 9

Boorstin, D.J. 1983. *The discoverers*. New York: Random House.

Katz, J. 1984. *The silent world of doctor and patient*. New York: The Free Press.

Kelly, G. A. 1963. The expert as historical actor. *Daedalus* (Themes in Transition) 92(3):529-548.

Sinclair, W. J. 1909. *Life of Semmelweiss*. Manchester University Press.

Stern, B. J. 1927. *Social Factors in Medical Progress*. New York: Columbia University Press.

Chapter 10

Dawes, R. M. 1988. *Rational choice in an uncertain world*. New York: Harcourt Brace Jovanovich.

Fallows, J. 1985. The case against credentials. *The Monthly* 256(6):49-67.

Chapter 12

Codman, E. A. 1918. A study in hospital efficiency, as demonstrated by the case report of the first five years of a private hospital. Boston:Todd Publishers.

Dawes, R. M. 1988. *Rational choice in an uncertain world*. New York: Harcourt Brace Jovanovich.

Lawson, I. 1974. Comments on the POMR. In *Problem-directed and medical information systems*, ed. M. F. Driggs. New York: Inter-continental Medical Book Corporation.

Lipp, M. R. 1980. *The bitter pill—doctors, patients, and failed expectations*. New York: Harper & Row.

Stravinsky, I. 1947. *Poetics of music in the form of six lessons*. Cambridge, Mass: Harvard University Press.

Weed, L. L. 1964. Medical records, patient care, and medical education. *Irish Journal of Medicine* 271.

Weed, L. L. 1969. *Medical records, medical education, and patient care.* Chicago: Year Book Medical Publishers, Inc.

Weed, L. L. 1975. *Your health care and how to manage it.* Vermont: Essex Publishing Company.

Weed, L. L. 1981 Physicians of the future. *New England Journal of Medicine* 304:903-907.

Zimny, N. J., and C. J. Tandy. 1989. Problem-knowledge coupling: A tool for physical therapy in clinical practice. *Physical Therapy* 69:155161.

Chapter 13

Bruggink, G. 1986. Character and safety. *NASA's CALLBACK.*

Huth, E. 1989. *The underused medical literature. Annals of Internal Medicine,* 110:99.

Weed, L. L. 1969. *Medical records, medical education, and patient care.* Chicago, Ill.: Year Book Medical Publishers, Inc.

Chapter 14

Anderson, C., D. Hogarty, and S. Reiss. 1986. *Schizophrenia and the family.* New York: Guilford Press.

Farmer, S. 1987. Medical problems of chronic patients in a community support program. *Hospital and Community Psychiatry* 38(7):745-9.

Ferguson, T. 1980. *Medical self care: Access to health tools.* New York: Summit Books.

Hall, R. C. W., et al. 1979. Differential diagnosis of somatopsychic disorders. *Psychosomatics* 381-9.

Weed, L. L. 1987. Medical education and patient care: Mistaken premises and inadequate tools, Part 1. *Physicians and Computers* 30-32.

Weed, L. L. 1987. Medical education and patient care: Mistaken premises and inadequate tools, Part 2. *Physicians and Computers* 32-35.

Chapter 15

Kaldenberg, D.O., B. W. Becker, and J. B. Hallan. 1990. Dentistry in the year 2000: Assessments from a Delphi panel. *Journal of American College of Dentistry* 57:20-28.

Monteity, B.D. 1990. *Personal Communication.*

Morris, A.L., and H. M. Bohannon, H.M. 1987. Assessment of private dental practice: implications for dental education. *Journal of Dental Education* 51:661-667.

Weed, C.C. 1982. Problem-knowledge couplers: philosophy, use and interpretation. Burlington, Vt.: PKC Corporation.

Select Bibliography

The following references provide background for PROMIS which were referred to in the introduction.

Cantrill, S. V. 1979. Computerisation of the problem orientated record. In *The Problem Orientated Medical Record*, ed. J. C. Petrie, and N. McIntyre. New York: Churchill Livingstone.

Esterhay, R. J., Jr., and P. L. Walton. 1979. Clinical research and PROMIS. In *IEEE Proceedings of the Third Annual Symposium on Computer Applications in Medical Care*. New York: IEEE Computer Society.

Gane, D. 1979. An example of the effects of computer usage on nursing practice. In *IEEE Proceedings of the Third Annual Symposium on Computer Applications in Medical Care*, 109-116. New York: IEEE Computer Society.

Gilroy, G., B. J. Ellinoy, G. E. Nelson, and S. V. Cantrill. 1977. Integration of pharmacy into the computerized problem-oriented medical information system. *American Journal of Hospital Pharmacy* 34:155-162.

Graves, S. 1973. Better records: First step to better quality. In *Applying the Problem-Oriented System*. New York: MEDCOM Press.

Graves, S. 1973. Records as a tool in clinical investigation. In *Applying the Problem-Oriented System*. New York: MEDCOM Press.

Hertzberg, R. Y., J. R. Schultz, J. F. Wanner. 1980. The PROMIS network. *Computer Networks* 4:215-228.

McNeill, D. G. 1979. Developing the complete computer-based information system. *Journal of Nursing Administration* 9:34-36.

Schultz, J. R., and L. Davis. 1979. The Technology of PROMIS. In *IEEE Proceedings of the Third Annual Symposium on Computer Applications in Medical Care*, 67:9. New York: IEEE Computer Society.

Schultz, J. R. 1988. A history of the PROMIS technology: An effective human interface. In *A History of Personal Workstations*, ed. A. Goldberg. Massachusetts: Addison-Wesley Publishing Co.

Walton, P. L., R. R. Holland, and L. L. Wolf. 1979. Medical Guidance and PROMIS. In *IEEE Proceedings of the Third Annual Symposium on Computer Applications in Medical Care*, 19-27. New York: IEEE Computer Society.

Wanner, J. F. 1978. Wideband communication system improves response time. *Computer Design* 85-91.

Weed, L. L., and PROMIS Laboratory. 1978. Representation of medical knowledge and PROMIS. In *IEEE Proceedings of the Second Annual Symposium in Computer Applications in Medical Care*, 368-400. New York: IEEE.

Weed, L. L. 1972. Background paper for concept of national library of displays. In *The Problem-Oriented System*, eds. W. Hurst, and K. Walker. New York: MEDCOM Press.

Wakefield, J. S., ed. 1983. Managing medicine. Washington: Medical Communications and Services Association

Further Reading

Nash, F. A. 1954. Differential diagnosis: An approach to assist logical faculties. *Lancet* i:875.

Index

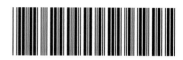